PSYCHOANALYTIC PSYCHOTHERAPY

Psychoanalytic Psychotherapy

A Practitioner's Guide

Nancy McWilliams

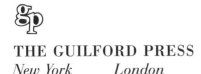

THE GUILFORD PRESS
New York   London

© 2004 Nancy McWilliams

Published by The Guilford Press
A Division of Guilford Publications, Inc.
370 Seventh Avenue, Suite 1200, New York, NY 10001
www.guilford.com

Printed in the United States of America

This book is printed on acid-free paper.

Last digit is print number: 9 8 7

Library of Congress Cataloging-in-Publication Data

McWilliams, Nancy.
    Psychoanalytic psychotherapy : a practitioner's guide /
Nancy McWilliams.
      p. ; cm.
    Includes bibliographical references.
    ISBN 978-1-59385-009-8
    1. Psychoanalysis.   I. Title.
    [DNLM: 1. Psychoanalytic Therapy.   WM 460.6 M478p
2004]
    RC504.M33 2004
    616.89′17—dc22

                                                      2003025342

For Art Robbins, with thanks

About the Author

Nancy McWilliams, PhD, teaches psychoanalytic theory and therapy at the Graduate School of Applied and Professional Psychology at Rutgers–The State University of New Jersey. A 1978 graduate of the National Psychological Association for Psychoanalysis, she also teaches at the Institute for Psychoanalysis and Psychotherapy of New Jersey, the National Training Program in Contemporary Psychotherapy, the Psychoanalytic Institute of Northern California, and the Minnesota Institute for Contemporary Psychoanalytic Studies. She has lectured throughout the United States and in Canada, Mexico, Russia, Sweden, Greece, Turkey, Australia, and New Zealand. Dr. McWilliams has a private practice in psychoanalysis, psychodynamic therapy, and supervision in Flemington, New Jersey, and is the author of *Psychoanalytic Diagnosis: Understanding Personality Structure in the Clinical Process* (Guilford Press, 1994) and *Psychoanalytic Case Formulation* (Guilford Press, 1999) as well as articles and book chapters on personality, psychopathology, psychotherapy, altruism, sexuality, and gender.

Preface

Psychology may be a science but psychotherapy is an art. Over the past century, having started as an effort to cure the baffling symptoms of patients with severe hysterical problems, psychodynamic therapies have been refined and expanded in attempts to reduce the suffering of an increasingly broad and diverse range of people. The impetus for this book is my sense that despite an abundance of good writing on the psychotherapy process, we lack an integrative work on psychotherapy that introduces students of the art to its essential features—across populations, across pathologies, across the sometimes radically differing paradigms currently in vogue in the psychoanalytic community, across the variations in human misery that express the idiosyncrasies of particular families in particular places in a particular age. That such a book is a product of its own era and culture is inevitable. I am hoping that nonetheless it will be more embracing and less narrow than most previous primers on analytic therapy. As with my previous texts, with this book I am trying to be helpful mostly to people in training, whether in psychology, counseling, psychiatry, general medical practice, social work, nursing, or faith-based practice.

In addition to trying to address the training needs of beginning therapists, I am hoping to start a conversation about therapy that traverses theoretical orientations and professional disciplines. Perhaps by discussing central aspects of psychodynamic practice across diverse patient populations, I can effectively represent the psychoanalytic tradition to colleagues who are put off by arcane terminology and the trappings of a historically much too smug fraternity. My personal experience attests to what some researchers have dubbed the "dodo bird" phenomenon (Luborsky, Diguer, Luborsky, Singer, & Dickter, 1993), the observation that the common features of effective therapies operate similarly, independently of the ideologies of individual practitioners (Weinberger, 1995; Luborsky et al., 2002). My colleague Brenna Bry is a Skinnerian. My language for what I do is radically different from hers, but when I watch videotapes of her work, I notice that I would intervene in much the same way she does. If I can capture some elements of these common features in ways that are less vague than concepts such as "personal warmth" and "empathy," I may be able to make what happens in psychodynamic psychotherapy not only comprehensible to novice analytic therapists but also interesting to colleagues of different explanatory leanings and to the educated nonprofessional reader.

My version of the dodo bird is not reductionistic; it does not negate the fact that there are effective, focused treatments for specific pathologies. We are, in the early years of the twenty-first century, in possession of cognitive-behavioral strategies that ameliorate many discrete disorders, medical interventions that transform psychoses and severe mood disorders, meditative disciplines that reduce anxiety and depression, and grass-roots-inspired movements like the twelve-step programs that have made addictions much more conquerable—not to mention countless other examples of particular weapons against particular ills. People who seek psychotherapy are generally looking both for specific expertise and for the kind of relationship that will allow them to unburden themselves and grow in a more general way.

Notwithstanding that some qualities are unique to a psychoanalytically oriented approach, much of its healing potential is shared by therapists of all sorts. Although my attitude about this derives from personal experience, it is compatible with some very stringently conducted research. Analyzing the work of Luborsky et al. (2002), Messer and Wampold (2002) observe that the current emphasis on "empirically supported treatments" is based on a discredited medical model and has contributed to an empirically unwarranted devaluation of the experiential, psychodynamic, and family therapies. They further conclude that specific, symptom-targeted strategies are effective "only insofar as they are a component of a larger healing context," and that (as we have known for a long time) more variance in outcome arises from differences among therapists than from differences among treatment approaches. Perhaps there is a contradiction in my being both passionate about the special value of a psychoanalytic sensibility and sincere in my appreciation for the contributions of competing perspectives. But much as Winnicott asked therapists to embrace paradox, I hope my readers will be sympathetic to my seeing things from several different angles at once.

Part of what has impelled me to take on the task of writing another textbook is having witnessed the confusion of my students as they try to translate their own understanding of effective therapy into interventions that help clients with borderline, narcissistic, antisocial, posttraumatic, and symbiotic character pathology. Currently, even in the private offices of experienced practitioners serving sophisticated clients, and in the college counseling centers originally established to address normal growing pains, most consumers of therapy are not suffering from what analysts consider neurotic-level problems. They are enduring miseries that represent developmental arrests, insufficiencies of internalization, severe attachment disorders, addiction, and other catastrophes of an unkind fortune. Many of the graduate students at Rutgers–The State University of New Jersey, where I teach, have been in conventional psychodynamic therapy of an uncovering sort, in which the traditional technique of attention to the transference and its historical antecedents has been deeply helpful. They have also been exposed to texts on psychoanalytic therapy that have aimed at teaching people how to work with clients who have good observing egos, self and object constancy, some sense of personal agency, and a vision of how they want to change. When they try to apply this version of help to their clients, they are dismayed to find themselves experienced as critical, attacking, mechanical, uncaring, or controlling.

Whether the technological, social, economic, and political changes in recent decades—or perhaps the rate of change itself—have produced new and more severe pathologies, or whether the "widening scope" of psychotherapy (Stone, 1954) has gradually attracted people who would previously have shunned treatment, or whether we can now see more primitive, characterological aspects of anyone's suffering better than we once did is a matter of debate. (All three factors are probably at work, but the first explanation seems highly likely to me, especially given the well-documented, staggering increase in the incidence of depression.) The clinical situation, however, is clear. More people need therapists for more severe, more emotionally disabling conditions.

It makes little sense to teach students how to deal effectively with the easiest clients, leaving them to learn by the school of hard knocks how to work with more challenging ones—all the while suffering from vaguely defined guilt that they are breaking textbook rules. It seems to me that instead of teaching novice therapists how to help "classical" patients and then how to make deviations from those techniques in order to help "preoedipal" or "understructured" or idiosyncratically structured individuals, a primer on psychodynamic therapy should emphasize the aspects of therapeutic engagement that apply to all clients. This is not to say that traditional texts on working with neurotic-level patients do not have a lot to teach, only that their focus on one kind of client has had certain unintended and inhibiting effects. I suspect the same thing will happen with the so-called empirically supported and evidence-based therapies.

Despite the fact that some well-placed analysts have been able to build practices with high-functioning analytic candidates, psychoanalytic therapy has never been just for the "worried well." Freud's early patients may have been comfortably middle class, but most of them seem to have had traumatic histories and quite disabling symptoms. My colleagues and students work in private offices, hospitals, clinics, jails, schools, institutions for troubled children, halfway houses, state child-protection agencies, corporations, emergency services, counseling centers, pediatric practices, and churches. They volunteer in catastrophic emergencies such as terrorist attacks and earthquakes. Working with therapists in other countries, I have witnessed the value of ingenious psychodynamic ways of addressing suffering in some very unfamiliar milieus.

It does seem to be true that the healthier the client is, the faster and better he or she makes progress in analytic treatment, but that is true for all therapies. Most short-term approaches, dynamic and otherwise, have developed criteria for exempting large numbers of more difficult and complexly disturbed patients from treatment by the method in question. Most of the "empirically supported treatments" have been tested using inclusion criteria—standards that the ordinary practicing therapist could never apply—such as the requirement that research subjects be cooperative and have no problems that are "comorbid" with what is being investigated. This sounds suspiciously like the return of the worried well. In the psychodynamic tradition there is a long, robust clinical track record with very challenging, polysymptomatic patients with personality disorders. Clinicians of other orientations, such as Jeffrey Young (e.g., Young, Klosko, & Weishaar, 2003), are now claiming promise for such clients via approaches that use a different language, but these treatments can look in practice surprisingly like psychoanalytic therapies and are beginning to take just as long.

Another reality with which beginning professionals in psychotherapy must contend, at least in the United States, is the changed mental health landscape. It is not unusual at this point for a therapist just out of a training program to be hired by an organization that expects him or her to handle a caseload of sixty patients with no provision for supervision or continuing education. Facilities that offer psychotherapy are in crisis about resources and are asking staff to do vastly more work than novice therapists used to be assigned, with virtually no support. The tips that therapists of my generation gained from mentors and colleagues in our first positions are not necessarily available. Thus, there seems to me to be a need for a book that covers the kind of lore we used to expect to be transmitted in the internship, on the job, and in the in-service training programs that were once a regular feature of mental health agencies.

I did not come to this task unambivalently. In fact, I resisted it for months despite the fact that a bite from the book-writing bug seems to have infected me more or less permanently. My editor and several other people had suggested that the logical successor to my writing on personality diagnosis and case formulation (McWilliams, 1994, 1999), would be a book on therapy. I protested that the whole point of my existing work was to challenge the idea that there is a basic "technique" of treatment, to which patients should be adapted à la Procrustes. Instead, I have always argued, the treatment approach ought to flow from a comprehensive understanding of the client and the nature of his or her problems. I felt, and still feel, that especially in the psychoanalytic tradition, the means of healing are too frequently given more weight than the ends (I am probably not the only therapist who has been told by an evaluator, "That was obviously very helpful to the patient . . . but was it *analysis?*"). Despite my dread that a book on therapy as a generic activity could be received as another technical ideal from which intuitively gifted students would feel guilty about "deviating," I began slowly to think about some essential features of relating therapeutically to other people, irrespective of their diagnoses, on which I could elaborate in an original and useful way.

In what follows, I have given special attention to those aspects of psychotherapy that are not typically covered in textbooks—for example, common boundary perplexities such as whether to accept gifts or give hugs, instances in which liability may be an issue, and the need for therapists to honor their own individuality in the arrangements they make and the ways they intervene with patients. As efforts to reduce medical costs have led to a brutal contraction of psychotherapy in the United States, pressure for work in the short term or on an infrequent basis has overwhelmed agencies, hospitals, counseling centers, and even independent practitioners. Thus, many of us in the daily business of trying to help people with complex psychological miseries struggle to do the bare minimum in an atmosphere of indifference to or skepticism toward our expertise. I hope to help students see the value of their efforts even in this nonfacilitating environment.

Perhaps to the surprise of readers with psychoanalytic experience, I have not organized the contents of this text under the traditional topics of the working alliance, resistance, transference and countertransference, interpretation, working through, and termination. This choice does not reflect any disdain for that way of structuring books about how to do therapy; rather, it expresses two observations I have made after years of teaching beginning therapists. First, there are already many such books, some of them excellent. Second, there are some things students need to know that are even more basic and fundamental to psychoanalytic practice than how to interpret transferences and resistances or how to understand the working-through process or when to consider ending treatment. They need to know how to maintain their own self-esteem, how to behave in a way that is both professional and natural, and how to protect their own boundaries from the incursions that their more desperate clients insist on attempting. I have tried to write a book that falls somewhere between a psychotherapy cookbook and the dense, epiphanic clinical poetry of the kind Thomas Ogden or James Grotstein or Michael Eigen write so well. I have always resisted the tendency to define psychotherapy by an invariant technique, but I also know that beginners need specifics and are not helped by vague statements to the effect of "It all depends." Most of what I cover here is ultimately about tone (cf. Lear, 2003).

The tone of this book has been affected by the political and economic pressures that currently conspire to devalue and marginalize the precious project of trying to understand oneself and grow into the most fully elaborated version of what one could be. Contemporary students of clinical psychology, the group I know best, come to training with all kinds of misinformation about the psychoanalytic tradition, including the unfounded impression that psychodynamic therapies have not been empirically supported. In this era of "evidence-based medicine," students of psychiatry who would rather listen to patients for fifty minutes than medicate them in lucrative but numbing fifteen-minute segments are even more isolated and besieged in their profession (see Luhrman, 2000; Frattaroli, 2001). And applicants to most social work programs know better than to tell their prospective teachers that they want to be therapists instead of administrators or social activists. Large segments of the public believe that therapy is about blaming one's parents, avoiding personal responsibility, and rationalizing selfishness. Therapists are neither well organized nor temperamentally disposed to battling their disparagers. So I am trying give moral and conceptual support to trainees who, despite all these circumstances, know that psychotherapy is the project to which they want to commit the rest of their working lives.

I am trying here to pass along some of what has been the oral tradition of psychotherapy practice. Most people learn how to help others from two sources that are much more influential than any text: their supervisors and their personal experiences in psychotherapy and analysis. Even when the wisdom that accumulates from these directions cannot be directly applied to a given client, therapists distill and extrapolate to meet individual needs as they understand them. Critics in academic psychology and psychiatry tend to approach the evaluation of therapy from the position that we need to do controlled empirical studies to learn what helps. People of a more introspective sensibility tend to assume that there already exists an art of helping people, an art that requires ingenuity and skill to apply to difficult patients and challenging problems, but one for which there is already ample expertise to be tapped in the knowledge base of experienced practitioners. Although I have a foot in both camps, my temperamental allegiance is with the artists more than the scientists. Perhaps it is more accurate to say that my vision of science encompasses clinical lore as a legitimate source of knowledge in addition to what can be learned from controlled studies. I deeply believe we need to be just as respectful toward more poetic, metaphorically expressed, experience-based clinical theory as we are toward more highly controlled research.

The American culture in which I grew up and now practice my profession often strikes me as having both the best and worst qualities of an energetic adolescent. Cherishing their revolutionary heritage, Americans tend to distrust established authority, value the new and provocative, and exuberantly dismiss the sensibilities of a previous generation. Revering one's ancestors or appealing to the wise tribal elders is culturally alien. Much of my own psychology is consistent with this cultural tilt, and yet, like my students, when I was in training I found myself hungering for the voice of authentic wisdom. Because of the American affinity for the new and revolutionary, psychoanalysis in its youth was too often uncritically embraced here; now in its maturity, it is too often uncritically dismissed. In this book, I would like to throw away some psychoanalytic bath water without losing the value of the psychoanalytic baby.

Such a bias probably speaks volumes about my own professional development. Despite my strong feeling that we need to do lots more research on psychotherapy and to pay attention to what researchers have already established, I have learned much more from passionate practitioners than from dispassionate researchers. Arthur Robbins (e.g., 1988, 1989), to whom this book is dedicated, was the first psychoanalyst I knew who taught psychotherapy as a highly individualized art rather than as the implementation of a set of demonstrated procedures, and his thoughtful discipline in addressing each clinical challenge seemed to me to reflect far more integrity than I saw in the work of those who claimed to teach a privileged and generalized "technique." I have also always felt a sense of kinship with Theodor Reik, (e.g., 1948), whose work originally attracted me to my profession, with

Frieda Fromm-Reichmann (1950), whose text on therapy was impelled by similar concerns to the ones that inspired this book, and with Roy Schafer (1983), who, notwithstanding his credentials as an empirical researcher, took pains to specify the more inchoate attitudinal dimensions of the psychotherapy relationship. These authors could also write engagingly, and they tried to make psychoanalytic ideas more rather than less accessible to people outside traditional analytic enclaves. I have learned from talented, compassionate therapists in all the main psychotherapy traditions—psychiatry, psychology, social work, and pastoral counseling—all of whom had more in common with each other than with colleagues in their discipline who had no interest in therapy.

I frequently talk here about what I personally say and do as a therapist. I do this not because I think my way is the "right" or best way but because students have consistently told me that they thrive on specific examples of what therapists do and say. Most of them get very little, if any, opportunity to watch experienced practitioners work, and they report that having concrete examples of how a professional behaves is helpful in the ongoing process of "trying on" different styles of intervention to see what suits their own personalities. When teaching about psychotherapy, I have learned to assign writers such as Martha Stark (1994, 1999) and Henry Pinsker (1997) because these quite different therapists provide the actual words they use with clients.

Notwithstanding my bias that training in an enlightened analytic institute is the best preparation for most therapeutic activity, this is not a textbook on psychoanalysis. Instead, it is a book about the psychoanalytic or psychodynamic therapies (I have never seen the point of making a distinction between "psychoanalytic" and "psychodynamic"), including psychoanalysis, the most intensive, freely exploratory, and open-ended therapy we have. Most therapists, and certainly most beginning therapists, do not have opportunities to do traditional psychoanalysis, however. Even if they have formal analytic training and an office in a city where analysis is part of the culture, the majority of practitioners have few opportunities to work with clients able and willing to come several times a week and to work in the depth that psychoanalysis requires.

This book emphasizes how helpful psychoanalytic therapies can be for less healthy clients and for those who cannot undertake analysis even if they are good candidates for it. Seasoned analytic therapists know that we help people to become healthier, to build inner scaffolding, to change their intrapsychic architecture. We do not simply "manage" clients, keep them in place, interfere with specific kinds of acting out. Patients embark on a growth process in therapy. Psychoanalytic therapies reduce emotional suffering, prevent disastrous enactments, improve resistance to illness, make life more meaningful, and provide solace to individuals who are very hard to console. I am hoping that long-term, well-designed studies will eventually vindicate our convictions about all this. In the meantime, this book represents an effort to distill some essential themes of effective clinical practice across the vast range of suffering people who need our help.

Acknowledgments

My editor has commented that my acknowledgment section is always long. Its length results from my trying to present not my own approach to diagnosis or case formulation or therapy but that of the psychoanalytic community as a whole, as I understand the tradition. Thus, my debts are extensive. This section follows the precedent, as I have been even more than usually concerned with generalizing about a disparate and long-lived field.

My deepest thanks go to those who have pored over the whole manuscript. Kerry Gordon, on whose psychoanalytic wisdom and personal integrity I depend, lent his exquisitely sensitive ear to my writing efforts in regular conversations over more than two years, critiquing each chapter as it emerged from my computer. He has not been even slightly proprietary about the many ways his influence now suffuses the book. Jan Resnick patiently confronted my tendency to universalize, subdued my culture-bound assumptions, and suggested substitutes for obscure American idioms. I appreciate the time and resources he expended in mailing or faxing me from Australia a detailed critique of each section. Sandra Bem reviewed and critiqued these pages with the invaluable dual vision of the serious scholar and the recently trained therapist.

Many friends and colleagues have read parts of the manuscript and given me their reactions. My husband, Carey, gave the early chapters his usual incisive attention and warm support; Mark Hilsenroth was generous in sharing his responses and informing me of areas in which recent empirical research bears upon my topic; Bryant Welch vetted the legal and ethical material. Sections of the book were also read and discussed helpfully by Karen Maroda, Spyros Orfanos, Louis Sass, Jonathan Shedler, and members of my Tuesday consultation group: Mary Altonji, Gayle Coakley, Marsha Morris, Diana Shanley, and Sue Steinmetz.

Several people who were in audiences to whom I presented parts of this book gave me encouragement and helpful suggestions. They include Mark Adams, Anne Appelbaum, Elgan Baker, Carol Munchausen, Mary Lorton, and Paul Mosher, among others I may have neglected to mention. For their response to the first two chapters, I thank the audiences that I found at the Cincinnati Psychoanalytic Institute, the Department of Psychology at Xavier University, the School of Psychological Sciences at the University of Indianapolis, the Indiana Society for Psychoanalytic Thought, the New York State Psychiatric Institute, the Department of Psychiatry at the University of Alberta Hospital in Edmonton, the Southeast Florida Association for Psychoanalytic Psychology, the University of Texas Medical Center, the Greater Kansas Psychoanalytic Society, the Vermont Association for Psychoanalytic Studies, the Tampa Institute for Psychoanalytic Studies, the Southeast Region of the American Association of Pastoral Counselors, the Karen Horney Institute, and my own psychoanalytic home base, the Institute for Psychoanalysis and Psychotherapy of New Jersey. I thank the faculty and candidates at the Postgraduate Center for Psychoanalytic Training for their warm reaction to parts of Chapters 10 and 11.

Many people have supported the basic concept behind this book, cheered on my progress in writing it, and suggested relevant material for me to read. They include Karin Ahbel, George Atwood, Louis Berger, Candis Cousins, Dennis Debiak, Michael Eigen, Carol Goodheart, Lynne Harkless, Hilary Hays, Douglas Kirsner, Stanley Lependorf, Lou Ann Lewis, Judith Felton Logue, Deborah Luepnitz, Jim Mastrich, Barbara Menzel, Stanley Messer, Linda Meyers, Nicole Moore, Lin Pillard, Art Raisman, David Ramirez, Kay Reed, Kit Riley, Arnold Schneider, Jonathan Slavin, Paul Steinberg, Diane Suffridge, Johanna Tabin, Floyd Turner, Fox Vernon, Drew Westen, Polly Young-Eisendrath, and my friends in Section III of the Division of Psychoanalysis of the American Psychological Association.

I am particularly indebted to those therapists in countries outside North America who have expanded my knowledge of psychotherapy in their cultures, especially Sofia Trilivas and Tanya Anagnostopoulou in Greece, Karen Batres in Mexico, Nina Vasilyeva in Russia, Margot Holmberg in Sweden, and Yavuz Erten, Guler Fisek, and Yasemin Sohtorik in Turkey. Tim Levchenko-Scott arranged a New Zealand lecture tour that exposed me to a different English-speaking culture (and therapy culture), and in Australia I have been grateful for the support, hospitality, and friendship of Jan Resnick, Liz and Trevor Sheehan, Len Oakes, and Judy Hyde.

I want to express my appreciation to Nadine Levinson, David Tuckett, and the Psychoanalytic Electronic Publishing Company, whose full-text compilation of articles from major journals on a CD-ROM has made research into the psychoanalytic literature infinitely easier. I also want to acknowledge all the researchers in psychology and psychiatry who are subjecting psychoanalytic concepts to empirical examination; we therapists are in their debt.

At the Graduate School of Applied and Professional Psychology at Rutgers, I am especially grateful for the support of Clay Alderfer, Nancy Boyd-Franklin, Brenna Bry, Cary Chernis, Lew Gantwerk, Stan Messer, Sandra Harris, Don Morgan, Louis Sass, Karen Skean, Jamie Walkup, and Seth Warren. I thank Michael Andronico and the alumni members of my diversity group: Carole Christian, Bob Lewis, Don Corr, and Jesse Whitehead. But my main sources of inspiration at Rutgers are the students, a remarkably diverse, capable, and dedicated group, who consistently raise important questions and have trusted me with their confidences about the subjective and emotional aspects of their training. Special thanks to Kate Chittendon and Christine Garcia for their permission to use anecdotes they shared, and to Sadia Saleem for her thoughtful feedback about a chapter.

I have learned the most about psychotherapy from my own therapists, Edith Sheppard, Theodore Greenbaum, and the late Louis Berkowitz. Second only to those experiences, the supervision and friendship I got from Arthur Robbins, to whom this book is dedicated, taught me more by example than any textbook could have. Other supervisors who have helped me include Bert Cohen, Stanley Moldawsky, Iradj Siassi, and Duncan Walton. My patients have been and continue to be excellent teachers and supervisors; I wish I could acknowledge them personally here. I am particularly grateful to the client I called Donna, whom I met in 1972 and still hear from, whose story is told in Chapter 9. Finally, I continue to learn a great deal from the members of my supervision and consultation groups, therapists notable for their willingness to expose their struggles to help people who are sometimes so devastatingly damaged that it is a wonder they are still walking around.

I want to mention also the most personal sources of my ongoing creative energy and satisfaction: my husband, Carey, who for over forty years has contributed to my intellectual development and supported my writing and other professional endeavors; my daughters, Susan and Helen, who have tolerated the misfortune of having a therapist mother with consistent good grace; and my friends outside the profession, who have provided some balance in a life that could otherwise have been completely consumed by my work, especially Deborah Maher, Fred

Miller, Velvet and Cal Miller, Susanne Peticolas and Hank Plotkin, Nancy Schwartz, George Sinkler, Jim Slagle, Rich Tormey, and Cheryl Watkins. Special thanks to Susan Burnham, Marie Trontell, Al Byer, and Pete Macor of TBC; to the Copper Penny Players; and to the late Mike Carney, whose sensitive intelligence and inimitable presence I will keenly miss.

Finally, I am indebted to Kathryn Moore, who originally sought me out, saw the potential for a book in my work, and sold The Guilford Press on the value of putting their resources behind my writing. She has been an ideal editor and has become a trusted friend.

Contents

PSYCHOANALYTIC PSYCHOTHERAPY

Chapter 1

What Defines
a Psychoanalytic Therapy?

We must not forget that the analytic relationship is based
on a love of truth—that is, on a recognition of reality—
and that it precludes any kind of sham or deceit.
                            —SIGMUND FREUD (1937, p. 248)

Psychoanalytic therapies, including psychoanalysis, are approaches to helping people that derive ultimately from the ideas of Sigmund Freud and his collaborators and followers. Perhaps such a genealogy could be claimed for almost all versions of the "talking cure," as most types of therapeutic encounter—even those that differ rather dramatically from Freud's way of working—have at least a distant connection with his influence.

It seems to me that the overarching theme among psychodynamic approaches to helping people is that the more honest we are with ourselves, the better our chances for living a satisfying and useful life. Moreover, a psychoanalytic sensibility appreciates the fact that honesty about our own motives does not come easily to us. The diverse therapeutic approaches within the psychoanalytic pantheon share the aim of cultivating an increased capacity to acknowledge what is not conscious—that is, to admit what is difficult or painful to see in ourselves. Unconscious phenomena may include a sense of weakness (risk of psychic decompensation, fragmentation, annihilation), vanity (vulnerability to shame, aspirations to perfection, fantasies of omnipotence, specialness, and entitlement), conflict (tensions between wishes and prohibitions, ambivalence, pursuit of mutually exclusive aims), moral deficit (self-deception, temptations to be self-righteous, blindness to negative consequences of actions), or the lust, greed, competition, and aggres-

1

sion that early Freudian theory unmasked so enthusiastically in the climate of a society considerably more decorous than the one we now inhabit.

Psychoanalytic clinical and theoretical writing has always specialized in exposing motives that are not obvious to us, on the premise that becoming aware of disavowed aspects of our psychologies will relieve us of the time and effort required to keep them unconscious. Thus, more of our attention and energy can be liberated for the complex task of living realistically, productively, and joyfully. Motives that tend to be relegated to unconsciousness vary from individual to individual, from culture to culture, and from one time period to another. It is probably no accident that in contemporary Western cultures, where individual mobility is assumed, where extended and even nuclear families are geographically disparate, and where the assumed solution to most relationship problems is separation—in other words, where longings to cling are unwelcome and signs of dependency inspire scorn—psychoanalytic researchers and theorists are emphasizing attachment, relationship, mutuality, and intersubjectivity.

If this account sounds somewhat moralistic, that is also not accidental. Several decades ago, the sociologist Philip Rieff made a scholarly and persuasive argument that Freud was essentially a moralist—not in the popular sense of the person who gets a rush from attacking others for engaging in specific sins, but in the more philosophical sense of being ultimately concerned with what is true:

> The tension between instinctual candor and cultural hypocrisy . . . must be acknowledged; the act of doing so describes for Freud the beginning of new health. . . . Psychoanalysis . . . demands a special capacity for candor which not only distinguishes it as a healing movement but also connects it with the drive toward disenchantment characteristic of modern literature and of life among the intellectuals. (1959, p. 315)

As Michael Guy Thompson (2002) and others inheritors of Rieff's perspective have argued, psychoanalysis as a field has, whatever its lapses from that ideal, embraced an ethic of honesty that takes precedence over other aims and regards therapeutic goals, including symptom relief, as by-products of the achievement of honest discourse. Thomas Szasz (2003) has gone so far as to as to define psychoanalysis as "*a moral dialogue, not a medical treatment*" (p. 46). For many decades, the ethic of honesty was personified in the image of a therapist who had presumably attained unflinching self-awareness in a personal analysis and who bore the responsibility for fostering the same achievement in the patient. In current analytic writing, there is more acknowledgment that participation in a therapeutic partnership requires *both* analyst and patient to become progressively more honest with themselves in the context of that relationship.

Bion (1970) observed that psychoanalysis is located at the intersection of two vertices: the medical and the religious (cf. Strenger, 1991). By "medical," he referred to the more objective, rational, technocratic, authoritative stance of the person trying to offer practical help to those suffering from mental and emotional disorders. The medical vertex is characterized by validated techniques, applied by an expert, intended to have specific, replicable effects. Recent efforts of Kernberg and his colleagues (e.g., Yeomans, Clarkin, & Kernberg, 2002) to develop manualized treatments for borderline personality organization exemplify this face of psychodynamic practice. Current writing on the neurology and brain chemistry of subjectivity and the changes that occur in analytic therapy (e.g., Schore, 1994, 2003a, 2003b; Solms & Turnbull, 2002) also belong to the medical axis. In noting the equally important "religious" vertex, Bion was calling attention to a dimension that is often depicted as existential, experiential, humanistic, romantic, collaborative, or discovery-oriented ways of seeking answers to (unanswerable) human questions.

Described empirically, approaches that have been labeled psychodynamic, at least in the short-term therapy literature, have a number of overlapping aspects. Blagys and Hilsenroth (2000), in an extensive review of the comparative psychotherapy process literature that examined replicated data across several studies, identified seven factors distinguishing psychodynamic from cognitive-behavioral treatments. The psychodynamic therapies were characterized by (1) focus on affect and the expression of emotion; (2) exploration of the patient's efforts to avoid certain topics or engage in activities that retard therapeutic progress (i.e., work with resistance); (3) identification of patterns in the patient's actions, thoughts, feelings, experiences, and relationships (object relations); (4) emphasis on past experiences; (5) focus on interpersonal experiences; (6) emphasis on the therapeutic relationship (transference and the working alliance); and (7) explorations of wishes, dreams, and fantasies (intrapsychic dynamics). The researchers noted that such differences are not categorical—they are not "present" versus "not present"; rather, they are dimensional. Hilsenroth (personal communication, June 22, 2003) compares such distinctions to a light with a dimmer switch instead of an on/off button; that is, they are employed significantly more by adherents of one philosophy of treatment. Thus, some of the features he and Blagys extracted (e.g., item 3) are shared by cognitive-behavioral practitioners, while some others (e.g., item 2) are not always features of psychodynamic practice—for example, in the work of therapists with a self psychology orientation or of those with a traditional ego-psychology view when treating clients they see as needing supportive rather than exploratory therapy.

I believe that what most practicing analytic therapists see as distinctive about the psychodynamic therapies (including psychoanalysis), what differentiates them from cognitive-behavioral and other non-psychoanalytic treatments, is not a matter of "technique"—that is, how frequently the person is seen, whether free association is encouraged, whether the therapist remains relatively quiet, whether the two participants talk about the patient's childhood, or even whether the therapist explicitly addresses transference reactions—but is instead the nature of the assumptions that underlie the therapist's activity. There is a certain mental set infusing psychodynamic thinking and practice. It is hard to describe, partly because it appreciates nonverbal and preverbal experience, but (as Justice Potter Stewart memorably quipped about a rather different topic) one knows it when one sees it. I will try to sketch it out in this chapter and the next by reference to several related topics.

Contemporary psychoanalytic scholarship has included increasingly frank attention to human spiritual needs and strivings (e.g., Gordon, 2004; Lawner, 2001; Roland, 1999). Bion did not go so far as to say so, but it is arguable that there is a rather substantial "theology" shared by psychoanalytic practitioners.[1] Among its articles of faith are, as noted earlier, the belief that knowing oneself deeply will have complex positive effects; that being honest (relinquishing defensiveness or replacing the false self with authenticity) is central to health and especially to mental health; and that the best preparation for doing analytic therapy is to undergo analytic therapy. In Chapter 2 I elaborate on this implicit belief system or overarching sensibility. Before going there, let me detour into psychoanalytic history to consider why so many people equate the psychoanalytic tradition with only one vertex, the one Bion called medical, and why, even within that vertex, they wrongly associate it with a narrowly defined version of therapy. My comments in the next section apply mostly to the United States, but given the subtle and pervasive ways that American attitudes can infiltrate or have unintended effects on other cultures, they may be of interest to readers in other parts of the world.

BACKGROUND INFORMATION

The Evolution of a "Classical" Psychoanalytic Technique

When psychoanalytic theory migrated across the Atlantic Ocean in the early part of the twentieth century, North American medicine was held in rather low esteem. Antibiotics had not been discovered, life expectancy was in the forties, a distressing number of women died in childbirth, twenty-five percent of children died in infancy, and doctors were regarded more as hand-holders than as miracle workers. Because medical training had not been standardized, many people practiced as physicians with certifications from diploma mills of dubious quality. In 1910, the Carnegie Foundation issued the infamous Flexner Report, describing the low and inconsistent standards that characterized American medical training. Wallerstein (1998) notes that by 1930, the effect of this exposé was a radical retrenching of training along the lines of a model that originated at Johns Hopkins: "The watchword was to exorcize the charlatans from the therapeutic activity and to make the proper medical degree, from the now fully upgraded schools, the hallmark of proper training and competence in the healing arts" (p. 5). Given their post-Flexner sensitivity to accusations of shabby standards, American doctors who became interested in psychoanalysis were determined that it not become viewed as a faddish, unscientific activity. They wanted to specify the technical procedures that defined it as a medical specialty.

Freud felt strongly that psychoanalysis should not be a strictly medical specialty, and eventually argued at length (1926) that the ideal preparation for doing psychoanalysis is the broadest possible grounding in history, literature, the social sciences, psychology, and the humanities, plus a personal analysis. A number of his most cherished analytic colleagues were not physicians, and although his own medical standing was a matter of great importance to him, he did not want to see psychoanalysis become "the handmaiden of psychiatry." Despite the fact that in one famous passage he compared analysis to surgery, he clearly saw it as something that could not be defined by an invariant technique, and he said so many times.

In the years when the Flexner report was disturbing American physicians, however, Freud was becoming increasingly troubled by reckless and misguided applications of his ideas. Self-described analysts were springing up, claiming expertise despite a lack of personal analysis or psychoanalytic training. And people were taking his name in vain. For example, he learned that a neighboring doctor, citing his work, had told a patient that her neurotic symptoms would vanish if only she would get a sex life. He was also becoming distressed to learn that some analysts were rationalizing sexual contact with patients. Understandably, he became concerned about what he called "wild" psychoanalysis, fearing that his cherished movement would be tarred with the brush of quackery. Freud appealed to readers to oppose glib impositions of his concepts, insisting that

> It is not enough . . . for a physician to know a few of the findings of psycho-analysis; he must also have familiarized himself with its technique if he wishes his medical procedure to be guided by a psychoanalytic point of view. This technique cannot yet be learnt from books, and it certainly cannot be discovered independently without great sacrifices of time, labour and success. Like other medical techniques, it is to be learnt from those who are already proficient in it. (1910, p. 226)

(It should be noted that at this point, the procedures Freud was recommending were designed to address only what were then called the "neuroses"—that is, hysterical conditions, obsessions and compulsions, phobias, and nonpsychotic depressions. Hence, technique could be characterized as more or less consistent across the problems for which analytic treatment had been devised. When psychoses, personality disorders, borderline states, posttraumatic conditions, addictions, and other nonneurotic problems were taken up, they naturally called for different approaches.)

Shortly after his 1910 article, as Freud was writing the papers on technique that were to become definitive of standard psychoanalytic practice (Freud, 1912a, 1912b, 1913, 1915), he was distressed to learn that some of his colleagues were having sexual relations with their patients. Before therapists became aware of how powerful a phenomenon transference is, it was perhaps not that obvious to would-be analysts that an affair with a patient would be considerably more destructive than a sexual connection that might develop between any two people in a professional relationship—for example, between an adult woman and her dentist or accountant. Consequently, Freud's comments on technique emphasize discipline and restraint and warn emphatically against exploiting feelings that may arise in treatment.

Mark Siegert (personal communication, November 12, 2003) suggests that in addition to worrying about the bad judgment shown by some of his colleagues, Freud was feeling defensive in the face of the accusations then being aimed at his ideas. His critics charged that rather than finding evidence in his patients of infantile sexual preoccupations, he was putting his ideas about sexuality into their heads. (This argument is strikingly similar, and probably involves a comparable patient population, to the contemporary concern among many thoughtful professionals that dissociative reactions and traumatic memories may be created iatrogenically by overly enthusiastic practitioners finding in their clients what they are already sure is there.) In response to such criticisms, it is understandable that Freud put so much emphasis on being neutral and avoiding all efforts to influence the patient's free associations.

The convergence of these concerns—the determination of American physicians to establish their scientific respectability, the impact of Freud's worry about irresponsible applications of his ideas, and a general determination on the part of Freud and others not to give ammunition to critics of the psychoanalytic movement—led to an effort by the American medical community to control analytic training and to define psychoanalysis *as a medical procedure*, a procedure as standardized as accepted surgical methods. There is an art to surgery, and it was understood that there is also an art to psychotherapy. But the accent was on uniformity of method, exactitude, and the systematic elaboration of the patient's psychology in the context of the analyst's neutrality, objectivity, and abstinence from gratifying any longing of the patient other than the wish for self-understanding. These emphases reflect the scientific values of the Enlightenment, with its idealization of the dispassionate scientist and its emphasis on freeing the rational from the irrational.

Some Consequences of the American Medicalization of Psychoanalysis

In the United States, until a 1986 lawsuit (*Welch v. the American Psychoanalytic Association*) opened the doors of all analytic institutes to nonmedical practitioners, most respected American psychoanalytic organizations were dominated by psychiatrists, who admitted psychologists and other "lay" professionals to their training programs only on the condition that they agree to use their psychoanalytic education for research rather than practice.[2] A benefit of the effort to claim psychoanalysis as a technical medical specialty rather than an interdisciplinary body of knowledge and praxis (Berger, 2002) was, given the vastly increased status of medicine in the postantibiotic age, that psychoanalysis piggybacked on the standing of medicine in general. Being a psychoanalyst became highly prestigious. Doctors who wanted to practice psychotherapy could do so with the confidence that they would be well regarded and well paid. Patients knew that in seeking analysis from someone affiliated with the American Psychoanalytic Association, they would be treated by a person with at least enough intelligence and sanity to get through medical school. It is also probable that a considerable amount of "wild" analysis was thereby prevented.

In addition, as it became common for people to cover their medical expenses via indemnity insurance, the definition of psychotherapy as a medical specialty permitted it to be eligible for third-party reimbursement. During World War II, when psychologists were recruited to do psychotherapy, it was not lost on them that they were doing the same work as psychiatrists. Soon they began establishing the doctorate as the preferable degree for practice as psychologist-therapists, and when they campaigned for licensing and inclusion in insurance plans, they argued "We're doctors, too!" Thus, the association between psychotherapy and medical science worked to the economic benefit not just of psychiatrists but also of psychologists.[3]

The costs of redefining psychoanalysis as a technical procedure comparable to surgery, however, have been steep. First, construing it this way contributed to the relative isolation of psychoanalysis in medical schools and free-standing institutes. This segregation reduced opportunities for analysts to learn from intellectuals outside their field and for other intellectuals to learn from psychoanalysts. It also conduced to a somewhat cult-like atmosphere in psychoanalytic training centers. Except in New York and a few other cities where analysts participated in university life, most undergraduate and graduate professors (other than those in medical schools) had no way of staying in touch with controversies and changes in psychoanalytic theory and practice. What they knew tended to come from intellectual familiarity with some of Freud's theories, or from their own experience as patients, or from the way analysis was portrayed by medical spokespersons or the media. Even today, it is common for authors of academic textbooks on personality and psychopathology to dismiss the psychodynamic tradition based on their reading of a small amount of literature from decades ago. One would never know from academic representations that psychoanalysis remains vital, regularly generating new paradigms that reflect advances in research, assimilation of different philosophical positions, exposure to non-Western cultural attitudes, and appreciation of new scientific theories.

Second, because of its high status as medical expertise, psychoanalytic training became greatly appealing to some professionals whose needs for prestige and recognition were more powerful than their wish to help or their feeling for others. In fact, it is probably not too much of a stretch to describe traditional psychoanalytic institutes, in what some have called the "halcyon years" of analytic preeminence in psychiatry, as magnets for narcissists. The education that took place in institutes became more than usually contaminated by narcissistically related processes such as idealization, splitting, envy, and punishment for those who fail to mirror the biases of their teachers (Kernberg, 1986, 2000; Kirsner, 2000). The sense of self-importance in some analysts in the mid- to late-twentieth century has been painfully evident and bears considerable responsibility for negative reactions to the psychodynamic tradition. According to Good's (2001) report of the findings of an American Psychoanalytic Association marketing task force, "We found out that other mental health professionals actually knew a lot more about psychoanalysis and psychoanalysts than we anticipated. We learned it wasn't so much that they didn't like psychoanalysis as that they didn't like *us*" (pp. 1, 6).

Third, the presumption that psychoanalytic treatment possesses medically demonstrated effectiveness contributed to the disinclination of many analysts to subject their ideas to conventional scientific investigation. Although there is much more empirical research on psychoanalysis and psychodynamic therapy than insurers, drug companies, and some academics like to acknowledge—Masling (2000, quoted in L. Hoffman, 2002) estimates that there are over five thousand empirical studies based on psychodynamic ideas—there is much less research on therapy outcome than there ought to be. Freud bears some responsibility for a dismissive attitude toward empirical research. Once when Saul Rosenzweig, an American psychologist, wrote to him saying that his ideas about repression had been validated in the laboratory, Freud's response was that his own evidence for repression had been sufficient; he considered the empirical testing of the concept gratuitous.

Partly, the disinclination of psychoanalytic therapists since Freud to conduct research is an issue of temperament: Few people who are attracted to the holistic, European philosophical traditions are interested in running carefully controlled studies. They tend to be introverted, introspective, and skeptical about what can be operationalized without distorting the phenomenon under consideration. People who want to be healers are more interested in being out in the imperfectly controlled world trying to help people. Partly, the disinclination to conduct empirical studies on psychotherapy outcome may have expressed a conviction about the value of psychoanalysis that comes from one's personal experiences as both patient and therapist—a conviction that can make conventional empirical evidence seem unnecessary or superfluous. But analysts' resistance to having their beliefs examined through the lens of the researcher also had something to do with the complacency that goes with being an elite. And in the current political climate in the United States, analytic practitioners are paying a high price for not having done more to subject psychoanalytic therapies to controlled investigation.

Fourth, the prestige commanded by psychoanalysis in its so-called heyday ensured that its language would be coopted in the service of very conventional social norms. For example, far too many American women were told by practitioners that they suffered from penis envy—not in the tone of a compassionate revelation that we all suffer primordial, inescapable envious feelings for anything we lack (breasts, child-bearing capacity, fertility, youth, riches, beauty, power, talent,

health . . .) but with the implication that any ambitions they had beyond being middle-class housewives and mothers were pathological. A
kind of pedestrian violence was done to the radical, unconventional,
tragic psychoanalytic message about unconscious desire in an effort to
enforce conformity, to tame and sanitize the soul rather than to plumb
it. The European psychoanalytic sensibility actually grafts rather badly
on to mainstream American attitudes; there is nothing in it that inherently values conformity or supports materialistic striving or equates the
"pursuit of happiness" with the bustle of commerce, the expansion of
markets, the assumption that scientific and technological progress will
resolve perennial human predicaments. In fact, as M. Thompson ob-
serves (2002), because of its insistence on talking frankly about phenomena that one's culture prefers to ignore, "psychoanalysis is unremittingly subversive" (p. 82).

Fifth, and most important from the perspective of this book,
American psychoanalytic clinical practice in the mid-twentieth century
became closely associated with the version of analysis that was regarded as standard technique within mainstream, medically dominated
training institutes. Despite the fact that Glover's (1955) midcentury sur-
vey of analysts showed striking disparities in how they actually practiced, the felt need to articulate a prototypical procedure was strong. In
the United States, many were distressed by the innovations of Franz
Alexander (Stone, 1961), who construed psychoanalytic treatment as a
"corrective emotional experience," a notion that they saw as opening
the door to manipulative ways of working with patients. A conservative
paper by Kurt Eissler (1953) on "basic model technique," which acknowledged a need for "parameters" in some treatments but specified
very narrow conditions for deviating from standard technique, was received as a welcome antidote to Alexander's innovations. Within psychiatry, what Lohser and Newton (1996) have called "a neo-orthodoxy
that is mistakenly considered to be traditional" (p. 10) came to domi-
nate practice. Bucci (2002) recently provided a succinct description of
"orthodox" procedure: "Psychoanalytic treatment was defined in terms
of adherence to standard techniques, focused on interpretation leading
to insight in the context of the transference" (p. 217).

This "classical" technique invoked—rather selectively—Freud's reflections on how he personally had come to conduct treatment. Freud's
ideas are notable for their tone of flexibility and respect for individual
differences, but they were condensed into a set of "rules" that supervisors handed down to trainees (e.g., "You never answer a patient's question; you explore it" and "Always analyze; never gratify" and "Coming
late must be interpreted as resistance" and "You can't tell the patient

anything about yourself"). Herbert Schlesinger (2003) writes of l
experience of psychoanalytic training in the 1950s:

> Perhaps most analysts were introduced to the mysteries of psychoana-
> lytic technique as I was: that it was not so much a cohesive body of struc-
> tured knowledge and practice as a loose collection of do's and don'ts.
> A chill in the heart warned me that to violate any one of them would
> ruin the analysis. (p. 1)

It has been my observation that the worst offenders in terms of defining psychoanalytic therapy as a list of unbreakable do's and don'ts
have been practitioners without analytic training or extensive personal
experience as analysands, who came of age professionally when psychoanalysis dominated psychiatry. Such clinicians have often had a stereo-
typed image of the way analysts practice and have affected all the trappings without the underlying substance of the tradition. What they
represented, with the rationale that it was orthodox or classical, has always seemed to me a perversion of psychoanalytic practice (cf. Ghent's,
1990, illuminating argument that submission is the perversion of a
healthy striving for the experience of surrender). Most fully trained
and seasoned analysts, medically affiliated or not, have been—and have
recommended being—considerably warmer, more natural, and more
flexible than such "rules of technique" suggest. And so was Freud
(Ellman, 1991; Lipton, 1977; M. Thompson, 1996).
    It is not surprising that people who know the psychoanalytic tra-
dition only from its caricatures as represented by untalented practitioners attracted to its status, or from nonanalysts identifying with
their fantasy of a perfectly sterile medical technique, define it as the
procedure in which the therapist says little beyond the occasional accusation that the patient is "resisting." It can also be confusing that
Freud himself was inconsistent in how he defined it. When he was
worried about people applying his concepts in a swashbuckling, undisciplined way, he tended to stress the care with which one applies a
particular set of technical interventions. When he was being simply
reflective about the essence of the process, he was known to say (e.g.,
1914, p. 16) that any line of investigation in which transference and
resistance are addressed can legitimately call itself psychoanalysis. In
a 1906 letter to Carl Jung, he made a serious comment—with which
anyone who has experienced a transformative personal psychotherapy
can resonate—that analytic treatment is essentially a cure through love
(McGuire, 1974, pp. 8–9).
    When students are taught psychoanalytic therapy as a prototypical

technique from which unfortunate deviations are sometimes required, they quickly notice how inconsistently such an approach actually meets the needs of their clients. Beginning therapists rarely get the reasonably healthy, neurotic-level patients who respond well to strict classical technique. They can easily develop the sense that they are "not doing it right," that some imagined experienced therapist could have made the conventional approach work for this person. Sometimes they lose patients because they are afraid to be flexible. More often, fortunately, they address their clients' individual needs with adaptations that are empathic, intuitively sound, and effective. But then they suffer over whether they can safely reveal to a supervisor or classmate what they really did. When beginning therapists feel inhibited about talking openly about what they do, their maturation as therapists is needlessly delayed.

Despite the fact that we all need a general sense of what to do (and what not to do) in the role of therapist, and notwithstanding the time-honored principle that one needs to master a discipline thoroughly before deviating from it, the feeling that one is breaking time-honored, incontestable rules is the enemy of developing one's authentic individual style of working as a therapist. It is more important to know the knowledge base and the objectives of a discipline than to be able to mimic its most typical procedures. Techniques that are good general practices are not always appropriate in a specific context. Since at least the inception of the self psychology movement, there has been a substantial psychoanalytic literature on the importance of making one's interventions patient-specific rather than rule-driven. It is my impression that effective analysts of all schools of thought appreciate this emphasis, and that they did so long before reflections on technical flexibility dominated the literature on practice (for one example, see Menaker's 1942 paper on adapting psychoanalysis to the dynamics of masochistic patients).

The contemporary relational revolution may be viewed, at least in part, as a grass-roots effort to affirm the substance rather than the trappings of psychoanalysis. Many of the most articulate spokespersons for the relational movement have made comments, often privately and sometimes in print (e.g., Maroda, 1991), about their memories of struggling to progress in treatment in the face of their own analysts' rigidities. Now with the voice of a movement, they have effectively been protesting the ritualization of certain technical "rules" that grew to have a life of their own in the twentieth century, often in defiance of evidence that for many clients, the imposition of those rules was deadening rather than liberating.

PSYCHOANALYSIS AND
THE PSYCHOANALYTIC THERAPIES

Psychoanalysis as it was practiced by Freud requires from the patient both a relatively secure attachment style and the capacity to be simultaneously immersed in and reflective about intense emotional experiences. It is therefore not the treatment of choice for most people whose task in therapy will mainly be to develop those capacities. Individuals with psychotic-level problems, active addictions, borderline personality organization, or significant antisocial tendencies are usually not good candidates for Freudian-style psychoanalysis. In addition, many people who could benefit from traditional analysis cannot afford the number of sessions per week that it requires.

Many writers make careful distinctions between psychoanalysis proper and the psychoanalytically based therapies that have been developed to treat individuals for whom analysis is either contraindicated or impractical. Some use the word "psychodynamic" for treatments that are less intensive than the procedure Freud invented yet depend on ideas that derived from his theories. In midcentury America, because of the unique cachet of psychoanalysis, many mental health professionals held the prejudice that even for patients with whom it is not feasible, the more closely one could approximate the technique of "real" psychoanalysis—the approach Freud (1919) had once described as "pure gold" as opposed to the "copper" of suggestion—the greater the value of the therapeutic experience for the patient. Hence, it became important to distinguish verbally the quality product from the knock-offs.

In accord with my inclination to emphasize continuities rather than discontinuities, I prefer to envision a continuum from psychoanalysis through the exploratory psychodynamic therapies in which transferences are invited to emerge and be examined in light of the client's history, then the transference-focused or expressive treatments that zero in on the here-and-now use of pathological defenses, and, finally, the supportive approaches for people who are in crisis or are struggling with severe psychopathology or are simply unable to afford treatments of more than a few sessions. At the ends of the continuum, the disparities are great enough to be legitimately considered differences of kind, but between four-times-a-week analysis and twice-a-week exploratory therapy, the difference seems to me to be one of degree (cf. Schlesinger, 2003). And although my experiences as both patient and analyst have led me to cherish traditional psychoanalysis, I regard the analytically influenced therapies not as a poor substitute for the real thing but as valuable in their own right and frequently the treatment of choice (cf. Wallerstein, 1986).

Because I feel it is more important to understand general psychological principles and the phenomenology of individual differences than to master technical skills in the absence of those bodies of knowledge, I will not be describing in this book how to conduct *particular* therapies that have been derived from psychoanalytic ideas. These are better learned from adherents of the various delineated strategies for specific kinds of clients and situations. Moreover, especially as they accumulate clinical experience, most analytic practitioners work flexibly, shunning technical purity and basing their interventions on their intimate knowledge of each individual human being (or couple or group or family or organization) whom they try to serve. But for newcomers to psychoanalytic ideas I should say a few things about the concepts that are central to most psychoanalytic treatments, including classical analysis. I first note Freud's contributions to our theories of clinical process and then mention more contemporary ideas about both psychoanalysis and the psychoanalytic therapies. (For a less abbreviated history of psychoanalytic clinical theory than what follows, as well as an examination of empirical research bearing on it, see McWilliams & Weinberger, 2003.)

Freudian Psychoanalysis

Freud invited his patients to recline and relax and to speak as freely as possible, reporting every thought and feeling as it made its appearance in their consciousness. He tried to listen with a trance-like receptiveness ("evenly hovering attention") for the themes that emerged in their free associations, to interpret their meanings, and then to convey his understanding to the analysand (the analytic patient). He soon discovered that as people tried to do this, they struggled against inhibitions about saying everything on their minds and against impediments to acting on the basis of their newer insights ("resistance"). He also learned that they persistently responded to him as if he were more like a past love object than he viewed himself as being ("transference").

When he felt that a patient's attitudes toward him were evoking in him strong feelings that went beyond an ordinary professional desire to help, Freud called the phenomenon "countertransference." He emphasized the importance of the analyst's not taking personal advantage of the powerful feelings that analysands develop in treatment, especially when those feelings involve sexual desire and evoke a countertransferential excitement in the therapist, and he cautioned analysts not to use the power of their role in the service of indoctrinating or rescuing their patients ("abstinence"). He also urged them not to intrude their own idiosyncratic personalities and agendas into the therapeutic setting and not to give in to "the temptation to play the part of prophet, saviour, and redeemer to the patient" (1923, p. 50n.). Instead, he exhorted them to try to act as mirrors of the patient's feelings and as blank screens onto which the person's internal images could be projected ("neutrality").

Resistance was initially regarded by Freud as a frustrating obstacle to be overcome. By that term he was not accusing his clients of being uncooperative; he was noting the power of unconscious efforts to cling to the familiar even when it had become self-defeating. Although in his early years of practice, he was known to complain to a patient, "You're resisting!," later he came to understand resistance as an inevitable process that must be respected and "worked through." Transference, too, was originally an unwelcome discovery to him, as it still is for many well-intentioned beginning therapists (even if one expects it, there is something disturbing about being the target of communications that seem to be aimed at someone else). Freud was troubled by the fact that while he was presenting himself as a sympathetic doctor, he was being experienced by his analysands as if he were a significant—and often problematic—figure from their past.

At first, Freud tried to talk his patients out of such perceptions by lecturing them about projection (attribution of one's disowned strivings to others) and displacement (deflecting a drive or affect from one object to a less disturbing one), but eventually he concluded that it is only in a relationship characterized by transference that significant healing can happen. "It is impossible to destroy anyone *in absentia* or *in effigie*" (1912a, p. 108), he pronounced, referring to how in analysis a person can bring about a different outcome to a problematic early struggle. What I understand him to have meant is that when the atmosphere of the patient's childhood emerges in treatment, with the analysand experiencing the analyst as having the emotional power of a parent, the patient becomes keenly aware of long-forgotten (repressed) feelings toward parental figures, can express what was inexpressible in childhood, and can, with the analyst's help, craft new solutions to old conflicts.

Freud saw his patients on successive days, five or six times a week. When therapist and patient are together this often, with one party urged to report uncensored thoughts and feelings while the other is relatively quiet, patients have more than passing transference reactions; they tend to develop what Freud called a "transference neurosis": a set of attitudes, affects, fantasies, and assumptions about the analyst that express central, organizing themes and conflicts dating from their experiences as children. Later practitioners found that a transference neurosis would also emerge in treatments conducted at a frequency of three or four times a week. Psychoanalysis became defined as the process by which a transference neurosis is allowed to develop and is then systematically analyzed and "resolved" (Etchegoyen, 1991; Greenson, 1967).

Resolution meant piecing together an understanding of the diverse effects of one's core conflicts, ultimately substituting knowledge and agency for unconscious tensions that had been manifesting themselves as psychopathology. Freud understood his patients' symptoms to be expressing conflicts between unconscious wishes (e.g., for sexual or aggressive self-expression) and an equally unconscious intolerance of those wishes—intolerance that represents the internalization of societal messages, conveyed by caregivers, to the effect that certain desires are inherently unseemly or dangerous. Paralysis of the hand, for example, a disorder that is inexplicable neurologically yet was common in Freud's era,[4] was interpreted as a neurotic solution to the conflict between the wish to masturbate and the horror of masturbating, both of which were outside awareness. By helping via free association to make such tensions conscious, Freud tried to foster a sense of agency (in this instance about managing sexual needs), in place of the paralysis that was handling the problem outside of consciousness. In other words, he was trying to substitute a mindful, reality-oriented process for an automatic, unformulated, somewhat magical one that operated at the price of symptom formation.

Freud tended to use ordinary, straightforward terms for the phenomena he described (see Bettelheim, 1983). Some of the simplicity and grace of his language, and hence the ease with which psychoanalytic theory can be understood, was lost in the English-language edition of his works, possibly because his writings were translated by his reputedly quite obsessional former patient, James Strachey. The medicalization of psychoanalysis also tilted its language toward mechanization and objectification. It has been a loss, for example, to have Freud's "it," "I," and "I above" represented by the Latin terms "id," "ego," and "superego." Personal pronouns thus morphed into abstract agencies with little subjective resonance. As Jonathan Shedler once commented to me, it is easy for most of us to relate to the distinction between "I" and "it" in ordinary speech: "I did this" is a different experience from "It came over me." The conflictedness of human psychology, the insight that the mind is not unitary but multifaceted and divided against itself, is a profound yet simple idea.

Gradually, the term "psychotherapy" came to refer to modified arrangements in which a transference neurosis is not cultivated but in which transference reactions are addressed, resistances are processed, and transforming insights are sought. The therapy client is not asked to lie down and say whatever comes to mind, but the therapist does invite the patient to speak as freely as possible about the problem areas that occasioned the treatment. While the two parties may try together to make sense of dreams and fantasies, as they would in analysis, they tend to keep focused on one or two central themes or conflicts. The therapeutic alliance is assumed to be internalized as a new model of relationship, as it is in analysis, even though the therapy partners do not search every nook and cranny of the client's psychic life. Recent research supports the value of psychoanalysis; in general, the more frequently and the longer one is seen in treatment, the better the outcome (Seligman, 1995; Freedman, Hoffenberg, Vorus, & Frosch, 1999; Sandell et al., 2000). Data from the comprehensive Menninger study (Wallerstein, 1986) suggest, however, that there are many individuals for whom psychoanalytic therapy is as effective as, or more effective than, psychoanalysis. This finding supports clinical observations to the effect that for some people, a less intense therapy is the treatment of choice.

Contemporary Conceptions of the Psychoanalytic Process

Clinical psychoanalysis, although invented as a therapy, has come to be defined as an open-ended effort to understand all of one's central unconscious thoughts, wishes, fears, conflicts, defenses, and identifications. People may seek analysis in order to pursue an agenda of personal growth or to develop a depth of understanding about universal issues with which their own patients struggle. Psychotherapy has more modest goals, such as relieving specific disorders, reducing suffering, and building stronger psychic structure. Analysis continues to be the most effective treatment known for resolving problems embedded tenaciously in one's personality, whereas therapy may adequately ameliorate more focal difficulties. Despite the convention of defining analysis as a treatment involving three or more sessions a week (usually on the couch), and psychodynamic therapy as twice a week or less (usually face to face), most psychoanalysts would probably agree that the critical difference between an "analysis" and a "therapy" is what happens in the therapeutic process, not the conditions by which the process is facilitated.

To accomplish the ambitious task of a full analysis, clinical experience suggests that patients must become comfortable enough to allow themselves, when in the therapy office, to "regress"—that is, to feel the intense emotions characteristic of early childhood. Many patients report that as they begin to feel more child-like in the therapy hour, they simultaneously find themselves feeling more grown up and autonomous outside it; thus, they experience the regression as contained and coexistent with significant growth. In the context of that circumscribed regression, the analyst gradually attains, in the mind of the patient, an emotional gravity comparable to the power of early caregivers. The emotional power of the analyst when the patient is in a transference neurosis conduces to both healing and prevention. Therapeutic regression is more apt to happen under conditions of frequent contact between therapist and patient, but experienced clinicians have noted that some people are able to undergo a deep analytic process in twice-a-week work, whereas others are not able to do so even after years of meeting five times a week.

The relational movement to which I referred at the end of the last section has brought a new language to the description of the psychoanalytic process. Relational analysts have drawn on diverse sources: the work of Freud's Hungarian colleague Sandor Ferenczi and his followers, Melanie Klein and the British object relations theorists, Harry Stack Sullivan and the American interpersonal movement, Heinrich Racker's writing on countertransference, Hans Loewald's conceptions of therapeutic action, Joseph Sandler's work on role responsiveness, Heinz Kohut's self psychology, Merton Gill's clinical theories, numerous philosophical writings on epistemology and hermeneutics, and many others. These influences converged in challenging the idea that the analyst is a neutral outsider who can comment objectively on the patient's internal dynamics (a number of psychoanalytic writers, starting with Schimek, 1975, have referred to this ideal as the doctrine of "immaculate perception").

Relational analysts have emphasized the interaction between the subjective experiences of both therapist and client and have pointed out that when they engage in a psychoanalytic process, *both* parties find themselves caught up in dynamics reminiscent of the client's early dramas. Countertransference is seen not as an occasional phenomenon but as a pervasive and unavoidable one; entry into the patient's subjective world tends to activate any compatible scripts from the therapist's life. Thus, a woman with a sexual abuse history and her therapist may find that they are subtly enacting familiar, reciprocal roles such as those that Davies and Frawley (1994) have noted as common in such dyads: "the uninvolved nonabusing parent and the neglected child; the sadistic abuser and the helpless, impotently enraged victim; the idealized rescuer and the entitled child who demands to be rescued; and the seducer and the seduced" (p. 167). "Enactment" (Jacobs, 1986) has consequently become a central concept in psychoanalytic understanding of the therapy process. Disclosure to the client of the therapist's feelings and mental images, in the interest of understanding what is being re-created in the clinical setting, is not uncommon among contemporary psychodynamic practitioners.

Acknowledgments that enactments are inevitable, along with the associated conception of the therapist's role as expressing a privileged understanding of mutually constructed contexts and meanings, have become standard features of psychoanalytic discourse. Some analysts continue see value in regarding the therapist as a relatively objective outsider, as Freud did, and therefore put their emphasis on transference as distortion. Relational analysts regard objectivity as impossible and therefore see the transference–countertransference matrix as constructed jointly by the two parties. One welcome side effect of the evolving relational sensibility is that psychoanalytic clinical writing has gradually became less pronunciatory and more explicitly confessional, with therapists describing the nature of their own emotional involvement in the clinical process. Relational analysts tend to depict psychotherapy in more egalitarian and democratic ways than their "classical" predecessors. In a recent article in *The Psychoanalytic Review,* (Eisenstein & Rebillot, 2002), for example, a patient and analyst scrutinize their work together in hindsight, noting the emotional changes that each made during the treatment.

Given the long history of the psychoanalytic movement and the disparate directions in which psychoanalytic clinical theory has gone, I should address the question of diversity within the psychoanalytic community and locate myself in that context. Some readers may be familiar with the passionate ways in which analytic practitioners may embrace their particular psychoanalytic orientation. Does one self-define as classical or relational? Intersubjective or self psychological? Freudian or Jungian or Kleinian or Lacanian? The historical stew of psychodynamic theory and practice, from Freud on, is peppered with enough conflict, disagreement and schism to rival some medieval heresy controversies. It can seem as if there is hardly enough in common among practitioners of divergent leanings for all of us to fit under one psychoanalytic umbrella. In *Psychoanalytic Diagnosis* (McWilliams, 1994) I commented that while theorists spar in the service of promoting their favorite paradigms, ordinary practitioners tend to be more synthetic, taking concepts from different and sometimes even epistemologically contradictory sources when they seem to hold out a way of understanding and helping a particular patient. Pine (1990) likened the different viewpoints in psychoanalysis to the proverbial blind men and elephant: "The complexity of the human animal is sufficiently great such that we gain in our understanding by having multiple perspectives upon it"

(p. 4). The perspective represented in this book is synthetic in the spirit of Pine's observations.

MY OWN ORIENTATION

The reader is entitled to know something about my own identifications, affiliations, allegiances, and assumptions. In deference to compelling arguments made by numerous contemporary writers that one cannot be unbiased but can at least acknowledge biases that are conscious, I will try to describe and account for my own point of view.

Re: Psychoanalytic Pluralism

I first became interested in psychoanalytic theory as a government major at Oberlin College, while writing a senior thesis on the political theory of Freud. My own dynamics are sufficiently Freudian that I found his writing utterly compelling. Several books by his protégé, the psychologist Theodor Reik, were in bookstores at the time, and I began to devour them. After graduating, I moved with my husband to Brooklyn, where it dawned on me that Reik was still alive and in Manhattan. I became intrigued with the idea of meeting someone who had been so close to Freud and had written so movingly about the human condition. I wrote to him asking if he would meet with me and advise me about a career in psychotherapy. Reik received me graciously and urged me to go into analysis. Eventually I went into training at the institute he had founded, the National Psychological Association for Psychoanalysis (NPAP).

My graduate work in psychology was in the department of Personality and Social Psychology at Rutgers University. I had chosen to study personality rather than clinical psychology at Rutgers because Sylvan Tomkins, whose work I admired, was teaching courses in personality, and because my overall fascination with individual differences went beyond a strictly clinical interest. Once I had completed my master's degree, I enrolled in NPAP and took courses there at the same time I pursued the doctorate. While I was a graduate student at Rutgers, first George Atwood and then Robert Stolorow joined the personality faculty and began their extraordinarily fertile collaboration. I loved their work, though I sometimes felt puzzled by their tendency to see what they were doing as a challenge to traditional psychoanalytic ideas. Their ways of thinking felt quite congenial to me, and not in essential conflict with what I had experienced in my own analysis or what I was learning in my analytic training.

At NPAP, what was generally considered "classical" was an orientation to treatment that came from Freud via Theodor Reik. It was on Reik's behalf that Freud had written his polemic to the effect that analysis should not become a servant of psychiatry. Having been excluded by the American medical institutes despite his mentor's position, Reik had started his own training program. His masterwork, *Listening with the Third Ear* (1948), which claimed direct descent from Freud's ideas, emphasized the artistic nature of the analyst's work, the value of letting oneself be surprised, and the virtue of moral courage, including the "courage not to understand." Most of my teachers and supervisors at NPAP in the 1970s embodied these attitudes. They taught me not just about Freud but about Ferenczi, Klein, Fairbairn, Balint, Mahler, Winnicott, Bowlby, Erikson, Sullivan, Searles, Kohut, and others. These thinkers were seen as carrying on Freud's work rather than replacing or contesting it. I was taught, as I will pass on in this book, that the criterion for whether an intervention has been proper or helpful is not the extent to which it follows a standard procedure but, rather, the extent to which it enables the patient to speak more freely, to disclose more genuine or troubling feelings, to deepen the work (cf. Kubie, 1952).

It was also frequently noted at NPAP, as it has been periodically in the psychoanalytic literature, that because psychopathologies differ from era to era and culture to culture, competing theoretical models arise from efforts to account for the psychologies of more typical therapy clients in any given time and place. Theorists derive their metaphors partly from working with a particular type of patient; thus, Freud, whose early work was with people with hysterical and dissociative psychologies, developed a model highlighting relations between different parts of the self experienced as in conflict, while Winnicott, who was fascinated by both infancy and psychosis (Rodman, 2003), created more holistic concepts such as "going on being." I rarely see anyone now whose psychology is best captured by the model of the id, ego, and superego in conflict, but in Freud's era, when stable patriarchal families and guilt-inducing child rearing were normative in Europe, such individuals were evidently abundant. I doubt that it is an accident that the self psychology movement arose in a time and place that creates as many problems for a consistent, positively valued self-concept as Western mass culture does. Similarly, the current popularity of relational paradigms makes sense in an age when authority is suspect and egalitarian models of relationship prevail (see Bromberg, 1992).

During my training in psychoanalysis I felt little pressure to declare allegiance to a particular point of view, and, impressed with Freud's willingness to revise his ideas, I regarded this openness as

quintessentially Freudian (which says a lot about my selective perception, given Freud's equally impressive tendency to ostracize people who
disagreed with him). I read not only Freud's papers on technique but
also some writing by people who had been in analysis with him, and I
admired his individualized responsiveness to his various analysands
(see Lipton, 1977; Lohser & Newton, 1996; Momigliano, 1987). On the
basis of an identification with him as a curious, flexible therapist, I
thought of myself as a Freudian.

It was not until several years after I had graduated from NPAP that
I came into contact with a different version of the "classical" analyst,
the one that emerged from the ego psychology movement as exemplified by Hartmann, Kris, and Loewenstein of the New York Psychoanalytic Institute. A colleague of mine who had trained at one of the "classical" analytic training centers often talked about "the rules" and
seemed to suffer spasms of guilt when he broke them, even when the
patient then flourished. He told me about a friend in his program who
had said, "What I love about psychoanalysis is that you always know
you're doing the right thing. Even if the patient gets worse or suicides,
you know you've offered him the best." This idea that the operation
could literally be considered a success even if the patient had died
seemed bizarre to me, and originally I chalked it up to a peculiarly
pathological narcissism in the psychologist in question. Over time,
however, I heard one after another story of psychoanalytic rigidity and
authoritarianism in the name of what was "classical." Eventually, I
learned not to call myself either Freudian or classical, because I was
typically misunderstood as an apologist for drive theory or a cheer-
leader for what then passed as orthodoxy in most institutes.

The truth is that I still think of myself as more Freudian than anything else, perhaps partly in appreciation of Freud's famous joke that
he was not a Freudian. I have been deeply influenced by analysts who
were self-identified as object relations theorists, Jungians, Kleinians,
self psychologists, intersubjective theorists, control–mastery practitioners, and relational analysts. Arthur Robbins, who was running experiential countertransference-focused groups (see Robbins, 1988) and
teaching about intersubjectivity long before that term appeared in the
analytic literature, was my most influential mentor. I value and identify
with contemporary relational analysts—not because I always agree with
their arguments but because they have palpably advanced the level of
honesty and the quality of dialogue in presentations of clinical work,
increased the level of respect with which patients and their struggles
are described, and brought back to psychoanalysis the excitement of
the search, the open dialogue, the spiritual quest.

Robert Holt once commented (Rothgeb, 1973) that if one ap-

proaches Freud's writing with an intent to debunk specific proposi-
tions, almost anything he said can be shown to be wrong, but if one approaches it with an interest in what can be learned, it will yield great
insights. I have always felt that to get the most from any theory, psychoanalytic or otherwise, one is best served by extending to its proponents
the respect one would grant a client. With patients, we try to understand where they are coming from, what problems they are trying to
solve, what contexts make their solutions reasonable. When one is genuinely empathic, it is impossible to dismiss even a psychotic person as
completely incomprehensible or hopelessly wrong-headed. Most theorists are struggling with their individual solutions to multifaceted human problems, and if we take their angle of vision, we can learn from
them much of value. If, however, we substitute their conclusions for
our own search for what is true, we will sell short our own capacities as
meaning makers. Thus, I remain skeptical of orthodoxies, especially
technical ones (cf. Pine, 1998), and agree with Roy Schafer (1983) that
although there are advantages to working wholeheartedly within one's
particular orientation, there are also advantages to questioning those
assumptions, and to appreciating the inevitable heterogeneity within
each school of thought.

Re: Psychoanalytic Therapy versus Other Approaches

I am often asked how I view nonpsychodynamic approaches to therapy.
Notwithstanding my devotion to psychoanalysis, I have come to respect
the evidence that there are numerous effective ways of helping people.
Overall, if one subtracts the distorting influences of insurance and
pharmaceutical companies, with their common interest in minimizing
the value of psychological interventions, I think the challenges to
psychoanalytic therapy from competing paradigms have been a positive development. A diversity of perspectives opens possibilities for
finding specific approaches to specific difficulties (e.g., pharmacological
management of bipolar symptoms, exposure treatments for obsessive–
compulsive symptoms, twelve-step programs for addictions, and family
systems therapy for dysfunctional relationships). Like most practicing
therapists, I am grateful for any approach, whatever its theoretical origin, that increases my effectiveness or provides me with resources to offer to individuals who seek my help.

Currently, the most academically sanctioned ways of addressing
psychological problems are the cognitive-behavioral treatments. The
intellectual forebears of cognitive-behavioral therapies are found in the
empirical–positivist tradition of American academic psychology rather
than in the European philosophical attitudes that influenced Freud. Al-

though representatives of the psychodynamic and cognitive-behavioral traditions may work more similarly than would be obvious from their theoretical rationales (Wachtel, 1977, 1997), their overall notions about the nature of suffering, the nature of change or help or "cure," and even the nature of "reality" diverge significantly. Some patients seem to prefer more focused and directed treatment, complete with homework assignments and systematically targeted symptoms, and some seem to be allergic to them. Many of the cognitive and behavioral therapies have demonstrated their effectiveness, at least in the short term and with the populations on whom they have been tested.

I do not think, however, that alternative approaches dramatically shorten the amount of time needed to help people with longstanding and far-reaching problems—that is, most people who seek therapy. It is worth noting that all mainstream approaches to psychotherapy, including psychoanalysis, have begun their respective journeys by claiming impressive accomplishments in a stunningly short period of time, and then all have lengthened as their practitioners have faced the complexities of the work. For Freud, a "psychoanalysis" could be as brief as a few weeks, but as he and subsequent analysts encountered the phenomena of resistance and transference and the intricacies of individuals' dynamics, analytic treatments began to extend over several years.

In the 1980s, therapists in the dissociative disorders field repeated Freud's journey toward progressively longer and more complicated treatments for individuals with posttraumatic symptoms: They initially described therapy for dissociative clients in terms of remembering and abreacting, as Freud once did, and they only gradually addressed the complexity of memory, the stubbornness of emotional habit, the importance of attending to the therapeutic relationship, the multiple functions of symptoms, and the consequent need for long-term treatment for complex trauma. Carl Rogers originally claimed that client-centered therapy could foster significant change in a few sessions, and yet humanistic therapists now work with their clients for years. As cognitive-behavioral practitioners wrestle with ongoing problems of relapse-prevention and expand their work into the treatment of personality disorders, the cognitive and behavioral therapies are also becoming prolonged. Eye movement desensitization and reprocessing (EMDR), once heralded as a quick fix for trauma, has expanded into a complex psychotherapy system of its own. We all keep learning the same lessons.

Different sensibilities appeal to different people, and different means of approaching problems operate within a larger arena of helping relationship common to all psychotherapies (Frank & Frank, 1991).

Clinicians practice in ways that make sense to them and that express their individuality. I would be reluctant to train anyone in psychodynamic therapy who is not temperamentally attracted to the *gestalt* I describe in the next chapter, just as I would be reluctant to give musical instruction to someone with a tin ear. (This comparison may be more than a felicitous simile; both musical aptitude and affective attunement seem to be distinctively right-brain phenomena, embodying individual differences in both genetics and infantile experience; Schore, 2003a, 2003b.) Correspondingly, as someone with a psychoanalytic sensibility, I would be hopelessly maladroit at practicing within a manualized cognitive-behavioral framework. (Too left-brained for me, I suppose.) Our talents and inclinations as practitioners are varied enough to encompass many different kinds of work. From my perspective as someone who cringes when authoritarian procedures are purveyed as the essence of psychoanalytic therapy, an accidental benefit of the fact that analysis is no longer intellectually dominant in medicine, clinical psychology, and social work is that only those students with genuine psychoanalytic affinities will now be likely to seek analytic supervision and training. I am hoping this change portends fewer instances of unimaginative, unempathic, dogmatic, routinized psychodynamic therapy in the coming years.

Even though medical metaphors pervade the clinical literature, the practice of psychotherapy is an art, and as such can be compared more aptly to disciplines of musical expression than to medical treatments. There is a science and a theory behind music, but when translated into performance, music offers its afficionados a particular mind–body–feeling–action experience. Music seems be registered by the brain in characteristic ways, irrespective of the particular musical preferences of the listener. Correspondingly, the question of which approach to therapy is globally superior seems to me as misdirected as the question of whether classical, jazz, rock, folk, or country music does a better job of nourishing the soul.

If I had not already come to this conclusion on observational and experiential grounds, I would have been drawn to it by Bruce Wampold's (2001) brilliant analysis of relevant empirical research. What Wampold calls the "contextual" or common-factors model of psychotherapy accounts far better for what we know about treatment outcome than the medical model that has influenced so much recent research and social policy. What are the implications for patients looking to make sense of all the competing voices in the mental health field? As Messer and Wampold (2002, p. 24) have concluded, "Because more variance is due to therapists than to the nature of treatment, clients should seek the most competent therapist possible (. . . often well known within a local community of practitioners) whose theoretical orientation is compatible with their own outlook." In the next chapter, I look at habits of mind that characterize those of us whose outlook is psychoanalytic.

NOTES

1. The late Herbert Strean told me (personal communication, March 17, 1976) that once, in a radio interview, he was challenged about whether psychoanalysis is not just "another religion." "Oh no!" Strean protested, "Psychoanalysis differs from all *other* religions. . . . " I have since heard a similar anecdote attributed to Ralph Greenson. The pleasure with which analysts describe this Freudian slip may say a lot about its truth.
2. Douglas Kirsner (personal communication, July 5, 2002) tells me that a critical component of this stance was the fear, documentable from 1938 on, that the immigrating European analysts, many of whom lacked medical training but had the luster of having worked with Freud, would successfully compete with American psychiatrists for patients.
3. I am grateful to Paul Mosher for calling to my attention this practical consequence of the medicalization of psychoanalysis.
4. When I recently taught in Istanbul, I learned that in Turkey, "Freudian" afflictions such as anesthesia of the hand ("glove paralysis") are still common. Daughters of traditional or fundamentalist Muslim parents who convey disapproval or fear of female sexuality seem to suffer the same problems that once plagued young women in sexually strict Viennese families.

Chapter 2

The Psychoanalytic Sensibility

Devotees of the British and French traditions have been known to point their pens at one another and say, in effect, "What *we* do is psychoanalysis, and what *you* do is not."

Having learned a great deal from both Winnicott and Lacan, I have come to think of them as representing, respectively, the comic and tragic values in the rich tableau of psychoanalytic thought. . . . In Winnicott we find a benign worldview and an ameliorism—a belief that health and happy families are possible, and that humankind can change for the better. In Lacan we are more apt to encounter a Freudian pessimism—a sense that there is something fundamentally unmanageable about human existence, making words like "health" extremely suspect. If collapsing these views into each other would be futile, disregarding one or the other seems almost phobic.

—DEBORAH LUEPNITZ (2002, pp. 16–17)

In this chapter I try to extract commonalities from a dizzying variety of approaches, all of which identify themselves as psychodynamic. There may not be one true, universal *technique* of psychoanalytic therapy, but there are universal beliefs and attitudes underpinning the effort to apply psychodynamic principles to the understanding and growth of another person. Mitchell and Black (1995) described such attitudes as including respect for "the complexity of the mind, the importance of unconscious mental processes, and the value of a sustained inquiry into subjective experience" (p. 206). Benjamin (2002) summarized them as a concern for "truth, freedom, and compassion for our

mutual vulnerability." Lothane (2002) recently noted that the psychoanalytic patient "seeks the Socratic goal of the examined life, both of
learning to know himself or herself . . . and to grow as a moral agent
who lives his or her life responsibly rather than impulsively" (p. 577).
Meissner (1983), in an article on psychoanalytic values, highlighted self-
understanding, authenticity, the valuing of values themselves, and the
quest for truth.

Buckley (2001) traces the psychoanalytic worldview to the ancient
Greek, specifically Platonic, "philosophical" model of the mind (as con-
trasted with other ancient models, the Homeric/poetic and the Hippo-
cratic/medical). Messer and Winokur (1984), appropriating the language of literary criticism, have labeled the psychoanalytic orientation
tragic, contrasting it with a behavioral outlook they depict as comic (in
a spirit similar to that of the Luepnitz quote above, though she was
pointing to differences of emphasis within psychoanalysis). "Tragic" de-
notes a sense that one has to come to terms with inherently flawed
and painful realities; "comic" captures the more pragmatic, problem-
solving view that changes can be made to bring about a happy ending.
Schneider (1998) has included the psychodynamic tradition with the
"romantic" (affective, intuitive, holistic) sensibility in Western thought,
as opposed to the hypothetical–deductive–inductive bias of most
American academic psychology and the logical positivist tradition in
general. While teaching recently in Istanbul, I was told that the Turkish
language has two different words for science: *belim*, referring to the
"scientific method" idealized by Western academic psychology, and
elim, referring to the pursuit of understanding by more observational,
introspective, and associative means (Yavuz Erten, personal communication, May 15, 2003). Psychoanalytic scholarship is appreciated as
within the domain of *elim*.

Different writers with a psychoanalytic temperament have identified themselves with phenomenology, existentialism, structuralism,
postmodernism, constructivism, skepticism, Buddhism, Christianity,
Judaism, and other philosophical, hermeneutic, and spiritual traditions. It is typical of psychodynamically inclined thinkers to locate their
habits of thought within a philosophical tradition and to challenge the
notion that therapy can derive solely from "objective" findings of conventional research paradigms or can constitute a compendium of
"techniques" isolated from orienting values, assumptions, and cul-
tural/historical contexts (see Messer & Woolfolk, 1998; Strenger,
1991). Some of what I summarize also characterizes orientations that
developed to extend or correct aspects of the psychoanalytic paradigm,
including (among others) Gestalt therapy, client-centered therapies and

the humanistic–experiential tradition generally, transactional analysis, existential approaches, psychodrama, and the art therapies. In what follows I have, rather arbitrarily, organized the elements of what W. H. Auden, in a poem mourning Freud's death, called "a whole climate of opinion" under the themes of curiosity and awe, complexity, identification and empathy, subjectivity and attunement to affect, attachment, and faith. These aspects are overlapping and therefore hard to isolate, and although it is impossible to describe a *gestalt* by breaking it down into component parts, I take each of these up briefly.

CURIOSITY AND AWE

Most fundamentally, psychoanalytic practitioners take seriously the evidence that the sources of most of our behaviors, feelings, and thoughts are not conscious. Given what we have learned about the brain in recent years, this conviction is increasingly shared by cognitive scientists and nonpsychoanalytic clinical psychologists and suggests the possibility of an eventual integration of approaches. Yet to the psychodynamically inclined, it is not just that these phenomena are *non*conscious but that there is a dynamic organization to the way we unconsciously register experience, an organization that prompts analysts to talk as if there is something called "the" unconscious, both generically and in each one of us. In any individual, this intrapsychic organization is understood to be the result of unfolding interactions between the growing child and the significant people in that child's world. Features of, and relationships with, these early figures, as experienced by the child, come to be internalized in stable ways.

    For anyone who has done analytic therapy for a long time, it becomes fascinating how nonaccidental are the "choices" people make. We rationalize what we do, but like the hypnotic subject inventing an explanation for why he or she unknowingly acted on a posthypnotic suggestion, we seldom, if ever, know all the determinants of our behavior. Perhaps this is most striking in the area of "choosing" a romantic partner (Mitchell, 2002; Person, 1991). Falling in love is one of the few common experiences that makes most people aware of how remarkably lacking in control they are over the emotionally powerful situations in which they find themselves. Children of affectively intense parents often seek intensity; children of negligent ones somehow find mates who ignore them. Daughters of alcoholic fathers bemoan their attraction to men with alcohol dependency; sons of depressed mothers may be drawn like moths to the flame of unhappy women. For that matter, sadistic people have radar for masochists, and pedophiles know the look in a child's eye suggesting a confusion or vulnerability to manipulation that makes molestation more likely to be tolerated.

People are often aware that they have a "type" of love object whose attractiveness feels irresistible, yet they seldom feel clear about why such a person is their type. We are always operating at many different levels besides the verbal, rational ones, sending elaborate signals to each other with facial expressions, tone of voice, tilt of head, tension of body, perhaps even odors of pheromones. Reviewing empirical work on sexuality, Money (1986) has documented our remarkably idiosyncratic individual "lovemaps." Proximity and chance certainly affect the connections we make, but when hearing clients' histories and witnessing their struggles, practitioners are repeatedly hit between the eyes with their unconsciously determined, remarkably repetitive, persistent interpersonal scripts. One man I treated, who as a child used to come into the kitchen each morning to see his alcoholic mother staring into space with a cigarette in one hand and a coffee cup in the other, fell "inexplicably" in love with a woman he first noticed in his college cafeteria, staring into space with a cigarette in one hand and a coffee cup in the other.

Some people take pains to find a partner who is the polar opposite of a problematic parent, yet find, as they start to build a life with the person who was supposed to be an antidote, that their earlier experiences are nevertheless eerily evoked in the new relationship. For example, a patient of mine whose father had been episodically violent fell in love with a committed pacifist, someone she felt was so wholeheartedly dedicated to nonviolence that she would never again have to live in fear. After a few months of marriage and more than a few heated fights, she became increasingly convinced that her husband's ideological pacifism expressed a not entirely successful effort to counteract his own violent tendencies. Once again, she was worrying that the man with whom she lived was dangerous. In therapy, she marveled at her having managed to "find" her father despite her diligent conscious efforts to lose him.

Those of us who work with dreams, along Freudian lines or others, are consistently awed by how much data can be condensed into a few images and a story line. Whether or not one analyzes dreams in a psychotherapy, it is hard not to appreciate Freud's conviction that his effort to make scientific sense of dreaming was his greatest accomplishment. There is so much extraordinary condensation in dream symbols that one cannot conceive of the brain's having that degree of power consciously. As Grotstein (2000) has elaborated, dreams show the activity of various cooperating "presences" in the mind: "the dreamer who

dreams the dream," "the dreamer who understands the dream," the actors, and the "Background Presence"—all intercommunicating and sym-
bolizing experience into a narrative that will "organize and unify the
data presented to the senses" (p. 24).

It is not difficult for a careful observer to see the evidence for unconscious processes in other people; it is harder to grasp the reality
that we ourselves are inhabited and moved by forces beyond our access
or control. For many of us who practice psychoanalytically, it was an incident in our intimate life or personal therapy that crystallized our ongoing sense of awe, that moved our appreciation of unconscious motivation from an intellectual deduction to a visceral conviction. Many
therapists remember, in the same, flash-bulb way in which people can
recall where they were when they heard about a plane hitting the
World Trade Center, a moment when the sense of pure wonder over-
powered the protest of their pride. For me it was when I realized that a
public figure with whom I was oddly mesmerized had the same nick-
name as my father. For a colleague of mine, it was when she dreamed
about a "Thomas Malthus" at a point in therapy when she was mourning the fact that in her family, love had been part of an "economy of
scarcity." She had no conscious knowledge that Malthus was an economic theorist who emphasized the limited nature of resources and
was stunned by the fact that unconsciously, she had obviously registered this information somewhere. For another friend, it was when he
discovered that his depression had begun thirty years to the day after
his father's death, a date he had not thought he knew.

The curiosity about how any individual's unconscious thoughts,
feelings, images, and urges work together is the engine of the therapist's commitment and the bulwark of the patient's courage to be more
and more self-examining and self-disclosing. The assumption that, as
therapists, we *don't know* what we will learn about a patient, is both realistic and healing. One frequently heard analogy for the role of the analytic therapist, a role that claims authority about process but uncertainty about content, is that of the trailblazer or travel guide. If one is
walking through an alien jungle, one needs to be with someone who
knows how to traverse that terrain without running into danger or going in circles. But the guide does not need to know *where* the two parties will emerge from the wilderness; he or she has only the means to
make the journey safe. Even though there are reams of literature about
dynamics that typically accompany various symptoms or personality
types, the thoughtful psychodynamic practitioner listens to each patient with an openness to having such constructions disconfirmed.
What Freud called "evenly hovering attention," what Bion and later
Ogden called "reverie," what Casement calls "unfocused listening" is

perhaps the *sine qua non* of the analytic attitude: the receptivity to whatever presents itself and the curiosity about the multitude of things it may mean.

The sense of awe is usually associated with religious themes, with the numinous realm, the place of the spirit. It is intrinsically connected with humility, the acknowledgment that human beings are, as Mark Twain observed, "the fly-speck of the universe" and that each of us is impelled by countless forces outside our own awareness and control. Awe involves the willingness to feel very small in the presence of the vast and unknowable. It is receptive, open to being moved. It bears witness. It could not be more different from the instrumental, utilitarian mind-set of the technical problem solver or from the pragmatic, can-do optimism of the man who believes himself to be completely in charge of his life. It is not antiscientific, but it defines scientific activity in much broader ways than the logical positivist who breaks huge, complex issues down into small and simple ones so that concepts can be easily operationalized and variables readily controlled. Awe allows our experience to take our breath away; it invites each client to make a fresh imprint on the soul, the psyche, of the therapist.

COMPLEXITY

Analytic thinkers regard intrapsychic conflict or multiplicity of attitude as inevitable. Most of us can find in ourselves wishes to be both old and young, male and female, in control and under someone's care, and so forth. Our adaptations to realistic limits are irreducibly ambivalent. The human animal was seen by Freud as insatiable, always yearning, never completely satisfied—partly because human beings often want mutually exclusive things at the same time. Post-Freudian analysts who see individuals as less influenced by drives and more motivated by the need for relationship still talk about paradox, ambiguity, dialectic, multiple self states, and the multifaceted nature of life and its challenges (e.g., Eigen, 2001; Grotstein, 2000; I. Hoffman, 1998). They regard reductionism of almost any kind as suspect. A comment like "She's just doing that to get attention" would not be an observation in a psychoanalyst's repertoire—at least not with the "just."

In 1937, the psychoanalyst/physicist Robert Waelder elaborated on two terms Freud had mentioned more or less in passing, the related concepts of "overdetermination" and "multiple function." The analytic community gratefully adopted them as ways of describing something that practitioners had long been observing. "Overdetermination" refers to the observation that significant psychological problems or tendencies have more than one cause; in fact, most have a complex etiology. A symptom important enough to instigate a trip to the therapist has typically resulted from many different, interacting influences, including factors such as one's constitution, emotional makeup, developmental history, social context, identifications, reinforcement contingencies, personal values, and current stresses. "Multiple function" refers to the fact that any significant psychological tendency fulfills more than one unconscious function, such as to reduce anxiety, to restore self-esteem, to express an attitude that is unwelcome in one's family, to avoid temptation, and to communicate something to others.

Thus, a woman who becomes anorectic may have developed that problem because of the interaction of the following contributants: (1) a background of parental overinvestment in her eating, (2) a history of sexual abuse, (3) a recent loss or disappointment, (4) a developmental challenge of which she is afraid, (5) an unconscious association of weight gain with pregnancy, (6) a history of having been shamed about her hunger or need for emotional nourishment, (7) a sense of having been neglected in her family, (8) an experience of having been admired for having lost weight, and (9) the repeated exposure to highly valued but unrealistic images of women's bodies. Her anorexia may unconsciously accomplish the following goals for her: (1) to achieve control over herself and others despite the efforts of others to control her; (2) to reduce her attractiveness to possible molesters; (3) to express grief; (4) to maintain a sense of being prepubertal, nonmenstruating, and nonadult; (5) to reassure herself she is not pregnant, (6) to avoid criticism for self-indulgence; (7) to get attention from her family; (8) to garner compliments; and (9) to conform to cultural expectations of beauty. Most analysts would say that is a short list for something as complex as anorexia, which may reflect many other influences and fulfill many other functions as well. For example, there now seem to be subcultures (modeling, dance) in which anorectic behavior is normative and assiduously reinforced.

When I was an undergraduate, one of my professors was an erudite Hungarian political scientist named George Lanyi. It was student lore that if one wanted to get a good grade from Professor Lanyi, it was unwise to suggest single-factor explanations for international political events. One had to look carefully at the countries in question and mention such things as their economic situations, the religious beliefs of their citizens, their historic allegiances and rivalries, the personalities of their leaders, the domestic agendas of their different internal factions, their theories about what constituted the greatest threats to their stability, their ideological heritages, their levels of development, their sense of national mission, their ethnic components, the vagaries of their weather, and so on. And it was always good to put a line in an international politics essay exam to the effect that no single factor could account for anything of major importance in world politics. A friend of mine referred to this orienting belief about the complexity of things as "Lanyi's balloon." He was contrasting it with "Occam's razor," the effort to account for any phenomenon with the simplest possible explanation.

Psychologists and medical researchers conducting conventional empirical investigations operate according to the principle of parsimony. And for research purposes, parsimony is a highly useful assumption. But it is not necessarily the truth (cf. Wilson, 1995). Both Occam's razor and "Lanyi's balloon" are fictions, ways of asserting a preference for either simplified or elaborated theories of causation. The tendency of psychoanalytic therapists to prefer complex, intricate explanations over simple ones may express both their clinical experience and the temperament that inclined them toward doing an in-depth, emotionally complicated kind of work in the first place. Certainly we may eventually learn that some psychological phenomena have single causes, but in the meantime the psychoanalytic prejudice is to assume complexity.

IDENTIFICATION AND EMPATHY

It is part of the psychoanalytic mental set to view a disturbance in any individual's functioning as expressing an extreme or currently maladaptive version of a universal human tendency. Harry Stack Sullivan's conviction that "we are all more simply human than otherwise" (1947, p. 16) suffuses psychodynamic thinking. In this assumption, analytic practitioners share a bias with humanistic, experiential, and client-centered therapists. Not that those of us who practice psychodynamically are not perfectly capable as individuals of feeling a defensive superiority to others, whom we may objectify with our diagnoses and implicitly devalue in our zeal to distance personally from their problematic dynamics; my point is that analytic theories consistently stress our common human developmental pathways, vulnerabilities, and strivings. The requirement of analytic institutes that their candidates undergo psychoanalysis themselves, about which I talk more in the next chapter, had the intention, among other aims, of increasing therapists' capacities to identify with patients' struggles by finding comparable issues in themselves.

There is a bias among analysts against categorization of human "problems in living" (Szasz, 1961) as categorical "disorders" unrelated to an understanding of the functions that such conditions fulfill for a psychologically complex individual. As I have elaborated elsewhere (McWilliams, 1998), psychodiagnosis as it is actually practiced by psychodynamic therapists is holistic, contextual, and dimensional. Seemingly discrete problems can rarely be well understood in isolation from the person in whom they exist. (In my experience, patients who have an Axis I disorder "not comorbid with anything else" must be from other planets.) An articulate expression of this bedrock analytic attitude appears in Roughton's (2001) article on his evolving understanding, over four decades, of sexual orientation as a dimension of human functioning that is independent of mental health or illness. In discussing specific sexual activities, he notes that "As in all psychoanalytic evaluation, it is the underlying psychic structure and the motivation and meaning—not the superficial similarity of behavior—that counts" (p. 1206).

While analytic therapists from Freud on have appreciated genetic, chemical, and neurological dispositions toward the serious psychopathologies, they have also looked for historical and current stresses that may cause such tendencies to erupt as problems. There is an implicit consensus in the analytic community that under the constitutional and situational conditions affecting the patient, the therapist would have become similarly symptomatic. By temperament and training, psychodynamic clinicians trying to understand the hallucinating schizophrenic, the determined self-mutilator, the starving anorectic—even the sadistic psychopath—look to the psychotic, borderline, body-obsessed, and sadistic parts of themselves. They also expect, when they work with anyone dealing with a difficult aspect of his or her personality, that their own similar issues will be activated. This tendency to identify with their clients, and to mine that identification for deeper and deeper feelings of empathy, contrasts with the responsibility felt by more biologically oriented psychiatrists and academic psychologists to take a more detached position toward people and problems. It is compatible, however, with the embracing attitude that tends to characterize both clinical social work and pastoral counseling as professions.

Freud set the tone on this. Although he could certainly be disdainful of people he was not interested in knowing better (including Americans as an aggregate, whom he considered naive, emotionally shallow, and excessively materialistic—he was known to refer to the United States as "Dollarland"), he extended empathy toward some groups that were highly improbable objects of identification for people of his era, class, and profession. When many other physicians were dismissing women with conversion and somatization disorders as frivolous malingerers, Freud took them seriously and tried to understand them. His famous 1935 letter to the mother of a gay man (quoted in E. Jones, 1957, p. 195), in which he insisted that homosexuality "is nothing to be ashamed of, no vice, no degradation, it cannot be classified as an illness" was certainly striking in its refusal to consign gay people to some lesser category of humanity (even if he did also view homosexuality, unfortunately for posterity, as an "arrest of sexual development"). And although the contemporary ear finds Freud's references to "savages" disturbingly racist, his main message was that people in civilized societies have more in common with those they typically dismiss as "primitive" than anyone had ever imagined.

In a highly influential work, Christopher Bollas (1987) made the now famous comment, "in order to find the patient, we must look for him within ourselves" (p. 202). The centrality of identification and empathy goes beyond a conceptual preference to the question of effectiveness. The main "instrument" we have in our efforts to understand the people who come to us for help is our empathy, the main "delivery system" of that empathy is our person. Whatever the benefit of more intellectual aspects of our understanding (our theories, research, and clinical reports), our capacity to "get" the patient (or more accurately, to *approach* an understanding that will inevitably fall short of completeness or perfect accuracy), and to convey our understanding to him or her in a useful way, rests mostly on our intuitive and emotional abilities. One of the chronic sources of both pleasure and fatigue in psychodynamic work is the need to keep moving back and forth, trying to go inside the patient's subjectivity and then trying to come out and reflect on the experience of immersion. Clients who feel their therapists are right but not empathic take their therapeutic medicine with a choking dose of shame, an affect that evokes compliance, oppositionality, or paralysis rather than receptiveness and emotional maturation. Clients who feel their therapists are wrong *but trying to identify* will not be shamed and will continue their engagement in the therapeutic process as they try to make themselves understood.

SUBJECTIVITY AND ATTUNEMENT TO AFFECT

Closely related to identification and empathy is the assumption that subjectivity, far from being the enemy of the truth, can promote a much more comprehensive understanding of psychological phenomena than objectivity alone. A theoretical physicist presumably does not fruitfully empathize with particles of matter (although Einstein did say that he simply tried to understand God's plan, and many unusually creative people do identify with inanimate objects), but the psychotherapist can use a disciplined subjectivity to draw testable inferences about a person's psychology. In fact, some psychoanalytic writers (Kohut,

1959; Stolorow & Atwood, 1992) have defined psychoanalysis as the science in which sustained empathic inquiry is the primary observational mode.

The perils of subjectivity are well known: We can easily distort in the service of our personal needs; we are all handicapped by our individual backgrounds, assumptions, and limitations; we cannot construct a cumulative science without objectively derived reliability and validity. But objectivity is full of liabilities as well. Researchers striving for objectivity tend to ignore data that cannot be operationalized, manipulated, or studied by randomized clinical trials; they tend to fragment complex, interrelated issues to make them empirically researchable; they have been known to be methodologically rigorous but substantively vacuous. The more we learn about infant–caregiver communication in the first year, the more we discover that there are many preverbally based communicative processes that are hard to observe, describe, and count. Rather, we feel them.

Between infant and parent in the first year, there is a dance of right-brain-to-right-brain communication essential to optimal neural development and the achievement of secure attachment, affect tolerance, and affect regulation (Goldstein & Thau, 2003). The scrutinized emotional experience of a disciplined clinician can reveal a lot about what a client is communicating via facial affect, body language, and tone of voice. Kernberg talks about patients transmitting on "channels II and III": nonverbal communication and countertransference evocation (Hellinga, van Luyn, & Dalewijk, 2001). Analytic therapists embrace their subjectivity, and they learn from their affective reactions a lot about what their clients are trying to say.

Some years ago a man came to the attention of neurologists because an injury had damaged his frontal lobes in such a way that he felt no emotion. Physiologically, he could have been the prototype for the "rational man" so idealized by Enlightenment philosophers and many contemporary researchers—a veritable Data or Mr. Spock (of the later and earlier *Star Trek* series, respectively). All his decision making was dictated by reason and logic rather than by such affective processes as sympathy, emotion, and intuition. The striking thing about this man's decisions is that they were often bizarre and sometimes glaringly self-defeating. Without emotionality, he seemed devoid of the capacity to understand the full meaning of his choices. Rather than being gloriously free of primitive contaminants that allegedly corrupt judgment, he was crippled by the absence of the sensibilities that make good judgments possible. This man had been a judge; after his injury he resigned from the bench because he understood that to render justice, one must be able to feel sympathy for diverse human motives. His predicament calls to mind the wisdom of Plato, who envisioned human reason as like the charioteer who needs not only the white horse of the will but also the dark horse of passion to move ahead (see Damasio, 1994; Sacks, 1995, pp. 244–296).

Early in his therapeutic endeavors, Freud learned that there is a difference between intellectual and emotional insight. That is, we can "know" something cognitively and yet not *know* it at all. To change, we need to appreciate our condition in a way that feels visceral as opposed to cerebral. That discovery has been made again and again by psychodynamic, existential, and humanistic therapists since Freud (see, e.g., Appelbaum, 2000; Hammer, 1990; Maroda, 1999). Drew Westen (personal communication, May 10, 2002) is probably right that as the cognitive-behavioral movement matures, we can expect its practitioners to start calling themselves something like "cognitive-affective-behavioral" clinicians because the same phenomenon will be impossible for them to ignore.

There is something about what we subsume under the label "affect" that is a prerequisite for meaningful understanding and genuine change. Experience suggests that most people do not separate, individuate, and come to a benign acceptance of the past without going through a period of feeling anger and even hatred toward the person or family or community or ideology from whose influence they are emerging. All known societies expect a grief process before a bereaved person resumes normal functioning. Overwhelming events cease to be traumatic once one can give voice to emotional reactions to them. Feelings have their own kind of wisdom. Empirical studies of emotion (e.g., Pennebaker, 1997) confirm the observation of generations of clinicians that affect plays a determinative role in the process of growth and change. Without the capacity to appreciate subjectively the emotional worlds of their patients, therapists would be missing a huge chunk of data, and their effectiveness would be severely compromised.

Practitioners, unlike those who consider mental health issues from a greater distance, have no choice but to deal with affect: A client's pain or hostility or excitement can flood the space between two people in ways that go far beyond words. Affects are contagious; they induce many complex emotional reactions in us. For a long time in the psychoanalytic tradition, therapists tried to defer to Freud's nineteenth-century scientistic bias to the effect that one should keep a cool head despite the emotional storms of one's patients, that anything other than a benign physicianly attitude is suspect, hinting of unworked-out emotional kinks in the analyst. Especially as therapists have worked with more "difficult" patients, however, we have abandoned this ratio-

nalistic ideal. Of course we need to ponder the implications of a patient's outburst and to restrain the natural tendency to act on our feelings while we do so. Of course we remember that it is the patient, not
the therapist, who is asked to give free rein to feelings in the office. As
several analysts have commented in recent years, we try to be our "best
self" with our patients, not our whole self. Psychoanalytic practitioners
have rarely endorsed the general wisdom of "letting it all hang out."
But we do pay close attention to our subjective responses to our clients'
emotions and value what we learn in doing so.

Emotions and affective dispositions may prove to be much more
consequential for human behavior than the instinctual drives in which
Freud embedded his comprehensive theories. Many contemporary psychoanalytic thinkers question assumptions about primal, universal instincts and emphasize affective organizations instead. Numerous writers (e.g., Fosha, 2000; J. Greenberg, 1986; Hedges, 1996; Nathanson,
1996; Spezzano, 1993; Tomkins, 1962, 1963, 1991) have offered comprehensive arguments about the primacy of affect, and contemporary
research in brain physiology and chemistry is beginning to make affective functioning much more comprehensible to us. In the meantime,
the subjective immersion of therapists, both voluntary and involuntary,
in the expressed and unverbalized emotions of their patients remains
one of the most important sources of information we have about what
is "the matter" with a person, how he or she experiences what is wrong,
what may have happened to create the problem, and what emotional
processes may be necessary in order to work out of the difficulty.

I would further conjecture that part of the psychoanalytic temperament involves an attraction to or pleasure in or inability to minimize
strong affect. There seem to be marked individual differences in
whether a person seeks and welcomes the experience of intense emotion or prefers to resist or subdue the more passionate parts of the self.
I have noticed that those graduate students at Rutgers who are most
naturally taken with psychoanalytic ideas are also frequently immersed
in the arts: poetry, music, theater, dance, and other repositories of powerful emotionality. One of my students characterized herself as an "affect junky." There are also individual differences in how much control
we each feel over our emotions. Some creative and influential psychoanalytic writers have described their personalities as schizoid, a disposition that includes a sense of "hyperpermeability" (Doidge, 2001) to
strong feelings. Those of us who have no choice but to be filled with
emotion may be attracted to psychoanalytic ideas because they give
voice to our affectively suffused experience and help us to make sense
of our intense, insistent inner lives. Along these lines, I have heard sev-

eral colleagues with this temperament make comments to the effect that they are "unfit" to do anything but psychoanalytic work. During the era when psychoanalysis wore the halo of medical prestige, many analysts may have been overly intellectualized and relatively impermeable to powerful emotions, but in recent decades, this kind of practitioner seems to have all but vanished from the therapeutic scene.

ATTACHMENT

Psychodynamic clinicians understand individual psychologies and psychopathologies as determined by complex interactions between lived experience and a person's constitutional makeup and normal developmental challenges. They view treatment as the opportunity for a new person, the therapist, to facilitate a benign maturational process that naturally unfolds in an atmosphere of safety and honesty. Working collaboratively, the therapist and patient find ways to help that process along when the patient gets stuck because of dangers that accompanied the developmental exigencies in his or her history. As the markedly oppositional client of one of my colleagues recently commented, in this case with considerable sarcasm, "I'm finally getting it. You think I need a new experience. And you think *you* are gonna be that new experience?!"

Although analytic therapists may hope to be ultimately assimilated by their patients as "new objects"—that is, as internal voices that differ significantly from those of people by whom their clients have felt damaged—they appreciate the fact that, because of the stability and tenacity of unconscious assumptions, they will inevitably be experienced as old ones. They consequently expect to have to absorb strong negative affects associated with painful early experiences and to help the client understand such reactions in order to move past them and learn something new that penetrates to the level of unconscious schemas. Most people in the psychoanalytic community have been struck by the wisdom in Jay Greenberg's (1986) observation that if the therapist is not taken in as a new, good love object, the treatment never really takes off, but if the therapist is not also experienced as the old bad one, the treatment may never end (see Stark's, 1999, fascinating reflections on this therapeutic tension).

Any therapist becomes impressed over time with how hard it is to find a way to talk with someone that avoids getting subsumed into that person's preexisting personal schemas. Psychoanalytic approaches to helping people share an orientation to treatment that assumes an intimate, highly personal, affectively rich relationship in which both parties slowly become aware of the nature of the patient's unconscious assumptions and work past them to new ways of seeing and acting in the world. Young-Breuhl and Bethelard (2000) write about the importance of "cherishment," the sense of being affectionately and personally cared for by a devoted other, in creating the possibility and the will for change. Many psychoanalysts, starting with Freud, have credited love with the major role in psychotherapeutic healing (e.g., Bergmann, 1982; Fine, 1971; I. Hoffman, 1998; Kristeva, 1987; Lothane, 1987; Shaw, 2003), even if what we mean by love is more like the Greek *agape* or the Japanese *amae* (see Doi, 1989) than the romantic love more commonly celebrated in our culture.

Although most of their contemporaries regarded both John Bowlby, who pioneered the empirical study of attachment in children, and Margaret Mahler, who developed the concept of separation from an early symbiosis, as suspect deviators from the Freudian paradigm, their work has had more influence on therapeutic practice than that of any of their disparagers. Their efforts to study human connections via infant–parent observation have inspired far-reaching empirical and theoretical efforts, rich with implications for psychotherapy (see, e.g., Fonagy, Gergely, Jurist, & Target, 2002; Greenspan, 1996). For example, Bowlby's postulating an evolutionary basis for attachment, in that it functions as a regulator of affect and a safety zone from which to explore, has influenced clinicians to appreciate the value of the therapeutic relationship itself over any interpretations issued by the therapist. Despite their notable indifference to many other avenues of pertinent empirical study, psychodynamic practitioners have been avid consumers of reports on attachment research, doubtless because relationship is the medium within which they work every day, and adapting oneself to each patient's attachment style is a continuing challenge.

As we learn more about attachment, we have new ways of understanding why the intimate emotional connection between therapist and patient has turned out to be so critical to healing (see, e.g., Meissner, 1991). That we are inherently social creatures who mature in a relational matrix and require relationship in order to change is suggested by the well-established empirical finding that the alliance between patient and therapist has more effect on the outcome of therapy than any other aspect of treatment that has been investigated so far (see Safran & Muran, 2000). It is odd that so many people see psychoanalytic therapy as an endless, intellectual rehashing of one's childhood experiences when, in fact, one of its core assumptions concerns the raw emotional power of the here-and-now therapeutic relationship.

FAITH

I have been ambivalent about writing about the role of faith in psycho-analytic therapy, for fear of offending readers who are uncomfortable with a term so rooted in religious and theological discourse. Moreover, because few analytic thinkers have written about faith in the context of psychoanalytic theory (notable exceptions include Charles, 2003; Eigen, 1981; Fromm, 1947; Kristeva, 1987; D. Jones, 1993), it feels as if I have fewer scholarly underpinnings to an argument about the place of psy-chotherapeutic faith than I have for other topics. I considered substi-tuting "belief," but that word is too cognitive and active (as opposed to visceral and receptive) to capture the phenomenon I want to convey. And "hope," another obvious candidate and one with perhaps a more established place in psychoanalytic writing (e.g., S. Cooper, 2000; Mitchell, 1993), connotes both less conviction and more of an expecta-tion of something specifiable than I think the psychoanalytic sensibility contains.

Ultimately, "faith" seemed the only accurate term for the attitude I am trying to distill here (cf. Fowler, 1981), notwithstanding the fact that many analytic practitioners who exemplify therapeutic faith are not theistic. Religious language does capture certain dimensions of ex-perience that secular language does not. It is not accidental that Freud, though a rationalistic atheist, chose the word *psyche*, which translates best as "soul," when theorizing about psychological experience (see Bettelheim, 1983), rather than writing about the "mind" or "brain." So I am using the term advisedly, asking even those readers with no affin-ity for the spiritual to consider that there is a kind of leap of faith we invite our patients to make, and a kind of keeping the faith that we as analytic therapists ordinarily demonstrate to them

What I mean by faith is a gut-level confidence in a process, despite inevitable moments of skepticism, confusion, doubt, and even despair. Analytic therapy has, as Lichtenberg (1998), and others have empha-sized, a kind of self-righting mechanism that iterates toward authentic-ity. Analysts have faith in the therapeutic project because they have experienced it themselves. They approach clinical material with an atti-tude akin to the "expectant waiting" that Quakers observe. They are loath to make predictions about just where the professional journey with any individual will go, but they trust it to take the therapist and patient into areas that will ultimately strengthen the client's sense of honesty, agency, mastery, self-cohesion, self-esteem, affect tolerance, and capacity for fulfilling relationships. In that process, therapists have learned that the specific problems for which a person sought treatment (e.g., anxiety or depression or an eating disorder) will disappear or become significantly less severe. Often the target symptoms remit very quickly, while the client decides to continue in the therapeutic endeavor in order to pursue related, more ambitious goals (including the emotional prophylaxis of future problems) that take on increasing value as the process unfolds.

Very often, the kind of change that the client originally envisioned is not the kind that occurs, only because what does occur is something the client could not have initially imagined. To move into areas that are emotionally new, the client must proceed on a kind of borrowed faith. If the practitioner proceeds with integrity, the client will eventually feel trust in the therapist as a person; the therapist, meanwhile, exemplifies faith in the client, the partnership, and the process. A woman coming to treatment may want to learn how to relieve a depression and instead learns to express previously unformulated feelings, to negotiate for herself in relationships, to identify the situations in which she is likely to feel depressed, to understand the connections between those situations and her unique history, to appreciate her tendency to blame herself for things that are outside her control, to take control over things that had previously seemed impervious to her influence, and to comfort herself instead of berating herself when she is upset. As the therapeutic process evolves, she gradually loses all the vegetative, affective, and cognitive symptoms of depressive illness. But more important, even though before the therapy she may have enjoyed long periods of freedom from diagnosable clinical depression and thus could conceive of feeling better, she could not have imagined the depth of authentic feeling that is now becoming a reliable feature of her emotional landscape.

Sometimes people come to treatment wanting help to get out of a relationship and instead find that they can behave in ways that make that relationship much more fulfilling than they had ever imagined. And sometimes the reverse happens: People contract for therapy with the hope of saving or improving a relationship only to decide eventually that the cost of doing so is too great, and that separation is their only tolerable option. The faith of the therapist is not attached to a particular expected outcome but to the conviction that if two people conscientiously put a certain effort in motion, a natural process of growth that has been arrested by the accidents of the patient's life thus far will be released to follow its own self-healing logic. This kind of faith assumes that the effort to pursue the truth of one's experience has intrinsic healing value.

Postmodern theorists and others have cast an unflattering light on scientific claims to "objectivity," "rationality," and efforts to discover "the truth" in the ways that an Enlightenment-era scholar such as Freud hoped to do. But whether or not we can find *the* truth about any matter, we can try to speak truthfully about it. As Edgar Levenson (1978, p. 16) memorably noted, "it may not be the truth arrived at as much as the manner of arriving at the truth which is the essence of therapy." The attempt to be emotionally honest is the wellspring of everything else that comes from analytic psychotherapy, and the cultivation of a relationship in which progressive approximations of emotional honesty are possible remains the central task of the psychotherapist. We may talk about this process in ego psychological metaphors such as the analysis of defense, or via self psychological appeals for accurate empathy, or in terms of relational notions about exploring subjectivity. We may hold as our image of a successful therapy Freud's notion of the person who has conquered repression, or Jung's notion of individuation, or Bion's ideal of living in O, or Winnicott's concept of the true self, or Weiss and Sampson's goal of abandoning pathogenic beliefs, or Lacan's idealization of the postsymbolic. Different psychoanalytic ideologies have different notions about where to locate the activity of forthright, clear-eyed acknowledgment, but they all share a commitment to the mutual search for what feels true. It is this effort in which the psychoanalytic community has invested its faith.

CONCLUDING COMMENTS

I hope I have conveyed in these initial chapters a sense of not just the figure but also the ground of psychoanalytic thinking and practice. I have tried to talk about the central values, assumptions, convictions, temperamental inclinations, explanatory biases, and emotional tendencies that characterize a psychodynamic orientation to psychotherapy. I have also offered some reflections on why those features of the tradition have often been less than conspicuous. Mainly, I have argued that what is distinctive about psychoanalytic ways of working is not a set of technical interventions but a body of knowledge, accumulated over years of practitioners' immersion in listening to their patients, understood in accordance with the mind-set I have sketched out.

It has not been conventional for textbooks to cover this ground, and periodically in the writing of these first two chapters, I have imagined critics from both inside and outside the psychoanalytic tradition telling me I have gone beyond the data or have misinterpreted gravely or have grafted my own sensibilities on to a discipline that they view very differently. I can only speak for what seems true to me. I have always taken pleasure in trying to put words to ideas that many people hold but few have articulated, and in this chapter I have done my best to do that for the often silent but always powerful, passionate under-currents in the psychoanalytic tradition.

It is my deep conviction that the attitudes I have discussed—curiosity and awe, a respect for complexity, the disposition to identify empathically, the valuing of subjectivity and affect, an appreciation of attachment, and a capacity for faith—are worth cherishing not only as components of a therapeutic sensibility but also as correctives to some of the more estranging and deadening aspects of contemporary life. Their opposites—intellectual passivity, opinionated reductionism, emotional distancing, objectification and apathy, personal isolation and social anomie, and existential dread—have often been lamented by scholars and social critics as the price we pay for our industrialized, consumer-oriented, and technologically sophisticated cultures. The cultivation of the more vital attitudes (cf. Sass, 1992) that undergird the psychoanalytic sensibility just might be good for the postmodern soul whatever one's orientation to psychotherapy.

Chapter 3

The Therapist's Preparation

> I see the quintessential task of the clinician as one of coming to know him- or herself sufficiently to be able to register the experience of the other in progressively more profound and also more useful ways.
>
> This process begins with our own discomfort at finding ourselves sitting in the chair that has somehow become designated as "the authority": the person ostensibly in charge of something we haven't even begun to comprehend.
>
> —MARILYN CHARLES (in press)

Although people vary a great deal in how they approach their first experiences in the role of therapist, anxiety is the norm. Many students describe a disturbing feeling of fraudulence, even the sense of being an impostor, a response that has been described in empirical studies of subjective reactions of new professionals (e.g., Clance & Imes, 1978). They worry that it will be obvious to those they try to treat that they are no more emotionally healthy, socially adept, individuated, intelligent, or free of psychopathology than their clients are. Fortunately for all of us, there is no evidence that one has to be a paragon of mental health (or any kind of paragon) to help people psychologically. To train an athlete, a coach does not have to be a superior athlete; similarly, to help a client, a therapist does not have to be more mature or normal or satisfied in life. In fact, it is arguable that, as Greenson (1967) observed, one is a better therapist for having suffered some significant emotional troubles. A clinician without an experiential reference for psychological suffering risks feeling insufficiently empathic with clients. Of course, it is a problem if one has exactly the same blind spots as one's patients, but there arc ways to deal with that via supervision and personal therapy.

Many novice therapists are troubled by doubts about whether they can carry out their role as well as a more experienced therapist would. There is legitimate consolation on this front, too. Despite the fact that most seasoned practitioners see themselves as having become increasingly skilled and competent over time, the empirical data on the relationship between training or experience and outcome have been mixed or complex (see Bergin & Garfield, 2000; Snyder & Ingram, 1994). The enthusiasm and dedication of the beginner make up for many of the deficits that will be filled in by experience. And the supervision sessions and class discussions typical of the early years of practice give the clients of newer therapists the benefit of ample expertise. Frieda Fromm-Reichmann used to try to assign the most "hopeless, untreatable" psychotic patients to the least experienced therapists at Chestnut Lodge, because those therapists did not know that they were hopeless and untreatable and consequently succeeded in helping them.

A great deal of what is therapeutic to patients inheres in the therapist role itself (about which I will have more to say in later chapters), at least when it is inhabited by people eager to do as well as they can. Long ago, the influential existential therapist James Bugental (1964) observed that one of the occupational hazards of our discipline is that as we develop increasing mastery of the art of helping people, we live with the accompanying guilt and regret that we were not able to be our more fully developed therapeutic selves with earlier patients. It is one of those painful human paradoxes that many of us with this vocation are forever poised between self-criticism for not being skilled enough and remorse over having been less skilled formerly.

It is doubtful that anyone embarking on a career as a practitioner can be adequately prepared for what it feels like to be in the role of therapist for the first time. Even individuals who are confident enough to trust that they have something helpful to offer cannot know who will walk into their offices; the uniqueness of every person makes it impossible *ever* to be fully prepared for the next new client. (Nor would one want to be; psychotherapy would be a dreary business without the surprises and challenges that each patient brings.) Yet perhaps there are some considerations that can increase one's comfort in the role, much as childbirth preparation classes increase one's readiness for another event that cannot be predicted with precision or emotionally imagined until it happens. In the first part of this chapter I discuss some matters that are not always obvious to the beginner that may make the transition into practice a bit easier. This section includes some observations and recommendations intended to help new therapists with challenges that commonly arise early in one's career. Later in the chapter, I make the argument that psychotherapy for oneself is the best preparation for doing psychotherapy with other people.

ORIENTING CONSIDERATIONS

On Making Mistakes

The bad news about starting out as a therapist is that one will invariably make a lot of mistakes. The good news is that making mistakes as a therapist is nothing like making mistakes as a surgeon or attorney or engineer. No lasting harm comes from most errors made by therapists—at least if they are picked up quickly, and that is what supervisors are for. In fact, mistakes (or what clients experience as mistakes) are inevitable, no matter how experienced one is, and they can be addressed in a conversation that has considerably more therapeutic power than the (strictly hypothetical) "ideal" response would have had (see Safran, 1993). And given that human beings have conflicting feelings about most important matters, there is often no response a therapist can make that is not frustrating to some part of the patient's wishes and needs. Conveying a sincere effort to understand, even if one is getting things wrong, is much more therapeutic than conveying the belief—or even persuading the client—that one *does* understand. Edgar Levenson (1982, p. 5) quotes Harry Stack Sullivan as exclaiming, "God keep me from a therapy that goes well, and God keep me from a clever therapist!"

I have a friend who has been in and out of mental hospitals several times for what has usually been diagnosed as schizophrenia. In reflecting on what staff behaviors were respectively helpful and unhelpful, he is emphatic in stating that even at his most psychotic, he could tell the difference between an "honest" mistake and a mistake made in the service of someone's effort to manipulate or dismiss him. Honest mistakes are not surprising or off-putting even to fragile and tormented individuals (who know they are hard to understand), but patients will not forgive malevolence or lack of caring. Mistakes of the heart are much more devastating than mistakes of the head. Self-serving acts purveyed as "for your own good" are particularly unpardonable. In appreciation of the fact that we are always getting it wrong when we try to comprehend someone else's psychology, Patrick Casement (2002) aptly titled his recent book on psychotherapy *Learning from Our Mistakes*.

In the graduate program where I teach, admission is very competitive. Applicants who are accepted have typically excelled academically, and many of them have held jobs in which their performance was exemplary. They are used to getting A's from teachers and rave reviews from supervisors. They tend to be perfectionistic, and few of them have had their aspirations to perfection seriously challenged. But in the human service professions, as in life in general, the pursuit of perfection is, to steal a biblical phrase, a snare and a delusion. There are only better and worse ways of trying to help another human being, and even the best interventions have pros and cons, upsides and downsides. Almost everything in psychotherapeutic technique is a trade-off. For example, deciding not to answer a client's question so that one can explore why it is being asked may illuminate an important aspect of the person's subjective experience, yet may inadvertently convey that the question itself and the client's conscious reason for asking it are "questionable"; electing to answer the question may convey respect at the price of learning what concerns inspired the question. Although there are still some teachers of psychodynamic therapy who insist that there is a "right" way to do it, both empirical data and a look around at the diversity among one's colleagues suggest that there are many different, comparably effective ways of facilitating the complex process by which people become more honest with themselves, less symptomatic, less self-defeating, and more agentic. One person's mistake is another's therapeutic ingenuity.

Jonathan Slavin (1994) has noted how appealing it can be to new therapists to adopt a more rigid style than their personalities and attitudes would predict. Speaking of the interns in his university clinic, he writes:

> These are bright, inquisitive individuals who usually bring with them no real familiarity with the technical literature in psychoanalysis but, very often a healthy skepticism about what they have heard about standard psychoanalytic practices . . . especially . . . the supposed distance, coldness, anonymity, and neutrality that they presume characterize a psychoanalytic stance.
>
> Thus, it is especially striking that when these individuals first begin work with patients they suddenly become imbued with a host of rules, and assumptions about rules, that play out some version of the very behavior about which they had initially expressed considerable doubt and antipathy. (p. 255)

He concludes that the sudden internal pressure to conform to a set of rules may reflect a reaction to the experience of being affected much more emotionally than one anticipated by the emotions and transferences of patients. In other words, the attraction to rigid ways of working may be a defense against anxieties about having one's own conflicts stirred up by clients' material, and specifically against fears that one will act out with the client. It takes some time to get used to the fact that subtle enactments happen inevitably, that no amount of rule observance protects a therapist from them, and that they constitute an excellent source of material to process fruitfully.

The transition to the role of a student who is learning an *art* is difficult for individuals coming from areas of study and practice in which there are clear "right answers." No matter how well they do with their patients, some supervisor will suggest an intervention that would have been slightly more attuned to a client's concerns, that would have accessed more affect or spared some narcissistic injury, or that would have avoided the ensuing quandary in which patient and therapist now find themselves. It is hard to hang on to one's self-esteem when one is repeatedly being told, however nicely, that one could have done better, but there is no other way to learn one's craft.

One way that some beginning therapists try to staunch the wounds that training inflicts on their narcissism is to become ideologically committed to some notion of the one "best" or "true" way to do therapy. They latch on to a supervisor who is opinionated about right and wrong interventions, or become devotees of a particular point of view, or slavishly follow the practices of their own therapist. There is probably nothing seriously harmful in this tendency, as long as they let time and experience thaw their rigidities. The stratagem does steep them in the wisdom of a specific point of view, from which they can later individuate with the confidence that they have been immersed in a particular orientation; they know it from the inside and can speak from experience about its strengths and weaknesses. In other words, it is as true of therapy as of other disciplines that one learns the craft before the art. That reality should be no cause for shame.

Possibly a better way to learn the craft, especially for clinicians who come to it with limited experience in the patient role, is first to learn how to do one of the more empirically tested and explicitly described psychoanalytic therapies. My colleague Mark Hilsenroth recommends the work of Lester Luborsky (1984) and Howard Book (1997) on the well-researched core conflictual relationship theme. These books are useful in teaching about what to interpret and how to interpret effectively. In the Appendix, I include an annotated list of texts on psychoanalytic therapy that may be of particular value to beginning clinicians.

Those of us with an oppositional streak and a touch of grandiosity may make a different adaptation to the insult of having our shortcomings as a therapist repeatedly called to our attention; namely, the silent conviction that our own sense of what is needed by a patient is probably superior to what is offered by our supervisors, teachers, therapists,

and textbooks. Skepticism toward authority, which often goes with a capacity for creative thought, has much to recommend it. When applied
to psychotherapy, this irreverent attitude has at least two advantages.
First, a novice therapist who has direct contact with a client sometimes
has a better feel for the person than an outsider—despite the outsider's
superior clinical experience. The intuition of a talented beginner about
what is going on with his or her patient is sometimes more accurate
than the once-removed inference of a supervisor. Learning to trust
one's gut is a critical part of therapeutic maturation. Second, in es-
chewing received wisdom and operating from the heart, the novice
therapist can feel personally integrated with the interventions he or she
is making. One's clinical style can thus be authentic, natural, and spontaneous rather than borrowed, out of character, and wooden.

There are, however, at least two significant disadvantages to this
otherwise appealing stance. The most obvious and emotionally salient
problem is that one will be relentlessly humbled. When I was starting
to do therapy, I repeatedly discovered the wisdom of certain generally
valued practices by doing something else and learning the hard way the
reason for the conventional rule. I have always resonated to Theodor
Reik's (1948) admission:

> That I only now, after thirty-seven years of analytic practice and theory,
> venture to speak on the subject of technique, is due to two peculiar
> characteristics which necessarily prevented me from appearing earlier
> in print. The first is an inability to learn from other people's mistakes.
> All the wisdom of proverbs and all exhortations and warnings are use-
> less to me. If I am to learn from the mistakes of others, I must make
> them my own, and so perhaps cast them off. And with this kind of men-
> tal stubbornness or intellectual contumacy, another is combined: I am
> almost incapable of learning from my own mistakes unless I have re-
> peated them several times. (p. xii)

The other drawback to the stance that one knows better than one's
professional elders is that there are some instances of individual ingenuity that trespass on professional ethics and risk-management practices, where doing something idiosyncratic can be disastrous for both
patient and therapist. In the area of conduct that can be construed as a
boundary violation, for example, well-intentioned acts can have serious
unintended consequences. The client who, in a state of dependent idealization, persuades a practitioner that the only possible way to reduce
her pain is with a hug has been known to make an ethics complaint
later, in a state of angry devaluation, about the therapist's seductiveness. Although I usually advise beginning therapists to trust their own

instincts and throw out the book when they have a deep conviction about what will help another person, in the area of what is accepted as ethical practice, it is foolhardy not to defer to the wisdom of one's predecessors. I talk about some of the more dangerous situations for therapists in Chapter 7.

On Being Oneself

As a psychotherapist, one is in a privileged role, a position with weighty responsibilities. But being in a role is not the same thing as playing a role. Even the most classical, "orthodox" writers on technique (e.g., Eissler, 1953; Fenichel, 1941; Freud, 1914; Sterba, 1934; Strachey, 1934), however emphatic they were about the value of neutrality and abstinence, did not intend for therapists to try to eradicate their natural warmth or to become robotic caricatures of human beings. As early as 1941, Fenichel expressed distress that many of his analysands were surprised by his naturalness and spontaneity. Glover (1955), another icon of orthodoxy, advocated a relaxed, forthright attitude and went on to attack colleagues who maintained a pretense that all arrangements (e.g., about time and fee) are made exclusively for the benefit of the patient.

Artificiality and posturing have no place in analytic therapy, mainly because they are discordant with the effort to foster an unflinching emotional honesty. It is natural to be anxious in a new role, and it is a common enough defense to cover anxiety with an adopted persona, but in the role of therapist, that defense is a handicap. Perhaps the best antidote to anxiety is the knowledge that psychoanalytic therapy does not require intellectual brilliance or sophisticated social skills or mastery of the literature on technique. Its most elemental ingredients are the therapist's genuine wish to help and nondefensive curiosity.

One of the most valuable things to be learned about practicing therapy is how to integrate one's individuality into the role of therapist. Anyone who visits a number of clinical offices will be impressed with the diversity in their appearance, all adequately professional but also uniquely personal. Individual therapists vary greatly not only in how they furnish and decorate their offices but also in how they dress, how close they like to sit to their patients, whether they maintain eye contact or take pains to protect their patients from feeling scrutinized, whether they write notes during sessions, how detailed a history they take during the first appointment, how they describe their cancellation policy, how they handle billing, how they tell patients that a session is over, and many other matters. There is not one right way to do these things, there are only ways that are congruent for particular practition-ers. Sometimes a supervisor will describe his or her own ways of doing things as standard practice, but claims of prototypicality sometimes mean only that they are practices that have worked well for that super-visor's personality, predilections, and circumstances.

Even under the conditions in which most beginners practice—namely, in a series of small, windowless treatment rooms containing two chairs, a clock, and a Kleenex box, where the clinic sets the billing policy and the administrator assigns the clients—there is room for the therapist's individuality. With all we have learned about the centrality of the therapeutic relationship to emotional healing, it has become even clearer that clinicians work most effectively when they relax and let their unique personalities become their therapeutic instrument. The more emotionally genuine the therapist is, the more the patient can open up without shame. Fluency in intervening will come with time, and in the meantime, one's basic humanity will get one through the rough spots.

I should stress that being oneself does not mean disclosing per-sonal information or giving advice in an undisciplined way. New-comers to the practice of therapy are often surprised (and self-critical, for "overidentifying") by the experience of a sudden, spontaneous sym-pathy for a client's problem—because they themselves have had a per-sonal challenge that was strikingly similar. It was an act of will for me, early in my work as a therapist, to inhibit the temptation to blurt out, "I know exactly what you're feeling!"—especially when the patient re-ported some fairly unusual life experience that, by chance, I had also had. And it was hard not to market my own solutions to a difficulty when it was one I had confronted and overcome, or to avoid confessing my sense of inadequacy when the patient described a conflict that I was suffering and had not resolved. But periodically we should remind ourselves that if helpful suggestions and sympathy from people with similar experiences were sufficient to work out a significant emotional problem, nobody would need a therapist. Good advice and warm iden-tification are not usually in short supply; most people who come for treatment are there because those resources have already been tried and have failed to help.

On Getting the Most from Supervision

Organizations that train people to be therapists differ widely in how much latitude trainees are given to choose their supervisors. Adminis-trators of graduate-level programs often assign students to members of the faculty for supervision (a problematic arrangement in my view, be-

cause students find it hard to be entirely forthright with those responsible for evaluating their academic progress) or refer them to a small
number of hand-picked therapists "in the field." Analytic institutes and
other programs at the postgraduate level typically afford considerable
choice. For those readers fortunate enough to have some autonomy in
this critical area, I would advise picking a supervisor at least partly on
the basis of whether the student can imagine feeling safe with that person. Supervision can be an empty ritual if the supervisee cannot be
open about what is happening in the treatment hours and about how
he or she feels about clients. (For interesting books on the psychology
of the supervision process, see Frawley-O'Dea & Sarnat, 2001; S. Gill,
2002; Rock, 1997.)

Especially in the early stages of training, it is more important to
work with someone who is not intimidating than to spend time with
someone brilliant or famous or influential in one's professional circles.
Even with the most supportive mentor, candor can be as difficult for
new therapists in the supervisory hour as free association is for new patients in the treatment hour. If new therapists cannot get comfortable
reporting to their supervisor what they actually did and said, they
should try to talk with him or her about their difficulty exposing their
work with all its warts. If the problem persists, the supervisee should
consider changing supervisors. Most students of psychotherapy are
highly self-critical people who second-guess their own reactions, and
sometimes that tendency impels them to stay far too long in a supervisory relationship that is just not working.

Supervisors are as varied and idiosyncratic as therapists. Most experienced teachers of therapy have worked out a style that integrates
their own personality nicely with their task. For supervisees who feel a
"good fit" (cf. Escalona, 1968) with the approach of a particular professional, supervision becomes a nourishing balance of support, stimulation, and challenge. After many years of hearing from my students
about their training experiences, I have concluded that the kind of
mentoring most likely to trap the novice therapist in a supervisory
blind alley is one in which the supervisor fails to differentiate supervision from therapy. In more advanced supervision, the experience of
working deeply with one's countertransference reactions can be highly
valuable, but early in one's training, excessive pressure for personal exploration and exposure is unwarranted. The supervisor's repeated incursions into the therapist's psychology, especially in the context of evasion of an explicit teaching role, tend to reinforce the therapist's
uncertainty rather than to provide a basis for the confidence necessary
to do the job.

The psychoanalytic version of this caricature of supervision is a perseverative inquiry into possible unconscious attitudes in the treater ("How did you *feel* about your patient's symptom? Does it remind you of anyone in *your* life?"). When this kind of questioning substitutes for information that grounds the new therapist in ways to help a client, it does more harm than good, even if the trainee learns something about his or her own psychology in the process. Students suffering this kind of supervision-as-therapy tend to become chronically self-questioning, unmoored, and demoralized, and usually it takes them much too long to reject the style of the supervisor because they keep finding evidence that, indeed, they have a lot of introspecting to do. The grains of truth in any observations by their supervisor about their own psychology are taken as evidence that they have to stick with the supervision until they are "cured."

Nonpsychoanalytic approaches to supervision can have comparable failings. At one point during my training, I contracted for supervision with a self-described Rogerian therapist who was a talented diagnostician but, as it turned out, not a very talented supervisor. My first session with her went something like this:

NANCY: I'm having trouble finding a way to like this patient.

SUPERVISOR: You're having trouble finding warm feelings for this woman.

NANCY: Yes, I'm even finding myself feeling angry at her.

SUPERVISOR: You are feeling angry!

NANCY: I need some help from you about how to understand her so that I can empathize.

SUPERVISOR: You really want help.

NANCY: You've heard her history. How do you understand her problems?

SUPERVISOR: You wish I could tell you how to understand her.

NANCY: Yes, she's very frustrating to me.

SUPERVISOR: You feel frustrated.

NANCY: Now I'm starting to feel frustrated with *you*—you're just reflecting. I already know what I feel, and I'd like to find a way to feel differently.

SUPERVISOR: Now you're feeling angry at *me*!

Not surprisingly, I fired this supervisor and found someone more willing to teach me about the kind of patient who provokes in a therapist the painful negative countertransferences with which I was struggling. It is not impossible that this practitioner's reflective way of working would be helpful to someone with a greater need for emotional mirroring, but I prefer to believe that her version of the humanistic, client-centered tradition, a parody of how a compassionate Rogerian would really behave, expressed her personal limitations as a supervisor. Either way, we were not a match made in heaven, and had I continued to work with her, I doubt that I would have learned much of value. By contrast, the next supervisor to whom I turned for help with my difficult patient was a social worker in analytic training whose first response to my description was, "What an impossible patient!"—a much more genuine, egalitarian expression of empathy. We went on to work together fruitfully for several years, and over time I came to be very fond of my patient, who never became "easy" but who eventually made significant gains in her treatment.

For those readers who are not granted by the authorities in their training programs the right to choose or change their supervisors, the outlook is cloudier but not bleak. If a therapist is lucky enough to be assigned a person with whom he or she feels "good chemistry," the supervision will be not only palatable but also vitally useful. If the trainee is given someone problematic, he or she will have to make the best of a bad situation. The latter is no picnic, but it is more than a rationalization to say that confronting adversity builds character. Specifically, the ability to find a way to learn from people with whom one feels significant disagreement or discomfort or lack of respect is an extremely valuable life skill. There is no supervisor from whom one cannot learn something of value. (Even my robotic Rogerian taught me something about what *not* to do in the supervisory role.) Indignation that one's superiors should be better can feel pleasantly righteous, but it does nothing to solve a problem. Making accommodations to the limits of real people is part of an incremental maturational process in which we slowly absorb the fact that the world is run by human beings, not by the wise parental figures we all wish were in charge.

Mark Hilsenroth (personal communication, August 19, 2003) tells his students that one of the best ways to help a supervisor give effective supervision is to ask, "What would be an example of how I might say (or do) that?" This effort to pursue the concrete is particularly useful when one is working with a person who makes vague pronouncements such as "You should have interpreted the resistance there" or "You need to get her to look at her omnipotence" or "You have to make that symptom ego alien." Helping a supervisor to be more effective in his or her role is not entirely different from helping a patient to get better. It requires a willingness to give sincere feedback about the best qualities of the supervisor and tactful, timely attention to the worst.

The most challenging problem that beginners may run into is a significant difference of opinion with a supervisor about a concrete clinical decision. In the United States, supervisors hold responsibility for the work of those they oversee—legal responsibility when the student is in training and significant liability even in later years when a therapist is credentialed to practice and is hiring the supervisor voluntarily. Consequently, there is an ethical imperative to defer to the supervisor's judgment. The problem with this bald reality is that occasionally one feels utterly sure, based on one's intimate knowledge of a particular client, that the supervisor is giving bad advice. Under such circumstances, there is no way the supervisor's recommendation can be carried out in a spirit of conviction. And without conviction, no therapeutic intervention stands much chance of working, no matter how appropriate it is in the abstract.

In this painful situation, one's first effort to cope should be to give voice to one's misgivings and try to persuade or be persuaded by the supervisor. Yet sometimes trying to talk out the disagreement simply highlights the fact that the two parties are irretrievably at odds. I remember in this context a problem I had with a psychologist who was supervising me on the treatment of a borderline woman who had canceled her last two sessions somewhat arbitrarily. He felt strongly that I should write her a letter in which I labeled her behavior as manipulative and unacceptable. I felt just as strongly that she would experience such a letter as critical, contemptuous, and insensitive to whatever fears were making it hard for her to get to the appointments. He believed that the naming of her manipulative behavior would motivate her to come back, whereas I thought it would drive the last nail into the coffin of the working alliance. (I later learned that such seemingly irreparable splits between two involved professionals, especially when they are framed in the mind of each party as morally right versus morally wrong, is a classic countertransference phenomenon associated with borderline psychopathology.) This supervisor was emphatic and opinionated like my father, whose rejection I had always feared, and I handled my discomfort in an immature way: I wrote such a letter, showed it to him, and then failed to send it.

This less than stellar behavior is emblematic of a kind of regression that can easily happen when one is in training. Sometimes, in the role of student, it is hard to maintain the emotional sense of being an adult: There is so much to learn, there are so many instances in which authorities call attention to one's limitations, so many devaluing com-

munications from clients who are afraid to attach, so many opportunities for shame at one's errors or ignorance. What is more, candidates
in training programs are often in personal therapies that have weak-
ened their habitual defenses, leaving them feeling a bit raw and vulnerable. Not uncommonly, they are being encouraged to regress in their
therapists' offices, and sometimes that regression leaks out into other
areas. Notwithstanding all these infantilizing forces, I want to state emphatically that it is possible to retain a sense of adulthood and personal
autonomy in the student role, and that the more one differentiates between being in a structurally subordinate role and being "reduced" to
the emotional position of the child, the better.

Most supervisors are grateful to work with people who convey the
sense of being a grown-up, take responsibility for their behavior, and
disagree without antagonism when they find themselves differing with
someone in an authority role. As I got to know better the supervisor
with whom I had behaved in this avoidant way, I realized that my transference had done him a disservice; he was capable of much more
thoughtful responsiveness than I had given him credit for. When I finally got brave enough to express disagreement in frank and direct
ways, he proved a little prickly but generally respectful, and the supervision hour became substantively enriching rather than an exercise in
overt submission and covert rebellion on my part.

From my own experience as a supervisor, I can attest to the psychology of the other half of the dyad when a supervisee behaves with
exaggerated deference, as if there is no room for our mutually working
out a resolution if we were to find ourselves at odds. In this situation,
the atmosphere of supervision becomes subtly pervaded with what
Benjamin (1995) would call a "doer/done to" tone. When months go
by before a student works up the nerve to tell me I have been belabor-
ing something unnecessarily, or teaching theory when the student
wants help with feelings, or giving advice with which he or she has
been privately disagreeing, I feel exasperated about the time wasted.
While I consciously appreciate that the supervisee may have adopted a
defensively accommodating style out of a need for approval, a stance
with which I can readily identify, I also have some gut-level narcissistic
reactions that I assume are not uncommon among supervisors. Whereas
I feel realistically supported in my self-esteem when I know I have tolerated learning about my shortcomings and have used the knowledge to
become genuinely useful, I feel implicitly accused of pathological narcissism when a supervisee hides behind compliance in the belief that I
cannot tolerate being questioned. (In fact, in the latter situation I feel
patronized, and my defensive reaction is the temptation to reverse the
dynamic and treat the supervisee less like an adult colleague and more

like a child.) Like therapy, psychoanalytic supervision flounders if it is not conducted in an atmosphere of mutual honesty. Because transferences toward supervisors can be powerful, it can take considerable moral courage to bring up a criticism, but it is worth the chance of learning that an authority may respond to negative feedback with grace.

It remains possible, however, that a supervisor is not only "wrong" but also too defensive to work out a difference of opinion in a spirit of mutual problem solving. One of my colleagues (Thomas Arizmendi, personal communication, December 15, 2001) remembers a supervisor from his internship who gave him very bad advice and treated his disagreement as if it were evidence of his ignorance of some obvious psychodynamic standard of care. He was treating an eight-year-old boy for aggressive and impulsive behavior in a clinic that had its offices on a busy city street. During the session, the boy angrily left the treatment room. My colleague, concerned about his patient's safety, followed him out. On reporting this to his supervisor, he was told that a therapist should never leave the "container" of the office, that he should remain there and leave it to the boy whether and when to come back. When he protested that the boy could run out into traffic, the supervisor only became more insistent that the "rules of treatment" required him to wait for his patient in the therapy room. Deferring to his supervisor's confident advice, he remained in his office the next time the client ran out, but his anxiety was overwhelming. At this point he consulted with the clinic director, who was horrified at the advice he had been given and resolved the problem by talking with the supervisor. Fortunately, his patient was not hurt the day my friend stayed in the office, but he still shudders that he acquiesced and feels lucky to have had someone to whom he could appeal.

Because I have heard numerous stories like this, I would not rule out the option of a supervisee's private decision to do something other than what the supervisor has directed, particularly when a pressing clinical situation gives him or her no time to get a second opinion. Especially in agencies with high turnover and financial stresses that make it prohibitive to pay for high-quality staff members, a beginning therapist may be better trained and more talented than the person to whom he or she reports. But the risks one takes in defiance are that (1) the supervisor has actually been right, or (2) whether or not the supervisor's solution would have worked, the therapist's will fail. Then there is no place to go to address the damage that one's independence has wreaked. Just as civil disobedience is an honorable response to unjust laws, noncompliance can be a justified response to bad supervision. But in each case, one must be prepared to take the consequences of one's stand. People who engage in civil disobedience in the name of a principle higher than the law willingly risk arrest in the service of their belief; the noncompliant supervisee must be analogously willing to take the consequences of acting contrary to a supervisor's recommendation. When I was running an early draft of this chapter past members of one of my consultation groups, three clinicians in that group recalled incidents from their own early professional experiences in agencies, in which they had been asked to do something by a supervisor, had refused on the basis of powerful moral convictions, and then had either been fired from their position or had quit.

These are very difficult waters for the beginning therapist to navigate. The more help one can get from experienced colleagues, the better. The natural wish that one can trust a mentor's judgment, combined with the self-questioning tendencies of most people attracted to this profession, can otherwise conspire to make novice clinicians compliant when their perfectly sound judgment protests, as in the case of my colleague. The tendency to psychologize about one's "oedipal rebellion" or "oppositionality" may complicate one's judgment about what to do; the beginner tends to worry that his or her independence of mind reflects some kind of sinister unconscious dynamism. Of course, the best insurance against the possibility that one's mature, healthy reactions will be corrupted by dynamics of which one is unaware is the maximum degree of self-knowledge in the therapist. Which brings us to the next topic.

THERAPY FOR THE THERAPIST

The better we know someone, the more we can help that person. For this reason and others, psychoanalytic therapists have always emphasized the importance of creating an atmosphere in which patients can feel safe divulging their most troubling secrets. The more someone feels that a therapist might understand the most frightening, hated, shameful aspects of private experience—the inner life and the lived life—the more possible it becomes to reveal them in the therapy relationship, to modify what is changeable, to accept what is not. To convey to the people with whom we work that we can bear hearing about things they may view as inexpressible, it helps to have "been there" emotionally.

Perhaps the most destructive affect a therapist can convey to a client is contempt. Unconscious contempt is particularly damaging because it tends to leak out around the edges of the therapist's conscious efforts to be warm and accepting and therefore feels all the more devastating on account of coming from a presumably supportive person. Analytic scholars (e.g., A. P. Morrison, 1989; Nathanson, 1987; Wurmser, 1981) have long noted that contemptuous attitudes function as defenses against shame. No matter how much self-talk we engage in to the effect that we should convey unconditional positive regard, when we are ashamed of aspects of ourselves that we see mirrored in our patients, we cannot fail to convey a subtle disparagement. No client can easily ignore or tolerate a therapist's disdain. Yet contempt is inevitable when we need to ward off the disturbing realization that the patient's problems are not so different from our own. Even floridly psychotic patients who have nothing overtly in common with the therapist can stimulate unconscious identifications that incite defensive devaluation.

The traditional prescription for ensuring that psychotherapy does not proceed in an atmosphere of condescension is for the therapist to undergo psychotherapy or psychoanalysis. This idea used to be so widely accepted—both inside and outside psychoanalytic circles—that it would be unnecessary to belabor the point in a text on therapy. Humanistic therapists have assumed that coming to terms with one's own deep feelings will deepen the therapy one is capable of providing. Many family systems practitioners recommend "working on one's family of origin" during training. But with the rise of the cognitive and behavioral therapies and biological psychiatry, a very different presumption has developed; namely, that one must master a set of skills, applying delineated, often manualized interventions to problems for which those techniques have shown short-term "empirical" effectiveness. Noting their radical difference from therapies based on relationship and the collaborative search for understanding, Louis Berger (2002) has labeled these approaches "technotherapies." Because young people interested in becoming therapists are increasingly introduced to the field via this technical mind-set, especially in university psychology departments and medical schools, it becomes important to articulate reasons for the traditional and enduring conviction among psychodynamic practitioners that therapists should get therapy themselves, whether or not they have problems in living that rise to the seriousness of a diagnosable disorder.

Irvin Yalom (2002) recently did so, in an accessible book offered as "an open letter to a new generation of therapists and their patients." After noting that the therapist's most valuable instrument is that therapist's self, he summarizes:

> Therapists must be familiar with their own dark side and be able to empathize with all human wishes and impulses. A personal therapy experience permits the student therapist to experience many aspects of the

therapeutic process from the patient's seat: the tendency to idealize the therapist, the yearning for dependency, the gratitude toward a caring and attentive listener, the power granted to the therapist. Young therapists must work through their own neurotic issues; they must learn to accept feedback, discover their own blind spots, and see themselves as others see them; they must appreciate their impact upon others and learn how to provide accurate feedback. Lastly, psychotherapy is a psychologically demanding enterprise, and therapists must develop the awareness and inner strength to cope with the many occupational hazards inherent in it. (pp. 40–41)

I concur, but I should also note a few qualifications. I have known some talented and naturally empathic therapists who seem very effective without benefit of personal therapy. They tend to have had supportive parents and naturally sympathetic personalities. I have also run into some fairly pedestrian practitioners whose work seems to have profited very little from their years on the couch—whether because of a bad fit between them and their therapists or because they had participated in a "training analysis" in a sheerly intellectual way or because they were complying with an institutional rule rather than coming to treatment with the same motivation as a person suffering significant psychopathology. And there is truth in allegations that it is self-serving for psychoanalysts to insist that all analytic candidates be analyzed (it creates a nice pool of patients for the trainers, a fact that has led some sardonic commentators to refer to psychoanalytic practice as a pyramid scheme). There is also validity to claims that a personal analysis functions as a socializing procedure, an initiation into a peculiar subculture whose shared convictions have more of an ideological than a scientific cast.

It has also been convincingly argued, most recently by analysts in the intersubjective and relational movements, that no matter how "well analyzed" any of us is, we cannot expect to find ourselves unaffected by the powerful psychological forces that assail us in a therapy session. The assumption of the utter objectivity of the thoroughly analyzed therapist has been pretty well put to rest in recent years. Although Freud hoped that his self-analysis had immunized him against emotional contamination by his patients' illnesses, reports of his behavior as a therapist are replete with what look suspiciously like unconscious enactments. Those of us analyzed not by ourselves (as Freud was) but by others have no better track records at resisting transference–countertransference inductions though, thankfully, we have discovered that therapy progresses anyway. Hence, despite Freud's (1912b, p. 96) hopes that practitioners could achieve "analytic purification" by undergoing personal treatment, a century of psychotherapy experience and some critical changes in our understanding of concepts such as "objectivity" and "neutrality" (Kuhn, 1962, 1977) have left little doubt that there is no such thing as an observed phenomenon unaffected by the observer's needs, no possibility in clinical work of keeping oneself out of the intersubjective emotional fray.

Notwithstanding these admissions, I want to speak for the tradition here, as I believe that in spite of all our frailties as human beings on both sides of the psychotherapy process, the best chance we have for increasing our capacity to understand, and thus our therapeutic range, is to know and accept ourselves as deeply as possible. Personal treatment may not innoculate us with "objectivity," but it can vastly increase our capacity to observe and make good use of the dynamics that inevitably get stirred up in our work. With all its hazards and limitations, personal treatment seems to me the best route to mature, empathic listening. Perhaps this conviction seems self-evident to many of my readers, but given the tenor of the times, I would like to add my voice to Yalom's and offer some thoughts about taking the time-honored injunction seriously.

In general, I would recommend analysis rather than therapy, meaning that more frequent sessions, use of the couch, and work with free associations and dreams is preferable to face-to-face weekly meetings—that is, when there are no individual reasons militating against analysis, such as significant borderline tendencies in the person entering treatment, or a trauma history that makes reclining seem too much like the position in which one was abused, or overwhelming practical problems such as lack of money or lack of access to anyone trained to do analysis. The classical theoretical basis for this recommendation is that greater session frequency and use of the couch are associated with the development of an analyzable transference, a phenomenon that intensifies the therapeutic encounter and attunes therapists to the experiences of patients who have intense transference reactions regardless of session frequency. The empirical basis for it is that several studies have suggested that increased frequency produces faster and more far-reaching therapeutic improvement (Freedman et al., 1999; Roth & Fonagy, 1996; Sandell et al., 2000; Seligman, 1995, 1996). If more intensive treatment is not possible, once-weekly therapy is still very valuable, especially if one is highly motivated.

Currently, insurance companies, aided by some academic critics of traditional therapy, have succeeded in setting a tone in which anything but weekly therapy (or less) must be justified by clinically dire circumstances. The basis for this stance is clearly commercial rather than empirical or clinical. It is vital not to let corporate interests corrupt our understanding of what makes sense clinically. Frequency is not a simple matter, however, even among analytic enthusiasts. In fact, it has been a thorny issue in psychoanalytic politics for decades. Freud started seeing patients six days a week, and then for practical reasons went to five and then to four. I am not aware that he ever complained that a significant loss in therapeutic momentum accompanied these changes, though he did note that any day the patient did not come created small amounts of defensiveness that in his six-day phase he dubbed "the Monday crust" (meaning that a small amount of repression had crusted over the previous openness). Some programs that train psychoanalysts require a minimum of two sessions weekly; others insist on four or more. No one has yet produced research data showing that analysis at five times a week is superior to analysis at four or three, yet there is some evidence that in general, three sessions a week are more effective than two, which are more effective than one (Sandell et al., 2000).

Appropriate or effective duration of therapy is almost as open a question as frequency of sessions. No one knows yet when or if the "average" patient (not that there is such a creature) reaches a point of diminishing returns, but there is some empirical data suggesting that most people will make significant improvement, change that goes well beyond symptom relief, by the two-year mark (Freedman et al., 1999; Howard, Kopta, Krause, & Olinsky, 1986; Howard, Lucgcr, Maling, & Martinovich, 1993; Howard, Moras, Brill, Martinovich, & Lutz, 1996; Kandera, Lambert, & Andrews, 1996; Perry, Banon, & Ianni, 1999; Lueger, Lutz, & Howard, 2000; Seligman, 1995, 1996). Most people in training to be analytic practitioners choose, once they have a good working alliance going with their own therapists and are seeing the benefits of psychotherapy, to remain in treatment considerably longer, examining aspects of themselves that might not have caused them any trouble in another profession but that are likely to get stimulated and stirred up in the course of working with patients.

In the clinical literature, Frieda Fromm-Reichmann (1950) has made the most eloquent and comprehensive argument that therapists should be analyzed. Even though her book is somewhat dated and assumes a strictly psychiatric audience, Fromm-Reichmann's comments about the qualities necessary to do psychotherapy are timeless. Her rationale for a personal analysis includes four elements. First, self-knowledge in the therapist can reduce the likelihood of acting out rather than reflecting on countertransference reactions (p. 6). Second, personal treatment increases the probability that the therapist will have an adequately secure and satisfying extraprofessional life, thereby enhancing the ability to listen and reducing the temptation to use patients for gratification of the therapist's narcissistic strivings, dependency needs, and sexual longings (p. 7). Third, effective treatment creates increased self-respect and realistic self-esteem that allow the clinician to absorb hostile and devaluing communications nondefensively, and thus to demonstrate how to maintain one's self-esteem in the face of provocation (p. 16). Fourth, a familiarity with one's own dynamics makes it possible to recognize comparable processes in other people (p. 42).

These are good reasons. I think there are some others, however, that Fromm-Reichmann omitted and that have not been particularly stressed in the literature. At the most basic level, it is important for a therapist to know viscerally how it feels *just to be in the patient role.* In the decades after Fromm-Reichmann wrote her textbook, self psychologists have made a convincing case for the utter centrality of empathy in the therapeutic process. The shortest route to empathy with someone in the role of patient is to take that role oneself. When I first went to an analyst's office, I was shocked to notice that despite my conscious embrace of the idea that there is no shame in seeing a therapist, I was hoping that nobody had seen me go in his door. No amount of intellectual facility prepares us for the sense of vulnerability and exposure that accompanies the role of the help seeker. Nor can we appreciate vicariously the nature of the sense of dependency, in both its positive and negative aspects, that simply comes with the territory of being a client. Adopting the patient role provides the best basis we can have for empathy, even when our own central dynamics are substantially different from those that one of our clients needs to address. And it is the best prophylaxis against contempt.

Just as important, the experience of psychotherapy gives us a model of how it works for which no textbook could possibly substitute. Candidates in analytic institutes uniformly comment that in their own training, their personal analysis gave them the richest source of knowledge about how to do sensitive therapy (they typically mention their experiences in supervision as the second most valuable part of their training; course work ranks a distant third). "I knew what to say because I knew what helped me in the same situation" is the kind of comment one frequently hears from therapists whose own treatment has benefited them. They report that the capacity to call on their own experience of being helped lowers their anxiety about doing the work, reduces their sense of fraudulence, and allows them to stay more uninterruptedly in the state that Csikszentmihalyi (1990) calls "flow." Readers who are interested in a more in-depth discussion of this phenomenon should not miss Tessman's (2003) fascinating qualitative study, *The Analyst's Analyst Within.*

I am convinced that it is a very different process internally, and comes across to the patient differently as well, to make ongoing, minute-by-minute clinical decisions on the basis of naturally stimulated identifications than to make them on the basis of a cognitive search for what one's supervisor or clinical theory or treatment manual suggests. Associating to times when one was in a state comparable to that of the patient and remembering what was deeply helpful feels like a natural, organic process that keeps the therapist in fundamental rapport with the client. It transforms comments that might otherwise come across as self-conscious and stilted into a more spontaneous, unrehearsed kind of talking. When it goes well, psychoanalytic therapy feels to both parties like a conversation from the heart, not the head.

David Ramirez (personal communication, August 24, 2002), when training interns and counselors at Swarthmore College, emphasizes that in psychodynamic therapy, the main instrument of healing is the personality of the therapist, not an impersonal technique *used* by the therapist (the truth of this observation in no way militates against skills training, of course). As with any instrument, the better one knows how it works, the better one can adapt it to each task. He points out that although students are often excited and grateful to learn that they can help others simply by relying on their own inherent resources, the painful part of viewing treatment in this quintessentially psychoanalytic way is that the sense of personal responsibility can feel crushing. If one can attribute difficulties and failures in therapy to the limitations of an external technique or to the inappropriate matching of technique to client, one's self-esteem is more protected than it is when one sees one's *self* as the instrument of change and growth. Usually, the more personal therapy one has had, the better one can use one's self, and the better one can recover and grow when one's narcissism is wounded because a treatment has gone badly.

I often wonder how beginning therapists decide when and how to intervene if they have not internalized a rhythm of interaction that emerges from a well-functioning psychotherapy dyad. Personally, I cannot imagine doing therapy without the internalizations that have come from my own experiences as a patient. Even when there have been unduly painful or destructive aspects of our encounters with therapy, we learn something important there: what not to do. Casement's (1985) emphasis on the ongoing process of internal supervision in the therapist, a welcome alternative to our tendencies to apply a favored theory to practice whether or not it fits, assumes a therapist who knows something from experience. Regardless of what they say about their personal theoretical bent or ideology, most analysts' actual behavior in the consulting room probably expresses some combination of identification and counteridentification with their own analyst(s).

Equal in importance to the mitigation of contempt, the experience of an effective personal therapy or analysis leaves us with a deep respect for the power of the process and the efficacy of treatment. We know that psychotherapy works. Our silent appreciation of the discipline can convey that assurance to clients, for whom a sense of hope is a critical ingredient of their recovery from emotional suffering. Sheldon Roth (1987) writes, "Conviction that the treatment works provides the therapist with a deep well of faith and hope in an endeavor characterized by ongoing uncertainty, doubt, and self-questioning." There are so many situations, especially early in treatment, in which the therapist has not a clue about what is right to say or not say, that I cannot imagine how beginning practitioners manage their inevitable demoralization without a personal exposure to therapeutic change and growth.

From the experience of our own therapy we also "get" the ubiquity and power of unconscious processes. Our struggles with our own resistances to change, our confrontations with the ways in which early cognitive and emotional lessons keep reinterpreting new experience as like older ones, and our awe at witnessing the nuances of our responses to our therapists eventually create in us a deep appreciation of how hard it is and how long it takes to make significant internal changes. This appreciation increases our patience and permits us to convey to clients both that we know we can help and that we are not surprised that it takes a long time to go as far therapeutically as each patient hopes to go. A gifted therapist *can* learn that psychotherapy is effective without personal therapy, simply by spending enough time doing it. After a few years with a few patients, it is hard to ignore the significant, far-reaching changes they become capable of making. But one learns this faster and with less difficulty from personal experience.

If Alice Miller (1975) was right that people who become psychoanalytic therapists often have a disturbance in their self-esteem related to their having been both congenitally gifted emotionally and used by their parents as a kind of narcissistic stabilizer or family therapist, then it is particularly important for them to give themselves a place where their feelings will be understood on their own terms rather than exploited in the service of others' narcissism. The fact that *The Drama of the Gifted Child* quickly attained an almost cult-like status among psychotherapists suggests that she was on to something important about the kind of personal history likely to point an individual in the direction of becoming a therapist—virtually all my colleagues found themselves identifying with her description. Miller's (1979) article applying her observations to the question of the therapist's therapy may be of interest to clinicians who have found themselves resonating to her generalizations.

Finally, the experience of being progressively more emotionally honest and expressive in one's own therapy increases the capacity to manage feeling states without resorting to either disavowal or impulsivity. Research on attachment has documented the extent to which our relationships, not just our earliest ones but our ongoing adult connections, provide the milieu that human beings require for feeling, expressing, and elaborating emotional experience (Fonagy et al., 2002; Tyson, 1996). Meanwhile, more and more clinical observers and researchers are noting the centrality of affect tolerance to mental health (Ablon, Brown, Khantzian, & Mack, 1993; Kantrowitz, Paolitto, Sashin, Solomon, & Katz, 1986; Krystal, 1997). As therapists, we have to absorb a succession of intense, toxic feelings while staying honest and inhibiting the "fight or flight" reaction stimulated by patients' facial expressions, tones of voice, and body language—phenomena that repeatedly activate painful implicit memories stored in our amygdala (see Coen, 2002). For empirical studies on the question of therapy for the therapist, see Norcross, Strausser-Kirtland, and Missar (1988) and Norcross, Geller, and Kurazawa (2000).

Jung (1916) wrote about a "transcendent function," the capacity to hold open one's subjective experience at times when there is an internal pressure toward action or defense. Winnicott's concepts of "potential space" and "play space" (Ogden, 1985, 1986; Winnicott, 1971) are other ways of talking about this learned ability to keep feeling from translating into impulse, to maintain the possibilities for creative and transformative experience by tolerating what is projected and internalized in the clinical situation. Bion spoke of the therapist as being a "container" of clients' affect. Much of our therapeutic success may come from a capacity to model the containment of emotion for people whose states of feeling have previously been unformulated, overwhelming, or dissociated. Personal therapy or analysis increases the likelihood that we can do this.

Like many people who entered analysis with the conscious belief that they were doing so to further educational and career goals, I was stunned to discover how radically the experience improved my life. Julia Kristeva, in an interview for *The New York Times* (Riding, 2001), made a similar observation: "I began psychoanalysis for professional reasons, to acquire an additional analytical tool. . . . Of course, once you lie on the couch, you also soon realize that you, too, have a need. I learned a lot about myself. Eventually, while the analysis helped advance my work on literature, on philosophy and even on understanding our century, I discovered that healing was also essential to me" (p. B9). This combination of a lesson in humility and a template for understanding the change process is hard to get any other way.

OTHER VALUABLE FOUNDATIONS OF PRACTICE

Finally, I would like to throw my weight behind the argument originally made by Freud (1926) and later reiterated by others (e.g., Chessick, 1969; Sharpe, 1930) that therapists are benefited by the broadest possible education in literature, myth, the arts, the humanities, the sciences, and the social sciences. Narrow training in one of the "tri-disciplines" (medicine, academic psychology, social work) from which therapists tend to be drawn does not usually include immersion in the profound questions about meaning, emotion, will, relationship, freedom, justice, and limitation with which the great philosophers, theologians, artists, and writers have struggled for centuries. It is with complete seriousness that Thomas Ogden (2001) writes that he looks as much to poetry as to psychoanalytic literature when he wants to deepen his understanding of human predicaments. The list of creative psychotherapists who have come to their discipline from an immersion in other fields includes such luminaries as Anna Freud (education), Robert Waelder (physics), Erik Erikson (art), Hans Sachs (law), D. W. Winnicott (pediatrics), John Bowlby (anthropology), Stephen Mitchell (philosophy), and, for that matter, B. F. Skinner (creative writing) and Carl Rogers (theology). My Australian colleague Jan Resnick (personal communication, December 30, 2002) writes that his background in philosophy helps "with the value of reflection, the pursuit of truth, the importance of inquiry, the need to avoid dogmatic opinionation, and a kind of mental discipline for holding a 'meta-perspective'—in other words, trying to gain a perspective upon my perspective (attitude, disposition, way of seeing my patients)."

Even if a would-be therapist feels no need to ponder the weighty topics that are traditionally understood to be the essence of the liberal arts tradition, he or she will quickly encounter patients for whom they are central preoccupations. Some of these clients will fill their therapy hours with reflections on their responses to films, books, and music, and although one need not be a polymath to be a good therapist, it is helpful to have some sense of the territory that organizes the enthusiasm and vitality of the individuals one is trying to reach. The same observation holds for basic knowledge of areas such as sports, business, investment, and other common human enthusiasms. For a therapist, no knowledge about important human pursuits is ultimately superfluous.

One of the best fringe benefits of being in this field is getting an education in the areas that impassion one's clients.

It is also advantageous to have had a breadth of life experiences and exposure to people of different ages, occupations, religions, ethnic backgrounds, cultures, socioeconomic levels, and sexual desires. A term of service in the Peace Corps or a job in a summer camp or an experience of immersion in another culture can be almost as good a preparation for one of the psychotherapy professions as a stint in an inpatient unit. Most therapists have, as part of the temperament that has inclined them toward their chosen profession, a vast curiosity about human nature in all its manifestations. The more opportunities they have had to pursue their interests in human heterogeneity, the less they will feel out of their depth when confronted with a particular patient.

Therapists from social minorities, who have spent their lives feeling marginal and uncomfortable with the rites and creeds of the prevailing majority, are actually advantaged here. So are people with a schizoid streak or a temperament marked by shyness. Being different creates a habit of reflectiveness about basic human questions that is an indispensable resource to a therapist. In addition, the experience of feeling like an outsider is good preparation for empathy with the pervasive sense of "not belonging" described by so many patients. Recent evidence that Abraham Lincoln may have struggled with homoerotic feelings (Katz, 2001) shed some light for me on his remarkable capacity to identify with, and speak eloquently for, the experience of the outcast and the slave.

In this area as in others, one's personal suffering can ultimately deepen one's work. In fact, psychotherapy is one of the few professions in which one's greatest misfortunes can be retooled into professional assets. Elvin Semrad, whom Sheldon Roth (1987, p. 7) called "the model of the devoted empathic therapist for a generation of Boston-trained therapists" stated that the source of his renowned capacity to bear the intense, painful feelings of his patients was "a life of sorrow, and the opportunity that some people gave me to overcome it and deal with it" (Semrad, 1980, p. 206). Fortunately, the work itself can be healing. Just as good teachers say they learn a lot from their students, most analytic therapists say that they are deeply helped by their patients. In the particular situation of psychotherapists from ethnic, racial, cultural, religious, or sexual minorities, practicing therapy can demolish the stifling assumption that there exists some kind of "normal" psychology that is beyond their reach given the "deviant" circumstances of their childhood and adolescence. Nothing is as effective as clinical work in making the point that diversity is the norm.

Heinz Kohut (1968) once encouraged the fourteen-year-old son of a colleague to write to Anna Freud about his interest in becoming a psychoanalyst, asking her what preparations he should make for such a vocation. Here is part of the letter this boy received from her in response, which I quote not only because of its inherent charm but also because I agree with it:

> If you want to be a real psychoanalyst, you have to have a great love of the truth, scientific truth as well as personal truth, and you have to place this appreciation of truth higher than any discomfort at meeting unpleasant facts, whether they belong to the world outside or to your own inner person.
>
> Further, I think that a psychoanalyst should have [an interest] in facts that belong to sociology, religion, literature and history . . . otherwise his outlook on his patient will be too narrow.
>
> You ought to be a great reader and become acquainted with the literature of many countries and cultures. In the great literary figures you will find people who know at least as much of human nature as the psychiatrists and psychologists try to do. (p. 553)[1]

CONCLUDING COMMENTS

Having argued for the value of well-roundedness in therapists, I want nevertheless to return to the theme with which I launched this chapter, namely, that whatever limitations characterize his or her background, a beginning therapist usually has the raw materials to do the work. There is much more uniting human beings than separating them. While it can be daunting to be confronted with a patient who is thirty years older than the therapist, or is only rudimentarily educated, or is given to racist or sexist or homophobic comments, or participates in eccentric sexual practices, or belongs to an exotic cult, psychological suffering is a great equalizer. Most people can be helped by even a young and inexperienced therapist, provided he or she approaches them with respect, admits mistakes, behaves with sincerity, and makes good use of supervision.

Not only can individual practitioners of any level of experience help patients with whom they seem at first glance to have nothing in common, analytic therapists can help people with such formidable and sometimes alienating problems as psychotic episodes, addictions, complex posttraumatic syndromes, borderline personality organization, and severe character pathology. There is wisdom about all these areas available in the long tradition of depth therapy. Most of us who have struggled to help difficult patients have been able to find supervisors, consultants, and literature that have brought a relieving glimpse of order out of the chaos of impotence and anxiety into which they typically plunge us. It may be a cliché that applicants to psychotherapy training programs want to be therapists because they "want to help people," but like most clichés, it is true. Clients will feel and respond therapeutically to a practitioner's genuine wish to be of help. That one can always help is a pipe dream, but that one is trying to help is an attitude that makes psychotherapy possible.

NOTE

1. I am indebted to Mary Lorton (personal communication, September 28, 2002) for letting me know about the existence of this letter.

Chapter 4

Preparing the Client

One of therapy's impossible tasks is to help build
resources that make it possible to tolerate therapy.
—MICHAEL EIGEN (1992, p. xiv)

Consistently, empirical research on psychotherapy identifies the achievement of a sense of comfortable collaboration between
patient and clinician as critical to the effectiveness of treatment
(Gaston, Marmar, Gallagher, & Thompson, 1991; Hovarth & Symonds,
1991; Safran & Muran, 2000; Weinberger, 1995). Before such research
existed, psychoanalytic writers, whose experience had led them to
appreciate the same phenomenon, had paid serious attention to this aspect of therapy. In 1915, Freud noted that an ordinary degree of confidence in the doctor, based on positive experiences with other authorities, is a necessary condition for a good treatment outcome. Calling the
phenomenon the "unobjectionable positive transference," he was implicitly contrasting this essential cooperative attitude with other transferences that typically surface in psychotherapy.

One way of viewing transference is as the Freudian term for what
behaviorists have called stimulus generalization. That is, we expect
from a new authority figure what we have experienced with previous
ones; we generalize from past experience. Freud was distinguishing the
unobjectionable positive transference (trust in the therapist, based on
positive experiences with authorities) from negative transferences (expectations of misunderstanding and harm by the therapist, based on
painful experiences) and from problematic positive transferences, such
as romantic fantasies and primitive idealizations. Both negative transferences and unrealistic positive ones interfere with the pursuit of therapeutic goals and therefore can be considered "resistances" to opening
up to another perspective.

Many who have written thoughtfully about psychoanalytic technique have emphasized the silent operation of this feature of the therapeutic relationship; that is, the sense of co-ownership of the treatment process without which no amount of brilliance on the clinician's part can make it work. Fenichel (1941), for example, noted the therapeutic significance of the "rational transference," and Nacht (1958) stressed the critical role of the patient's perception of the analyst's supportive "presence." In midcentury, the terms "therapeutic alliance" and "working alliance" were introduced by Zetzel (1956) and Greenson (1967), respectively, to highlight the importance of the therapist's appreciating and, if necessary, cultivating this sense of mutual effort. Greenson's term, with its implication of two combatants allying against the psychopathology of one of them, seems to have captured the psychoanalytic imagination, though the less adversarial word "rapport," first used by Freud in 1913, also describes this dimension of psychotherapy. Most recently, Meissner (1996) has done a scholarly and thoroughgoing study of this concept, and although I respect the counterarguments, I agree with him about the value of talking about the therapeutic alliance as an aspect of the professional relationship that is conceptually separable from transference and countertransference.

People come to practitioners with a wide range of attitudes, backgrounds, and prior experiences of trying to solve their problems—alone and with other professionals. In the initial sessions, clients may arrive in a high state of affective arousal (mortifying shame, paralyzing fear, grim hostility, desperate need), or they can be tentative and subdued. Individuals from families and subcultures in which psychotherapy is accepted and valued may arrive with attitudes ranging from eager anticipation to arrogant entitlement. Those who are sent by others (friends, relatives, physicians, employers, the court system) are likely to be suspicious and defensive; one often feels a stony resistance behind an overtly compliant exterior. Some, including many adolescents, can hardly get themselves to talk. Consequently, the art of establishing a working alliance cannot be reduced to a few boilerplate procedures; the therapist must rely on empathy, intelligence, intuition, tact, and an understanding of different kinds of character and circumstance to draw the person out and interest him or her in the possibilities that psychodynamic therapy offers. There is some emerging empirical evidence, however, that structured clinical training positively affects the alliance (Hilsenroth, Ackerman, Clemence, Strassle, & Handler, 2002).

If I had to identify the most common failing of novice therapists, I would say it is the tendency to try to "do therapy" without first securing an alliance. Beginners frequently attempt to carry out technical procedures before their patients have been helped to understand and accept

why their therapist is acting in a certain way or adopting a particular focus. They may do this because they assume the client will understand
their good intentions intuitively or because they are eager to get deeply
into the work or because they have not yet been given supervisory help
with how to explain the therapeutic process to their patients. For example, a critical part of psychodynamic technique is the repeated investigation of how the client is feeling toward the therapist and how he or
she imagines the therapist is feeling. Analytic therapists pursue this
topic because we know how much projection goes on between people,
and we want to understand what prior experiences or inner states the
patient may be projecting. If the clinician asks a question such as "How
are you feeling about me?" or "How are you imagining I feel about what
you've said?," the client who has not been given a rationale for such
queries may sensibly conclude that the therapist is seeking either praise
or reassurance. Not surprisingly, most people are not inclined to cooperate with such a narcissistic agenda and fail to see the point of exploring their answer. When told why we ask that sort of question, however,
most people are quickly appreciative of the value of this kind of inquiry.

Psychotherapy is a peculiar kind of conversation. It is not like social discourse, nor is it like a visit to an expert who gives explicit advice,
nor is it like studying with a teacher or mentor or spiritual advisor. Patients often have no prior experience with which they can compare it,
and especially if they feel vulnerable, exposed, and prickly when seeking help, they are susceptible to numerous misunderstandings of what
the therapist is trying to do. Some sophisticated clients, because of previous treatment or because of being reared in psychotherapy-savvy families and subcultures, understand immediately why a clinician might answer a question with a question, or decline to disclose personal
information, or ask about dreams, or urge the patient to express feelings, or ask about the patient's reaction to the therapist, or inquire
about his or her sex life when the person came to treatment for something else. But most clients, perhaps all to some extent, need some explicit education about and/or socialization into this strange process.

Many primers on psychotherapy do not devote much space to the
question of conveying to a patient how to participate productively in
the clinical process. (I suspect that the enduring popularity of Ralph
Greenson's 1967 textbook on psychoanalysis has a lot to do with its being an exception.) But some authors seem to take it for granted that
most potential patients arrive at one's office already knowing something about the nature of therapeutic collaboration. Or they may assume that once the practitioner gets the process going, its nature and
advantages will become self-evident to the client. Perhaps these were

reasonable expectations in the so-called heyday of psychoanalysis, when Eissler's (1953) "basic model technique" was sufficiently normative that most educated people in Western cultures, especially those in the United States, shared an image of what happens in psychoanalytic treatment. Innumerable cartoons, jokes, media characterizations, and other references to Freudian rituals attest to the universality of these ideas. But contemporarily, there is a bewildering diversity of accepted ways of working therapeutically, and even within the psychoanalytic world, there are widely disparate ways of conducting treatment. Clients cannot be expected to know what is going to happen between themselves and a mental health professional. Even if they have had prior treatment (and especially if they have had the minimal interventions that health maintenance organizations like to call therapy), their expectations may be vague or inaccurate or unrealistic. For this reason, I am devoting a chapter on how to prepare the patient for his or her role in the therapeutic partnership. I have organized the pertinent issues under the topics of safety and education.

ESTABLISHING SAFETY

Aristotle commented (trans. 1997) that "mere life" is a precondition for the "good life." As Sullivan (e.g., 1953) was among the first to note, we must have our security needs met before we can pursue the question of satisfaction of other needs. Freud, who may have taken his sense of basic security more or less for granted (Breger, 2000), emphasized satisfaction issues (finding avenues for drive discharge, reducing guilt that interferes with reasonable ways to meet needs) much more than safety issues, but for many patients—possibly most—security questions are a first-order concern in psychotherapy. In the following sections I address issues of both physical and emotional safety.

Physical Safety

For most clients, physical safety is not an issue, but in the case of those for whom it *is* an issue, it is urgent and primary. We cannot bring psychological help to people who are in acute physical danger, or who feel threatened in their basic sense of security, until we establish minimal safety. With psychotic patients, who can be consumed with anxieties about fragmentation and annihilation (see Atwood, Orange, & Stolorow, 2002; Hurvich, 1989) therapists may have to express an appreciation of their fears that professionals will harm them (see FrommReichmann, 1952; Karon & VandenBos, 1981). Even well-medicated patients with psychotic tendencies harbor such fears. Bertram Karon (personal communication, August 23, 2002) begins an interview with a withdrawn patient with schizophrenia by announcing, "I want you to know that I will not kill you and that I will not allow other people to kill you." Often, it helps to ask a frightened client if there is any way the therapist can behave that will reduce the fear of obliteration (sitting farther away, not staring, leaving the door open, not taking notes, etc.). Respectful negotiation of the conditions under which the psychotic person can feel safe enough to talk may consume weeks, months, or even years.

Such conversations prepare the client for the collaborative process of self-exploration that we think of as therapy proper, yet in another sense they *are* the therapy. Just as addressing breaches in the therapeutic alliance strengthens that alliance (Safran, 1993), negotiating about safety creates a safer atmosphere. The attainment of a sense of safety is a significant therapeutic accomplishment. Learning that an authority can adapt respectfully to one's personal needs can be a liberating revelation to clients with psychotic tendencies, whose parents and other caregivers seldom knew how to cope with their idiosyncracies. Such negotiations can also be crucial to developing a working alliance with severely traumatized patients, who may go into temporary dissociative states in which they fail to distinguish current circumstances from traumatic memories. Eventually, sometimes after many years, even very disturbed individuals should come to experience their therapist's office as a sanctuary. During times in treatment at which the work seems to get stuck or derailed, a renegotiation of the working alliance, with special attention to restoring a sense of safety to the relationship, will be necessary to get both parties back on track. Safety can be a valuable issue to explore at any juncture where the process feels stuck or "off" or unproductive to one or both parties.

With severely depressed patients in danger of acting suicidally, it is critical to intervene authoritatively on behalf of their safety. One may need to hospitalize them and/or to have repeated, frank discussions with them about procedures to be followed if they are seriously tempted to act on suicidal ideas. For several reasons, such procedures should not depend on the therapist's constant availability. For one thing, the therapist could be temporarily unreachable or incapacitated, in which case having urged a person to call when suicidal can be a formula for disaster, when the patient is traumatically disappointed by the therapist's inability to keep an implied promise. For another, offering oneself as an on-call rescuer feeds an idealization that can make the patient feel (by contrast to the confident and generous clinician) even more helpless and defective and hence increasingly suicidal. Finally, such an arrangement is too burdensome emotionally not to generate resentment in the therapist. It is hard to give wholehearted help to a person one is resenting; emergency services are much better safety nets than one's own good intentions. When the clinician believes hospitalization is necessary, he or she should not hesitate to insist on it. If the patient has limited insurance and a balky case manager, the therapist may have to be aggressively protective, making noises to managed care bureaucrats to the effect that "I am putting it in my records that you are refusing, against my professional advice, to keep this acutely suicidal patient in the hospital."

Similar considerations apply to individuals with exigent life-threatening problems, such as anorectic patients who are ominously underweight, severely self-mutilating clients, drug addicts at grave risk of overdose, alcoholics who drink and drive, and people who pursue anonymous, unprotected sexual encounters. Sometimes one has to take an extratherapeutic measure, such as hospitalizing gravely anorectic people until they attain a certain weight, and sometimes one can only address self-destructiveness within the treatment context, such as when one persistently insists that the client examine a pattern of sexual risk taking. The first order of business in working with people who put themselves at risk is to keep them alive. Before agreeing to provide outpatient treatment for such patients, some experienced therapists require specific commitments, such as an agreement to participate in Alcoholics Anonymous and to achieve a certain period of sobriety. Others consent to meet with self-harming clients as long as it is understood that the therapist will insist on talking about virtually nothing else until the patient finds a way to reduce the threat to his or her survival (see Isaacson, 1991; Levin, 1987; Richards, 1993; Washton, 1995, 2004).

My experiences with "contracting for safety"—that is, getting suicidal patients to make a pledge not to hurt themselves as a condition for therapy—have been unimpressive. My general sense is that such contracts are often urged by the professional or employing agency as a way of reducing liability and assuaging the anxiety of the therapist, and that they have little effect on ensuring actual safety. Not that reducing one's liability is an unseemly practice in this litigious age, but a number of suicidal individuals have told me that they eventually caved in to pressures to sign an agreement not to kill themselves while privately retaining suicide as an option. In fact, some have said that their willingness to keep on living has depended on their knowing that if the psychic pain were to get too bad, they would have an out. Given that psychodynamic therapy is based on honesty, and that colluding in a fiction for purposes of risk management is hardly an expression of can-

dor, the therapist may have to tolerate a patient's refusal to give a guarantee. Otherwise, one is teaching that dishonesty is the price of
relationship, a lesson that cannot fail to corrupt psychotherapy at the
core. Especially when the patient will not swear off lethal intentions,
one should repeatedly, even relentlessly, investigate the current suicidal
risk and be willing to hospitalize an acutely self-destructive person.

At the same time, there is a great deal one can do in an atmosphere of mutual candor to increase the probability of the client's staying alive. Part of any experienced therapist's repertoire is a conversation about the resources available to suicidal patients to maintain their
safety. Clients are usually willing to engage in problem-solving discussions about friends they might call or visit if their affect becomes too
intense, activities that may distract them from the pressure of self-
destructive urges, and crisis services and hotlines that are available
around the clock. I have known instances in which a patient carried
around a list of emergency phone numbers as a kind of transitional object (Winnicott, 1953), a portable substitute for the calming presence
of the therapist. Taking the risk seriously and talking frankly and cre-
atively about harm avoidance generally strengthens the working alliance and makes the client feel fully heard.

One's diagnostic impression of the patient's general personality
and specific disorder has profound implications for the assessment of
lethality. A person with a bipolar disorder or major depression who reports suicidal urges will appreciate the therapist's understanding the
power of the wish to die, while the individual with borderline personality organization may be threatening suicide because this is the way he
or she has learned to evoke serious attention and concern. In borderline clients, "parasuicidal gestures" are common in the context of separation from someone or something important to them. Sometimes simply talking about how grief-stricken they are about a loss is enough to
remove the threat of suicide. In fact, if one moves too quickly into doing the usual crisis-intervention inventory of plans, means, and availability of means, the person with more borderline tendencies tends to
feel "unheard" (because the therapist is not addressing the loneliness
and pain that the suicide threat was intended to convey) and may proceed to escalate the threat to ensure a hearing. Some people who express suicidal ideas want to communicate their literal wish not to go on
living, whereas others are giving metaphorical expression to an already
existing sense of internal deadness. Desperate individuals in either category are usually grateful when a therapist's sincere interest in the nature of their experience takes precedence over an anxious rush into
"management" procedures.

Despite the fact that expressions of suicidal intent from borderline patients may not indicate that they are actually at death's door, a therapist cannot be casual about the risk. Even parasuicidal gestures must be taken seriously. Borderline patients with a self-dramatizing tendency have been known to make attempts that cause their death more or less "inadvertently"—for example, by overdosing on a medicine they think will work slowly (allowing time for them to be discovered, taken to a hospital, and dramatically revived) but which instead causes abrupt heart failure. Borderline clients who will not agree to refrain from flirting with suicide need to be confronted with the fact that they are evidently not ready to commit seriously to therapy. If the therapist does take such a client into treatment, the person must be told what the specific consequences will be each time he or she acts self-destructively (see Clarkin, Yeomans, & Kernberg, 1999; Yeomans et al., 2002).

Finally, some patients present a threat to the safety of the therapeutic dyad. Both they and their therapists must be protected from their potential homicidality. The best predictor of violence is previous violence; clients with histories of harming others need to get the message that they will not be allowed to harm the therapist. Some individuals with such histories have dissociative psychologies and are terrified of entering a hostile state of consciousness in which they could attack a professional whom they otherwise value. Others are essentially psychopathic and cannot be trusted to resist opportunities to exert their destructive power. Others have such an extreme problem with affect regulation that in the heat of the moment they fail to differentiate between hostile feelings and aggressive actions. *The therapist's sense of safety is as important as the patient's.* One should not see anyone with a history of violence in an isolated office or after others have left the building. A clinician who sees markedly disturbed or unpredictable people should never accept an office arrangement in which the patient is between the clinician and the door; anyone who has felt "trapped" in an office with three-hundred-pound raging paranoid schizophrenic knows that such sessions are endurable only if a clear escape route is available.

I have advised several solo practitioners who have found themselves working with someone who reveals a destructive potential to call their local police departments and have a "panic button" installed under their desk or chair so that they can get immediate help if the patient starts to threaten them. They tell me that their awareness of having this option keeps them calm and contributes to a sense of safety in both themselves and their patients. Something about having such a recourse available makes it unlikely that it will ever have to be used. Concerns of this sort depend, of course, on the nature of one's practice. A colleague of mine who evaluates many dangerous, sadistic, and high-profile offenders with antisocial personality disorder works in an office with bullet-proof glass. Most of us do not need to be this careful. But even those of us whose clientele consists of highly motivated, self-referred customers occasionally find ourselves working with someone who gives us the shivers. It is important to respect the information coming from the gut and to treat it with the seriousness it deserves. Denial is not an adaptive defense in a therapist.

Once I was asked by a friend who is a defense attorney to interview a man he represented who had been charged with murder. This client had just been arrested for killing his wife in what his lawyer sincerely believed was a tragic accident. According to the accused, she was threatening to kill herself with a gun, which went off as he tried to wrestle it out of her grip. On the possibility that my friend's confidence in his client was misplaced, I asked my husband to sit in my waiting room during the interview so that I could yell for his help in the unlikely event of my being attacked. Whether or not my apprehension was warranted, the knowledge that I had that protection available made it possible for me to do a much better interview than I otherwise would have. (As it happened, I ended up endorsing the attorney's belief in this man's probable innocence. It became evident that he had deeply loved his wife, a woman who sounded flagrantly borderline and who had been in treatment for suicidal depression. It appeared that he had been doubly traumatized—first by her death at his hands and then by the intimidating police investigators. I had worried, however, that my friend could have been taken in by a skillful psychopath.)

Emotional Safety

The more subtle issue of emotional safety is probably relevant to every psychotherapy patient. Depending on the person's history, he or she will be worried, consciously or unconsciously, about different possibilities for a repetition of painful experiences. Will the therapist be bored? Critical? Contemptuous? Indifferent? Shocked? Afraid? Skeptical? Seductive? Incompetent? As Weiss, Sampson, and the Mt. Zion Psychotherapy Group (1986) have documented empirically, clients have a sense, going into the therapy process, of what they need, and they proceed to "test" the therapist to see whether he or she is capable of facilitating their plan for emotional recovery. Usually it is not hard to discern a person's paramount fears about committing to the therapeutic partnership. It is important to find ways to demonstrate that one understands the client's worst apprehensions about what can go wrong in a relationship of dependency, thereby conveying that one will try not to make those fantasies come true. Many therapists address the working alliance explicitly as an issue of "goodness of fit" between therapist and

patient (Schafer, 1979; Kohut, 1984). One of my colleagues, for example, makes a point of telling new clients that the fit accounts for at least
fifty-one percent of what happens in treatment; he then encourages
them to let him know after a few sessions how they are experiencing
the relationship.

Sometime the therapist knows immediately what stumbling block
the patient is expecting. It does not take the proverbial rocket scientist
to deduce from the belligerent question, "So how long have *you* been
practicing?" that the person is worried about inexperience, or from the
comment, "Oh shit, they gave me a woman," that gender is an issue.
With more contained clients, the simplest way to evaluate the presence
or absence of a nascent working alliance is to ask the person, near the
end of the first session, "How are you feeling about working with me?"
or "Are you finding yourself comfortable talking with me?" Such questions can be followed up by exploration if the person discloses negative
reactions, such as "I wasn't sure I'd feel comfortable with a man [white
person, non-Asian, secular therapist, gay therapist, student, older person . . .]" or "I find myself wondering if you can understand the importance to me of being a serious Buddhist" or—the most dreaded but
probably inescapable message to a beginning therapist—"I worry that
you might be too young [or inexperienced] to help me."

If the person assures the therapist that he or she is perfectly happy
with the connection but the therapist senses a potential problem, it is
valuable to make a comment as early as one can that communicates this
possibility. For example, "Given how you describe your mother, as so
intrusive and controlling, I'm surprised that you can open up to this extent with a woman," or, "You may find that as our work goes on, the
fact that you have been mistreated by so many white males may make it
harder for you than it now feels to be comfortable with me; please let
me know if that starts happening," or, "It's going to be interesting to
see if we find ourselves inadvertently repeating the pattern you describe, of self-involved parent and desperate-to-please child. These repetitions can happen in this kind of therapy."

The reader may notice that these sample comments are not explicitly reassuring. That is, the therapist is not saying, "I'm sure I won't do
what your mother did; I'm just not an intrusive, controlling person."
Anyone who has practiced psychodynamic therapy for any length of
time knows that one cannot avoid being pulled into emotional repetitions of painful earlier relationships. We can, of course, guarantee that
we will not physically attack or sexually exploit a patient, but beyond
these reassurances about our overt behavior, we are on uncertain
ground. The emphasis of relational analysts on processing "enactments" (rather than issuing dispassionate interpretations) is one of

only many indications of the general psychoanalytic appreciation that familiar patterns get repeated, often in remarkably subtle ways, in psychotherapy. Despite our omnipotent wishes to the contrary, we know that coexisting with the client's realistic perceptions of the therapist as different from disappointing childhood love objects, there is always a more powerful, insistent dynamic that grafts current objects on to the internal working models (Bowlby, 1969, 1988; Bretherton, 1990; Main, 1998) of previous relationships. The power to foster healing lies not only in the therapist's opportunities to be experienced as an authority who differs from previous objects of attachment but also in his or her willingness to tolerate, name, discuss, explore, and express remorse for the inevitable ways in which old patterns get transferred to and repeated in the therapeutic partnership.

As analysts have noted at least as far back as Wilhelm Reich (1932), it is particularly important to deal with negative transferences in the earliest sessions; otherwise, the patient may not come back. Higher-functioning clients often need a sense of permission to put words to what may seem "impolite" or "inappropriate" to say in other contexts. Patients with severe personality disorders, borderline features, or psychotic tendencies also need to feel that they can vent their distrust and malice safely, although with such clients the therapist rarely has a compensatory sense of connection with a less antagonistic part of the person. The more the therapist can exemplify a tolerance for hostility and even contemptuous devaluation, without the need for retaliation, the more likely the patient is to feel safe.

Many particularly unhappy individuals will exhibit their worst selves right away, to test the therapeutic waters. Without submitting masochistically to verbal abuse, therapists must be able to convey that their self-esteem can withstand such attacks, and that in spite of the fact that it is no pleasure to be reviled, it will eventually be possible to bring meaning together out of the patient's hostility. A comment such as "Wow—you certainly are good at enumerating all my defects!" or "It must not be easy to be going to a therapist that you see as such an idiot" or "You and I are going to have our work cut out for us, given how much you distrust me" is probably the best one can do to accept the negative feelings without either counterattacking or colluding in diminishing oneself.

Under ideal circumstances, the therapist is clearly, in the minds of both parties, hired by the patient. As the therapist's employer, the patient has the ultimate responsibility, assuming that nothing disastrous happens to either participant, to determine the frequency of appointments and the length of treatment. The clinician offers his or her expertise to that decision, advising the client about the pros and cons of more-than-once-weekly treatment (frequency intensifies affect and ensures continuity in intellectually defended people but may provoke malignant regression in those with profound conflicts about closeness) and about the wisdom of whether to terminate (how much of the wish to end therapy seems to be an avoidance of something important and how much seems to be a healthy urge to try one's wings). Under less than ideal circumstances, both participants must contend with limits on both the frequency and length of their collaboration. When treatment is arbitrarily limited, it may not go on at short enough intervals or for a long enough time for the client to achieve a sense of safety. Under such conditions, the best a therapist can do is to find ways to convey understanding and acceptance of the person's insecurity, to encourage him or her to vent feelings of distrust and anxiety freely, and to avoid taking the patient's wariness and suspicion personally.

I mentioned earlier the importance of negotiating, with psychotically disturbed people, the conditions under which they can tolerate being in therapy. This process can also be important with other clients. Some individuals will tell their therapist exactly what they require to feel safe: "I need to be able to pace if I get too anxious" or "If I can't talk easily, I want you to try to draw me out" or "I have to sit closer to the door." Sometimes these concerns appear as questions: "How do you feel about patients calling between sessions?" or "Given my unpredictable schedule, can we just set up appointments week to week?" Sometimes in response to these concerns, the therapist can simply assent; at other times, negotiation is in order. In such negotiations, therapists must be careful not to be so empathic with the patient's request that they neglect to honor their own individuality and personal requirements. It is the therapist's responsibility to protect his or her "conditions of labor" (i.e., the circumstances under which it is comfortable to practice). For example, "I'm willing to take calls between sessions, but not after nine o'clock at night, and I typically will be able to spend only a minute or two talking," or "I appreciate that you can't control your business trips, but I need predictability in my own schedule. Could we establish a regular weekly meeting time and have an agreed-upon "back-up hour" to reschedule if you have to cancel?" This exemplification of self-respect is itself a therapeutic communication, especially to depressive and self-defeating clients who always put their own needs last, and to pathologically entitled ones who need to come to terms with the fact that the world does not always defer to their wishes.

Sometimes a patient will ask outright, "Can you help me?" Unless the therapist feels that the client has come for an untreatable problem (an organic disorder that has been misunderstood as psychological, for example), it is perfectly appropriate to say "I think so" or "I'm going to

do my best" or "If both of us give it our best shot, I think we can do it."
It would be misleading and presumptuous to say a simple yes, given the
importance of the client's sincere cooperation. Even a master therapist
cannot bring about change alone. With patients who may be helpable
but for whom the prognosis is guarded—for example, those with severe
narcissistic problems or significant antisocial tendencies or a history of
failed therapies—the best one can do is a response such as "I don't
know. I'm going to do my best, but I think it's going to be hard going.
What's your own guess about whether this can work and what might go
wrong?"

Readers familiar with the second chapter of *Psychoanalytic Case Formulation* (McWilliams, 1999), in which I described my own approach to
an initial interview, know that I believe that a patient who is deciding
whether or not to work with a particular therapist is entitled to information that helps in that decision. This idea can be unwelcome to neo-
phyte therapists, who face the unattractive prospect of queries such as
"How much clinical experience do you have?" or "Am I your first patient?" or "How do I know you know what you're doing?" The evasions
of the "classical" tradition would be a comfort now (What is your fantasy about my training? Perhaps you are worried that I am too inexperienced to help you? What comes to mind about your need to grill me
about my competence?), and at many points in treatment an evasive, exploratory response may be appropriate, but in the initial meetings the
consumer has a right to know the professional's credentials.

Perhaps the best one can do in these interactions is to give an honest but encouraging answer and explore the client's worries. For example, one could reply, "Not a vast amount of experience yet, but I make
up for that in my enthusiasm," or "Yes, you're my first official patient,
which gives you the honor of being the one I'm most determined to do
well with," or "Perhaps the issue of knowing what I'm doing is better
judged after rather than before we've done some work together, but in
the meantime, if you think what I'm doing isn't helpful, I hope you'll
tell me." These kinds of answers should be followed by questions investigating how the patient feels about what he or she has just heard, and
about the implications to him or her of having a less experienced clinician. One very useful line to have handy is, "I'm willing to answer that
question, but first, I'm curious what thoughts and feelings are behind
your asking it."

Some individuals believe that no one can help them who has not
been through some experience that has been central to their own suf-
ferings. They may ask questions such as whether the therapist has undergone sexual trauma, or had a religious epiphany, or tried psyche-
delic drugs, or been diagnosed with a major mood disorder, or brought

up a difficult child, or had an abortion, or suffered from an addiction. The clinician can empathize with this sentiment while commenting that no two people have *exactly* the same experiences, even when their lives contain similar features. "I'm hoping to learn from you what it was like *for you* to go through what you did, without imposing my preconceptions on it" is a useful comment. I am frequently struck by how helpful a caring therapist can be to someone very different; for example, one of my colleagues talks with awe about a chaste Catholic nun he knew who had a remarkable capacity to help clients with their sexual problems. Still, there are instances—often involving race, gender, religion, ethnicity, and sexual orientation—in which a general commonality is important enough to the patient that the two parties to the intake interview may be better off agreeing to pursue a referral to a therapist whose experience is more analogous to that of the patient.

When a client's questions feel unduly intrusive (Where do you live? Were you ever sexually abused? How often do *you* masturbate? Do you have a personal relationship with Jesus Christ?), one can simply say, "I'm sorry—I'm not comfortable answering a question about such an intimate part of my life, but I'm very interested in why that question is important to you." Different therapists draw the line in different places when it comes to how much they divulge; each of us needs to find a way to address our patients' concerns respectfully without feeling painfully exposed or invaded. If a client becomes angered by the therapist's refusal to talk about private matters, chances are that he or she needed a good reason to rage about the limits that life and other people impose on one's personal agendas, and to observe whether the therapist can tolerate the outburst. As any thoughtful parent of a toddler or teenager knows, fury about limits is an important and inevitable part of maturation, a part that many contemporary clients, reared by indulgent or negligent or overstressed authorities, appear to have missed.

EDUCATING THE PATIENT ABOUT THE THERAPY PROCESS

Some patients, as noted previously, come to psychodynamic therapy with a pretty accurate sense of what to expect and what to do in the client role. But most people need to be educated about the process. Despite the fact that virtually all therapists develop little speeches and stories that address the patient's need to understand what he or she is signing up for, there is not much written about this aspect of treatment in the literature on technique. Left to themselves, most practitioners probably draw on the ways their own therapist made the process comprehensible to them. In supervision and consultation groups with their colleagues, practitioners often enjoy trading analogies and allegories they can use to make the therapy process less of a mystery to their clients. Perhaps because it seems to penetrate parts of the client's mind other than the prefrontal cortex, a good metaphor is worth a hundred intellectual explanations. I mentioned in Chapter 1, for example, the utility of comparing psychotherapy to trailblazing.

Other analogies are ubiquitous in the field; every therapist develops a stable of favorites to call on when an educative intervention is called for. Freud, like many charismatic teachers, was a particular master of metaphor and parable; his capacity to convey meaning with stories, jokes, and allusions was so highly developed that the *Standard Edition* of his work has a whole index devoted to his analogies. Many of his psychoanalytic heirs have followed his lead in this style of teaching. Different clinicians find different ways, however, congruent with their personal backgrounds and personalities, to explain the rationales for different aspects of therapy to people with no background in the psychodynamic enterprise and no basis for automatically accepting this unique kind of professional relationship.

Informed Consent

It may also be a good idea for some of the therapist's educative role to be carried out in writing. Many clinicians currently practicing, often thanks to the grueling experience of having been investigated by a professional board at the instigation of a vindictive patient, ex-patient, or relative of a patient, have their clients sign a statement of informed consent that spells out the nature and methods of psychoanalytic therapy. In the United States, practitioners who do any of their work electronically must by law have the client sign a consent form acknowledging the practitioner's policies with respect to patient privacy. Certain individuals are at special risk of spiraling into a malignant psychotic regression and accusing the therapist of mistreating them. When one is working with a client with severe dissociative symptoms or serious childhood abuse or striking borderline features or pervasive hostility or unrelenting suicidality or a history of suing authorities, it is advisable to have him or her literally sign on to undergo psychodynamic treatment. As Bryant Welch notes, on the basis of having represented numerous colleagues in legal actions:

> There is nothing wrong or inherently unjust about the increase in litigation against psychotherapists. To a significant extent, it is an appreciation of the fact that psychotherapy is important, and when done

improperly, can have a devastating impact upon people's lives. . . . [But] it is a fantasy to think that only the culpable are brought before licensing boards or become the targets of malpractice litigation. Being a good person and a competent therapist does not guarantee that one will not be forced to defend the profession, often with the very right to continue practicing at stake. Anyone who works with borderline patients, families, children, or very sick patients is at risk. It is that simple, and it is only at one's peril that one denies this fact. (Hedges, 2000, p. xiv)

Examples of such documents, relevant to different therapy and supervision arrangements and conveniently sized for copying, can be found in Lawrence Hedges's (2000) useful text on risk management. In *Psychoanalytic Case Formulation* (McWilliams, 1999) I appended a prototypical informed consent form. Hedges's book contains examples of contracts that spell things out in much more detail, with an eye toward protecting therapists from the worst that can befall them from embittered clients. In the recent rush of practitioners in the United States to become compliant with new federal regulations about electronic transmission of clinical data, various professional organizations and individual practitioners have drafted documents of this sort. More ominous than threats to practice from dissatisfied customers or legal bodies, I have been hearing lately, both from enthusiasts of empirically supported treatment and from promoters of medication, enough rumblings about psychoanalytic treatment being viewed as "unethical" that there may be wisdom in protecting ourselves this way from our more doctrinaire colleagues of other orientations, as well. (Why should they be expected to treat us any better than some of our dogmatic psychoanalytic predecessors treated the early behaviorists?)

Addressing Early Obstacles to Full Participation in Treatment

Although there is a huge clinical and empirical literature on "analyzability" and "treatability" (Bachrach,1983; Bachrach & Leaff, 1978; Doidge et al., 2002; Ehrenberg, 1992; Erle, 1979; Erle & Goldberg, 1979; Paolino, 1981), most of it concludes that we cannot predict which patients will do well in psychodynamic therapy. Despite many recent efforts to correlate preferred treatment approach with type of problem (what works, under what conditions, for whom—see Roth & Fonagy, 1996), there is still so much variance attributable to uncontrollable factors such as the personality of the therapist that we can say very little about who is a particularly good candidate for psychodynamic therapy and who would probably do better in another modality. Most analytic therapists thus proceed on the basis of the belief that it is always worth a try to see if a particular patient can become responsive to psychodynamic help—assuming the person knows what else is available and how practices differ. Clients are often very good judges of what kind of treatment will be helpful to them.

Most analytic practitioners, though, would probably say that the very concrete person is hard to treat dynamically, and that the individual who insistently asks the therapist to "tell me what to do" or "just make me normal" is particularly challenging to one's clinical skills. There may be a better fit between such a person and one of the cognitive-behavioral treatments, in which concrete skill training may be stressed and in which the clinician is more accepting of a teacher-like role. But before transferring the person to a colleague trained in cognitive-behavioral treatment, most of us with psychodynamic biases will see if we can engage this sort of patient in the kind of work we value, in hopes of nourishing the stunted capacity the person may have for introspection, reflection, and self-propelled emotional growth.

Resistance is a key concept in psychodynamic therapy. Among many professionals, the term has come to be used rather promiscuously to refer to any lack of cooperation with the therapist. But the original Freudian concept of resistance assumes a largely unconscious phenomenon more akin to the resistance described by physicists than the resistance of willful obstinacy. With the term, Freud was identifying an intrapsychic process rather than an interpersonal one—though, of course, resistance can be felt interpersonally by whoever is trying to exert influence on another person. The concept captures the fact that our psychic structures do not assimilate new experience easily; rather, they redefine it as old experience. Resistance in therapy sometimes has conscious elements but is not always an act of negation. One cannot decide not to be resistant any more than one can decide not to perspire when it is hot. It is worth noting that resistance is not just the adversary of the psychotherapist but also a powerfully protective phenomenon. If human beings did not have intrinsic resistance to being influenced in new directions, we would be infinitely more vulnerable to activities such as brainwashing and demagoguery. For obvious reasons, however, it is an old clinical maxim that the therapist must address as early as possible any resistances that may impede the client's committing to treatment.

Sometimes the ostensibly resistant patient is not resisting in the classical psychoanalytic sense (i.e., suffering unconscious fears of participating and thereby changing) but, rather, has no mental picture of what a mutual therapeutic engagement looks like. In such instances, raising a person's consciousness about what kinds of interaction are possible sometimes brings about a rather abrupt shift from a confused, resistive state to a willingness to cooperate. People from subcultures that encourage deference to authority, or distrust ambiguity, or regard reflection about one's motives as base self-indulgence may need the therapist to address explicitly the rationale for engaging in a collaborative exploratory process and to differentiate that process from behavior deemed unacceptable by the person's culture of origin. The effort to socialize a person into the role of patient requires the therapist not only to elicit the fears and expectations that are in the way (traditional resistance analysis) but also to give the patient information that at least intellectually challenges those internal voices. Such information will not resolve the conflict, but it may make it ego alien. And before any entrenched attitude can be deliberately changed, it must become acknowledged as problematic.

For example, artists, scholars, and passionate activists often harbor a fear, based on a keen intuitive sense of the kinds of dynamics that propelled them into their vocation, that if they lose their neurotic features, they will lose their inspired ones. The poet Rilke refused to go into psychoanalysis because he felt it would destroy not only his demons but his poetic muse. It is valuable to encourage clients with such reservations to express their worries, but emotional expression may not by itself reduce their trepidations. They may also need to hear an opposing point of view. In the face of reluctance by creative and committed individuals to take chances with their psychological equilibrium, the therapist can legitimately say that the general psychoanalytic experience has been that one's creative energies increase with treatment, as they become divested of some of their conflicted aspects. Gordon Allport (1961) seems to have been right that patterns that originated in and that were once fed by unconscious conflict can achieve functional autonomy.

Beginning therapists are not, of course, expected to know how to address all the possible reservations different individuals have about entering treatment, but there is nothing wrong with helping the client to name his or her apprehensions in one session, then talking with one's supervisor, and then responding to the substance of the patient's concerns in the next meeting. One can simply comment to the client, "I've been thinking about what you said last time about your misgivings about participating in this process, and I've had a conversation with a senior therapist about it, who says that it's a common worry, but that in her experience it's not a realistic danger. Evidently, creative people who have undertaken psychotherapy usually report that it has only enhanced their existing strengths." Notwithstanding the beginning therapist's understandable reluctance to call attention to the fact that he or she depends on the expertise of more seasoned colleagues, patients ordinarily feel touched that their therapist has given extracurricular thought to their feelings and has taken their concerns seriously enough to seek answers to their questions.

I want to reiterate that I am not contending that such educative interventions resolve a person's deep and longstanding conflicts (in fact, I regard it as the chief limitation of cognitive therapies that their partisans underestimate the resistances to the therapist's efforts to challenge and reframe existing ideas), but I am arguing that they may permit the reluctant or uncomfortable client to decide to give therapy a chance.

Encouraging Spontaneous, Candid, Emotionally Expressive Speech

As I have related elsewhere (McWilliams, 1999), I typically spend the first session with a new patient trying to get a sense of his or her presenting problem (including its history and the person's prior efforts to deal with it) and to establish myself as a potentially helpful presence. In the second meeting I take a detailed history. After that, I make a statement along the following lines:

> "I think that's enough information for me to a have a context for what you want to work on. From this point on, I'll follow your lead. If you can come in and talk as freely as possible about any aspect of this, or anything else that's on your mind, I'll try to listen for the more emotional side of it and see what I can say that might cast some new light on what you're talking about. For a while, I'll probably be pretty quiet, as I try to catch up with your own understanding of your problem. The most important thing for you to keep in mind is to try to be as open and honest as you can. Feel free to talk at any point about how you feel the process is going and whether you feel I'm being helpful or not."

If the person is in analysis, I explicitly encourage free association, approaching it pretty much the way Freud did (1913, p. 135: "Say whatever goes through your mind . . . and [try not to] leave anything out because, for some reason or other, it is unpleasant to tell it"). If the client is seeing me less than three times a week, some more limited focus on the presenting problem is required, but the same support for trying to speak honestly applies. Some people need quite a bit of encouragement to talk freely, and they may persistently ask, "How is this supposed to help?" I usually reply something along the lines of, "It's hard to solve a problem before one really understands it. I don't think we know enough yet about why you're suffering this depression (anxiety, compulsion to act self-destructively, dissociative reaction, obsession, phobia, problem with your partner, etc.) at this time." In other words, I implicitly convey my assumption of overdetermination. Or sometimes I simply say, "First we have to try to understand this." In either case, after addressing the content of the concern, I attend to patients' feelings of frustration or anger or impatience or fear or whatever they tell me fueled the question.

Sometimes I tell people that while I am impressed with how much they have struggled to make sense of what they are experiencing, and while they seem to have a lot of good theories about how their problems came about, I am nonetheless struck with the disjuncture between their intellectual knowledge and their emotional mastery. I explain that a big part of my job is to help them link their cognitive life with their emotions. I add that this is why I will be persistently asking them how they *feel* about what they are saying and wanting them to tell me about their immediate emotional experience, not just what they have struggled with during the week. It seems to relieve most people when their therapist acknowledges their areas of competence, such as their intellectual facility or their having managed to continue functioning despite a severe depression, because it reminds them that they have not been reduced in the mind of the therapist to a pile of pathology.

Most people know that analysts (and humanistic therapists in general) press clients to express feelings, but sometimes they have no idea why. Here is another area where therapists may strengthen a working alliance by giving rationales, often metaphorical ones, for their behavior. Babette Rothschild (see Rothschild, 2000), when working with victims of trauma who are terrified of being overwhelmed by toxic affect, literally shakes up a carbonated beverage and shows how the pressure in the bottle can be safely reduced by twisting the cap and letting the air out a little at a time. My colleague Michael Andronico talks to parents about the value of mirroring their children's feelings by comparing that process to draining a pool. When I work with very cerebral clients, I am fond of citing some of the empirical work on emotions (e.g., Frey, 1985; Pennebaker, 1997), because I have found that patients with intellectual defenses are more willing to try to find and express their feelings when they have a "good reason" to do so. Over time, the bulk of the therapist's work with affect involves helping patients to name and formulate feelings (see McDougall, 1989; D. B. Stern, 1997), helping them to tolerate and contain intense states of arousal (Maroda, 1999), and helping them to acknowledge, embrace, and even enjoy emotional reactions that they have previously considered shameful (Silverman, 1984). First, however, there may be a legitimate need of the patient for information about why the therapist seems so fixated on the topic of feelings.

It never hurts for the therapist to ask, periodically, "How do you feel this is going?" Sometimes one gets a monosyllabic answer like "Fine," and sometimes one learns things one would never have suspected about the client's reactions to the treatment. Occasionally, one even learns that the patient is feeling very pleased with what feels like enormous progress and is surprised that the therapist did not automatically know how well things are going. It also may be useful to ask the person occasionally, at any point in the process, whether there is anything the client notices that he or she is having trouble talking about, especially if one is sensing a certain stiltedness in the person's discourse. Questions such as "Is there any way in which I could make it easier for you to talk freely in here?" reinforce in the patient's mind, whatever the active transferences to the contrary, that realistically, the therapist's aim is to be of help in the process of self-exploration.

Recommending the Couch

This section will not be of much immediate relevance to beginning therapists, but I find that newcomers to the profession have a lot of curiosity about "the Couch," especially if their own therapists have recommended that they lie on one. In view of the fact that there remains a hint of mystique about this quaint relic of early Freudian practice, I would like to demystify the analytic couch a bit and in the process illustrate the principle of educating patients about their role.

Contemporary analysts differ as to whether they use the couch. Some dislike using it because they find that being out of the client's line of vision allows their mind to wander away. Others do not recommend it because in their own analyses they disliked being on the couch. Others feel it gives graphic reinforcement to patients' sense of being in an "inferior" position in the therapeutic relationship. Others infer from research on parent–infant eye contact and affective communication that psychotherapy should be face to face in order to correct early failures of emotional mirroring. I like to use it, and I do so in the traditional way, sitting behind the patient (more accurately, I lie down, too, in a recliner chair in which I can stretch out almost flat). Mainly, this arrangement relieves me from the tiring activity of monitoring my facial affect hour after hour. It also frees me up to close my eyes and join the patient in the trance-like state that free association induces, a meditative frame of mind that Freud called "evenly hovering attention" and that Ogden (1997) has framed as "reverie." Working with the client out of eye contact also allows me to become tearful when I am moved or to grin when something strikes me funny without worrying that my reaction will distract the person. (Freud originally introduced the couch for similar reasons; he said he got tired of being stared at.) Having some clients with whom I can lie back instead of sitting forward also spares my back the damage that can be caused by constant sitting (see Chapter 12).

What I tell patients when I recommend that they use the couch consists of three parts: (1) I like to work that way, because I find it less tiring; (2) they will probably discover, at least eventually, that the supine position relaxes them and allows them to enter a slightly different, more free-flowing and less intellectual state of consciousness; and (3) they will probably find themselves, once they cannot see my face easily, having much clearer images of what they imagine or fear I am thinking and feeling. I add that those fantasies about my attitudes will give us a lot of information about what kinds of expectations they carry around all the time but do not notice because they can instantly disconfirm them by looking at others' facial expressions and body language. Finally, I state that if they find they do not like using the couch, they are welcome to move back to the chair. It has been my experience that although most people approach lying down with a certain amount of trepidation, the majority of those who try it find that they prefer working that way.

Introducing Work with Transference

As I noted earlier, if a therapist simply launches into an effort to get the patient to express fantasies of what the clinician is thinking and feeling, without explaining why, the client is likely to conclude that this line of questioning is motivated by the therapist's neurotic needs for affirmation or reassurance or admiration. The only experience most of us have with someone who repeatedly asks how he or she is being perceived is our interactions with very narcissistically preoccupied individuals who are so anxious to be validated that they have no mental energy left over for genuine interest in others—like the football player in the joke who, having spent an hour going over every play he made in a recent game, announces, "Enough about me. How do *you* think I played?"

The assumption that the therapist is narcissistically needy is itself a transference, and certainly can be interpreted ("Sounds like you took my question as evidence that I'm pretty self-centered"), but before a transference interpretation can be useful, it must be understood as not *necessarily* representing an objective state of affairs. In other words, the therapist has to give some kind of rationale for this peculiar line of inquiry before the patient will get interested in the fact that he or she continues to see it as representing the therapist's narcissism. Although contemporary relational theorists have rightly emphasized how accurately patients can perceive the actual unconscious motives of their treaters (Aron, 1991; I. Hoffman, 1983), and although as R. D. Laing (1960) noted, there is always an element of truth in the patient's projections (what therapist is without narcissistic anxieties about how he or she is doing?), there is also great value to the more traditional understanding of transference as projection and distortion based on the history and needs of the patient (see Chodorow, 1999; Jordan, 1992). Beginning therapists tend to be more impressed with the distortion aspects of projection, because it makes such a dramatic impact on them—for example, when they take pains to be supportive and are instead experienced as critical or even sadistic. For patients to be able to rethink their automatic ways of understanding other people, they first need to see them as ideas that have derived from their particular lived experience.

When I first notice that a client looks surprised or irritated by my asking about how he or she feels about me, I will make a comment something like:

> "You look startled when I ask you about your reactions to me, including negative ones that wouldn't be appropriate to express if we were in a social context. But therapy is based on the idea that the thoughts and feelings you have with others will come into this relationship. When they do, we can have a close look at them, in the safety of a professional office. So please try not to inhibit any responses you have to anything I say—or anything else about me—no matter how much you would normally withhold them."

I find that this makes sense to most people, though it does not, alas, prevent patients in the borderline spectrum from embracing powerful convictions that I am fundamentally like the images they are projecting on to me, thus inducing in me exactly the feelings they are convinced I already have. In other words, this kind of education about the process will not protect the therapeutic dyad from intense projective and introjective identifications in patients who use these mechanisms as their main ways of communicating. But even the most attacking borderline client deserves to know the conscious, therapeutic rationale for the clinician's actions. Moreover, I have heard years later from such patients that even though they fought me tooth and nail as I endeavored to let them know why I behaved as I did, some part of them was taking in my stated rationale.

Here is another nice example of this kind of intervention, from Elio Frattaroli's (2001) recent polemic on the value of psychotherapy. His patient Mary has just realized that she is having a powerful reaction to him that is identical with previous reactions to male authorities. She has asked him what this means and he answered:

> "Well, we don't really know what it means yet, but it does make sense that sooner or later you would develop the same sort of problem with me that you've had with other important men in your life. That's what's called transference. Whatever problem people come into analysis to talk about, they end up repeating the problem in their relationship with the analyst. And that's actually good, because when we're experiencing the problem together, it puts us in a much better position to understand it than if we simply talked about how you've experienced it in the past." (p. 188)

Notice that the therapist here is not simply interpreting the patient's feeling toward the analyst as a transference; he is teaching her about transference in a way that allows her to be pleased about the emergence of her disturbing feelings rather than ashamed of reacting as she has. This active, educative reduction of shame is healing in itself and is arguably as important as whatever the client learns about his or her interpersonal repetitions. It is an integral piece of the therapeutic art that many skilled clinicians practice but about which comparatively few have written.

CONCLUDING COMMENTS

I have tried to cover here some aspects of relating to patients, especially new ones, that are often skimmed over in the literature on technique, aspects that are nevertheless fundamental to the therapeutic project. Some writers (e.g., Adler, 1980; Dewald, 1976; Greenson, 1971; Paolino, 1981) have discussed such issues under the rubric of the "real relationship," and others have approached the topic as I have here, as part of the therapeutic alliance. Perhaps authors of textbooks on psychotherapy assume that individual supervisors will suggest ways that beginning practitioners can explain their behavior to their patients, but I have found that sometimes supervisors are so concerned that the student learn a standard technical approach that they unwittingly ignore the more elementary transactional details of therapeutic engagement.

I am continually impressed, both from comments my own clients have made about other therapists and from books and articles in which patients talk about their experiences in treatment (e.g., Kassan, 1999), by how often people will simply comply with what the therapist is doing without understanding it. Many individuals, for example, describe having been uneasy with their former therapist's silence or passivity. But typically, they never complained, assuming that this style was somehow just an impenetrable part of clinical culture. Their therapists probably never knew about their unhappiness in the silences. If the therapists had said something about their own intentions to avoid intruding on the patient's capacities to figure things out, and if they had, in addition, invited their clients to be candid whenever they found themselves uncomfortable with any aspect of the relationship, some patients would probably have felt better during the silent spaces of therapy, and others would have been able to persuade the therapist to respond more actively to their need for more conversation.

Some of the most helpful comments my own analyst ever made involved educating me about what to expect in the therapy process. Such interventions freed me up to become more open and also supported my feeling that however neurotic I might be, I was also a person going through a process that had certain predictable features. When I first became aware, for example, of how I tended to regress when my therapist was on vacation, I regarded this pattern as my unique personal shame. He called my attention to the specific losses and separations in my past that had sensitized me to his absence, but more consequentially for my self-esteem, he also commented that there is something about being in the patient role, especially if one enters it wholeheartedly, that makes such reactions to separation from the therapist virtually inevitable.

From my perspective, an overriding reason for trying to help clients to understand the reasons for their therapists' behavior is that this kind of comprehension reduces their feelings of being manipulated and increases the chances that they can be honest. The more patients feel that the therapist is hiding behind some kind of arcane ritual with no defensible rationale, the less they will invest in the process. Conversely, the more they feel that the therapist is forthright about what is going on and why, the more they can take the risk to do something similar and disclose their own private motives. Partly because he came to realize that some patients had been withholding information from him, Freud eventually tried to ensure honesty by pledging his patients to follow the "basic rule" of free association. I doubt that setting rules is effective in reducing people's resistance to being deeply known, especially if they have had mostly negative experiences with authorities and rules. But when therapists themselves speak openly and nondefensively, they naturally invite and inspire this possibility in their patients.

Chapter 5

Boundaries I: The Frame

> I propose to call the *psychoanalytic situation* the sum total of phenomena involved in the therapeutic relationship between the analyst and the patient. This situation includes phenomena which make up a *process* and which is studied, analysed and interpreted; but it also includes a *frame*, that is to say "a non-process" in the sense that it represents the constants, within whose limits the process occurs.
>
> —José Bleger (1967, p. 518)

All of us who practice psychotherapy must make decisions about the conditions under which we work best and the arrangements and agreements we need to do so. Some aspects of therapy are essential (e.g., the therapist listens, the therapist protects confidentiality), and some are optional and widely varied, reflecting the special needs of a particular practitioner or therapy dyad (e.g., the therapist works only on weekdays, the therapist charges for canceled meetings, the client is welcome to e-mail the therapist). When Freud eventually (and somewhat reluctantly) wrote about technique, he described and gave rationales for many of the more optional procedures he had adopted over a long period of trial and error. Other therapists since Freud, especially those who have worked with patients substantially different from the neurotic group to whom he tailored his approach, have also written about their ways of working and their recommendations about technique and optimal conditions of treatment. For example, Fromm-Reichmann (1950) elaborated on extending psychoanalytic therapy to psychotic clients; Kohut (1971) pioneered a way of treating people with prominent narcissistic dynamics; Davies and Frawley (1994) discussed ways of working with adult survivors of childhood sexual abuse.

As I described in Chapter 1, it has been irresistible to many mental health professionals, especially during the period in recent American history when psychoanalytic prestige was at its height, to make some of Freud's personal parameters into unchallengeable "rules." This tendency is understandable, not only because it has been easy for psychoanalysts to idealize Freud but also because most of his practices are reasonable and have operated fairly well as general rules, especially with neurotic-level patients. Freud presented most of them not as rules, however, but as recommendations. Lohser and Newton (1996) have further noted that the best translation of the German word that Freud's English translator rendered as "recommendations" is "bits and pieces"—in other words, unsystematic reflections. There was wisdom in Freud's tentativeness about technique and conditions of practice: Psychoanalytic therapy was new and still in development; he was aware that he worked in a particular social, cultural, and historical context; and he appreciated that his ways of working reflected his own idiosyncracies. In a letter to Ferenczi he commented,

> I considered the most important thing was to emphasize what one should not do. . . . Almost everything positive that one should do I have left to "tact." . . . The result was that the docile analysts did not perceive the elasticity of the rules I had laid down and submitted to them as if they were taboos. Sometime all that must be revised without . . . doing away with the obligations I had mentioned. (quoted in Lohser & Newton, 1996, p. 15)

Much of what Freud was trying to articulate in his papers on technique concerned dimensions of what was later called the therapeutic frame (Bleger, 1967; Chasseguet-Smirgel, 1992)—that is, the ground rules, the reliable circumstances under which the therapy takes place. The arrangements Freud made with patients were those that worked for him as a particular therapist. For example, unlike many contemporary clinicians, Freud would never have considered forbidding smoking in session, because he could not have imagined working without his beloved cigars. In this chapter, I emphasize those aspects of the frame that express the personal requirements of the individual therapist more than those that time and experience have shown to be necessary for all patients. Intelligent reflection on those more universal norms can be found in most textbooks and from most supervisors.

Although some psychoanalytic writers maintain that there is only one basic frame, and that they can specify its dimensions (e.g., Langs, 1975, 1979), I have seen too much variation among practitioners to be so confident. I know what my own boundaries are, but I know many very effective practitioners whose rules and procedures differ from mine (see S. Pizer, 1996; Shane, 2003). Such differences may derive from their work situation, their client population, their personal circumstances, their temperament, their identification or counteridentification with their own therapist or supervisor, or some combination of these factors. Over time, sensibilities also change. Several analysts in the British group used to knit during sessions, a practice that most people today would consider disrespectful to the client. Gabbard (1998; Gabbard & Lester, 1995; Guthiel & Gabbard, 1993, 1998) has made a useful distinction between "boundary crossings," which may further the therapy, especially as they are examined routinely, and "boundary violations," which may significantly injure the patient and are usually not processed with care. It may be crossing an ordinary boundary to lend a client a book, but it is a boundary transgression to pour one's soul out or offer a glass of bourbon or make sexual overtures to a patient. Most people have a pretty good intuitive feel for the difference.

Beginning therapists often have very little latitude to define their own preferences about boundaries. They typically work in settings in which the clinic, agency, counseling center, school, or hospital makes the rules. When a clinician accepts employment or placement in an organization, he or she implicitly agrees to adopt its established methods of determining the fee, billing the patient, deciding what hours the office can be open, coping with emergencies, handling phone calls for the therapist, and similar issues. But because so many central psychodynamic issues get raised, examined, and enacted in the context of these practical arrangements, it is not an insignificant matter to think carefully about them and to understand the rationales that created them.

It is also important even for beginners not yet considering independent practice to think about their personal boundary preferences. A clinician who has practiced for many years in an institutional setting may be an exemplary therapist, but he or she will face important new issues when developing a private practice. In my view, the fact that one has reliable boundaries is more important than what those boundaries are. Both patient and therapist need to have the security of working under conditions that make sense to them, and both deserve the protection from anxiety that predictable parameters provide. Edgar Levenson (1992), who has devoted his career to articulating a morally egalitarian psychoanalytic vision, argues that the frame is needed just as much by the therapist as by the patient. I agree. And like Levenson, I do not make the assumption that the therapist is or must be emotionally healthier than the client or that it is only the client's anxiety that has to be reduced when the two participants are negotiating a therapeutic relationship. The boundaries we set reflect legitimate efforts to make ourselves comfortable enough to do the very demanding work of psychotherapy.

SOME GENERAL OBSERVATIONS
ABOUT THERAPISTS AND BOUNDARIES

Although one occasionally hears stories about therapists who are so unbending that they undermine their own work (by losing patients who object to their inflexible policies, by engendering a child-like compliance in those who stay, and by reinforcing prior pathogenic experiences of clients with unempathically rigid caregivers), it has been my observation that the much more common problem for most therapists is to stand firmly by a reasonable set of arrangements. People who are drawn to this profession tend to have soft hearts, and given the choice about whether to frustrate a suffering person or ignore a boundary in an effort to communicate warmth and understanding, they will usually do the latter. Sometimes this is the right decision, especially in the case of neurotic-level patients who had authoritarian parents and who are testing to see if *this* caregiver can be more accommodating. But sometimes it is a problematic and even dangerous decision, and it can be hard to tell the difference.

The Frame and the Question of Deviating from It

Early in treatment, often in the first session, most clients will subject the therapist to a test—sometimes consciously but usually unconsciously (Weiss, 1993; Weiss et al., 1986). Naturally, most individuals coming to a therapist are at some level asking themselves, "Can I trust this person not to hurt me as I've been hurt before?" and implicitly devising means of investigating that question. Sometimes the therapist will not even know he or she is being tested and will pass the test simply because, in the context of the client's life, commonplace kindness or consideration is extraordinary. One of my patients decided I was an acceptable therapist when I turned down the air conditioning after she had said that my office felt cold to her. Her mother, she later explained, would have attacked her for differing with her about the temperature in the room. Sometimes it is even the therapist's failings that make him or her acceptable to a client. One man was touched that I forgot to bill him after our initial meeting and decided on that basis that I might be trustworthy, because he felt that my casualness about money was so different from his parents' acquisitiveness.

Early tests about the therapist's capacity to avoid the failings of childhood caregivers often concern boundaries. One way for therapists to have a sense of what constitutes passing or failing a test, respectively, is to listen carefully to the personal history for themes of specific parental limitations. Usually, ordinary kindness, interest, and warm professionalism are sufficient to pass most such tests. But in addition, therapists learn to behave with more disciplined predictability when interviewing patients who emphasize that their parents were out of control, and they learn to trust their own spontaneity with those who say their caregivers were painfully rigid.

Frequently, however, one feels tested very early and cannot tell whether "passing" requires flexibility or inflexibility about boundaries. For example, a woman with a history of incest asks whether the therapist can extend sessions a few extra minutes if she is in the middle of remembering and grieving a particularly painful episode of sexual abuse. Is she needing the clinician to demonstrate responsiveness to her emotional concerns, unlike the nonprotective parent who allowed the incest to go on? Or, is she needing the therapist to be firm about the time boundary, unlike the sexualizing parent, who ignored limits and broke the rules? It is often hard, in the millisecond in which one has to decide what to say, to figure out how to respond. And sometimes no possible answer will be "right." Many people, especially those in the borderline range, are remarkably skilled at putting therapists into binds in which any response will be cause for outrage or hurt.

There is very little about therapeutic boundaries that is simple. Once the frame is clear to both parties, the security of the therapeutic couple depends on observing a mutually understood set of boundaries consistently. But, somewhat paradoxically, it is also true that the most moving and healing moments in treatment are often the times when the therapist does something exceptional, stepping out of the frame and responding to the patient with a spontaneous gesture (Winnicott, 1960). When patients and ex-patients are asked about the most pivotal incidents in their treatments, they tend to talk about moments when their therapist surprised them, often by deviating from the frame.

A friend of mine, a woman with some depressive and dissociative problems, was in analysis with a man skilled with dissociative clients and mindful of their special need for clear boundaries. Typically, he neither interrupted her nor touched her. (Even if that had not been his ordinary style, it was called for in light of her sexual abuse history.) She tells me, though, that once when she was going through a particularly intense phase of self-hatred, she began hitting herself. Her analyst grabbed her hand and exclaimed, "Don't you hurt my patient!" She remembers this as a turning point in her analysis, a kind of epiphany to the effect that her therapist, unlike either parent, was actively on the side of her self-care. After this incident, as she allowed herself to identify with his startlingly protective attitude, she found herself behaving with much more self-respect. Another colleague worked for several years with a strictly trained analyst who rarely spoke to him except to inquire, clarify, or interpret. He was deeply moved when, at the end of a session before he was to face a daunting professional examination, his analyst simply wished him good luck.

For such moments to have any power, they must be genuinely spontaneous, and they must be exceptions to an established pattern. This means there has to be a pattern. Irwin Hoffman (e.g., 1992) has been particularly articulate about how one cannot "throw away the book" until one knows the book so well that it is no longer needed. Therefore, despite my recognition of the immense power of the exceptional therapeutic act, I will be stressing the importance of consistency. In other words, when in doubt, it is better to be conservative. The persuasiveness of contemporary relational arguments in psychoanalysis has left some readers with the idea that as long as what they do is authentic, it will ultimately not be a problem (see J. Greenberg, 2001). But sometimes even a sincere, loving departure from the norm is not experienced that way by the client. And it is worth noting that the leaders of the relational movement are trained analysts, conducting psychoanalysis and intensive analytic psychotherapy. Their moving depictions of extemporaneous deviations often refer to events that happened with their patients after months or years of very consistent, conventional therapeutic work. Clients cannot be expected to appreciate the special meaning of a spontaneous moment unless it can be seen as an exceptional event.

This tilt toward conservatism also applies to therapists working for others, in workplaces where the rules have been decided by current or former administrators. Despite the stability of the conventions in institutional settings, clients often put pressure on practitioners to subvert the rules of the organization. It can be harder emotionally to defend someone else's parameters than to speak for one's own, especially if one's own rules would have been different. Therapists who feel critical of their agencies may be tempted to join their patients in making the institution the target for rebellious behaviors, especially if they sense, consciously or unconsciously, that otherwise the patient's insurrections might be aimed at the therapist. Although an institution may, from an employee's point of view, deserve a certain amount of hostility, it is rarely in the patient's interest for the therapist to promote departures from its procedures. There is nothing wrong with describing the rules apologetically and still insisting on compliance.

Psychological Disparities between Clients and Therapists

I also want to address the problems created by characterological dissimilarities between therapists and their patients—specifically, how the depressive personality style so common in mental health professionals may make it harder for many of us to respond therapeutically to people whose basic psychologies are substantially different from our own, especially if depression is part of their presenting problem and invites our immediate identification.[1] According to my informal observations, most people who are attracted to being psychotherapists like closeness, dislike separation, fear rejection, and suffer guilt readily. They tend to be self-critical, to be overly responsible, and to put other people's needs before their own. They feel more unentitled than deserving. They try to avoid feeling greed, anger, and other "selfish" states of mind and become disturbed when they notice evidence of their own competitiveness or hostility. They favor the defense of reversal, attempting to nourish the child in themselves vicariously by taking care of the child in their client. They identify with victims rather than with oppressors, with children more than with parents. One of my colleagues, for example, has announced his intention to found the "Bill Taylor Home for Kids Whose Parents Are Slugs or Worse."

Psychotherapists get pleasure in giving but are often inhibited about taking, fearing that their hunger will antagonize. When other people go out of their way to extend themselves to them, they are deeply touched because, privately, they see themselves as undeserving. When their patient makes progress, therapists tend to attribute it to the person's motivation and capacity to grow, but when a patient is not doing well, they blame themselves. As I noted in Chapter 3, the immense popularity among psychotherapists of Alice Miller's (1975) portrait of the "gifted child" suggests that people in the mental health community deeply identified with the picture Miller painted of the young empath who sacrifices personal authenticity for the sake of supporting a parent's self-esteem or maintaining a family myth. Therapists put a high value on genuineness and honesty and try, sometimes to a fault, to behave with scrupulous integrity.

My colleague Pat Miller told me the following story, which she swears really happened. As she was coming back to the United States from a trip abroad, she went through Customs Inspection and then noticed that she was wearing a bracelet bought in Europe that she had not declared. She went back to the customs official and said, "Excuse me, but I just realized I didn't declare this bracelet, and it may put me over the limit and require a fee." The officer looked at her in disbelief and exasperation, shook his head, and responded, "Lady, are you a psychotherapist?" Speechless at this triumph of intuition, she nodded, then collected herself and inquired why he had asked the question. "Because they're the only ones who ever do this!"

When patients of a depressively organized person complain in various ways of not getting enough, the therapist is temperamentally inclined to try to provide more. It is easy to project one's need, longing for closeness, and inhibition about asking for care on to the patient, who is then seen as hungry, lonely, and subjectively undeserving. From such a perception it is a natural leap to try to extend oneself to provide what is needed. Questions that activate this dynamic often arise around boundaries, including fees, scheduling, endings, cancellations, telephone availability, e-mail contact, emergency procedures, gifts, invitations, and special requests. Patients may ask for lower fees, the freedom to run up a bill, extra sessions, longer sessions, or unusual plans for handling insurance. They may call the therapist's cell phone when upset. In the case of individuals for whom it is out of character to seek special prerogatives (e.g., a depressive client who for the first time calls between sessions or a counterdependent client who has finally taken the risk of asking for something), an appeal of this sort can indicate significant therapeutic growth. In such instances, a request for something atypical may be honored by a therapist as a way of conveying support for new and more self-regarding behavior.

But all too frequently, someone who makes a request for a personal exemption, especially early in the therapy process, is enacting a sense of grandiose entitlement, or seeing whether the therapist can be conned, or looking for an opportunity to feel justified anger, or testing the therapist's boundaries for fear that they are too permeable, or some combination of similar motives. In these situations, the depressive tilt of the therapist may prompt a misunderstanding of the patient's communication. The client may in fact be hungry, but he or she may also be feeling entitled, resentful, spiteful, and determined to provoke a fight—all qualities that may be less immediately obvious to the clinician, who is conflicted about such feelings and whose empathic radar is set to detect need, not hate. Or the client may, despite consciously asking for evidence of the therapist's caring, be terrified of solicitude, because childhood care always came with a hefty emotional price tag. If the practitioner assumes that the patient needs to feel cared about, needs to test the therapist's willingness to go the extra mile, he or she may try to be accommodating. For the entitled person, or the psychopathic one, or the client who seeks to discharge intense anger without feeling crazy, or the person who needs reassurance that the boundaries will not bend, such a response will foster not trust but malignant regression.

It can be very confusing, and eventually quite infuriating, for a therapist to be trying to demonstrate what a good, thoughtful, concerned professional he or she is, only to have the client escalate a series of unreasonable demands in an effort to find out the *real* location of the boundary. Some clients need to see the therapist as having a capacity for toughness as well as flexibility and as possessing the strength to look after his or her own welfare. In addition, the setting of an appropriate limit can convey that the practitioner does not view the client as so pathetic or desperate as to be unable to take "no" for an answer.

When my older daughter was two, she threw a tantrum at some limit I set. Exasperated by her rage, I initially tried dealing with it by saying, "I can understand why you're angry, Susan, but. . . . " "DON'T UNDERSTAND!" she yelled, at the top of her lungs. It became immediately clear to me that she needed someone to come up against, to fight, and that my "empathic" stance only made her feel she had to give up her honest feelings or else hate herself for torturing a loving person. It may also have been true that even at two, she could sense the reaction formation in my effort to stay reasonable and supportive when she was giving me such a hard time, and that in some primitive way she was insisting that I be more honest with myself.

SPECIFIC BOUNDARIES AND THEIR VICISSITUDES

The frame may vary depending on whether the therapy is more exploratory or supportive. Its parameters may also be somewhat different for different patients, depending on a therapist's degree of realistic flexibility and understanding of each person's unique psychology. For example, I have let some very conscientious clients who ran into a sudden financial problem have a reduced fee or owe me money for a period of time, but I would not be so accommodating with anyone who had tended to act out around the fee or who had borderline features or whose history suggested some masochistic tendencies (for the rationale on holding the line with borderline and self-defeating clients, respectively, see the relevant sections in *Psychoanalytic Diagnosis*, McWilliams, 1994). Some therapists are much more comfortable having consistent policies across their client population, and it is certainly easier to remember and explain one's basic ground rules if they do not change. Again, boundaries are as important for the therapist's well-being as the patient's, and it is never a good idea for a therapist to make an arrangement about which he or she has misgivings, no matter how reasonable it seems to be from the client's perspective.

Privacy and Inviolability

Patients have the right to be the center of the therapist's attention for the entire session. They should also be able to count on not being interrupted during their scheduled appointment. It may once have made sense for some clinicians to take telephone calls during sessions, but in these days of answering machines, voice mail, and nonring phone options, interruptions may be avoided almost completely. An aspect of the confidentiality to which the patient is entitled is a soundproof setting or at least a therapist's best efforts to reduce the possibility that the therapeutic conversation will be overheard. Other people in the building should be told—the easiest method is a "Do Not Disturb" sign—not to knock on the door during sessions and not to make noise that may penetrate the office walls and distract the therapist and client. Sound machines in waiting rooms may help with basic privacy. The therapist's regular and cellular phones should have the ring off, with calls taken by voice mail. Although it is up to clients whether to take calls that come in on their own mobile phones, many therapists ask patients to consider turning their own phone off so that the treatment hour will not be interrupted.

On the rare occasions when the practitioner is dealing with a professional or personal problem dire enough to warrant interrupting a session, the patient should be informed at the beginning of the hour, with an apology, that because of highly unusual circumstances, today the therapist has to leave the phone or the beeper on. Whatever time is taken from the person's session for dealing with such an emergency should be made up as soon as possible. I have found clients very generous about exceptional circumstances like this (in fact, they enjoy the role reversal involved in taking care of the therapist in a small way), as long as they have experienced enough consistency in the protection of their privacy to know that the therapist is asking for a singular deviation from the norm.

Practitioners differ in the ways they ensure that they are not distracted during treatment hours. Some focus their attention by taking notes. Others find note taking during sessions diversionary (Freud recommended against it on the grounds that it interfered with the analyst's primary process thought and sensory receptiveness) and therefore write summaries between appointments rather than in the presence of the client. Some drink coffee, and there are probably a few who still smoke, whereas others feel strongly that the therapist should relinquish all "oral supplies" during a treatment hour. I sip herbal tea all day and reload my cup between sessions. So far, none of my patients has felt that my tea drinking interferes with my capacity to listen, and neither do I.

Occasionally, privacy issues create challenging dilemmas. For example, a man comes for treatment, and during the initial interview the therapist realizes that he is a friend of, and has a complex and somewhat competitive relationship with, a current patient who has troubling issues about sibling rivalry. Although the two men socialize frequently, the prospective client does not know that his friend is seeing a therapist—let alone *this* therapist. The clinician realizes it would be a mistake to take this man into treatment because if the current patient learns about the arrangement, he will feel betrayed. Given the simultaneous demands on therapists to be honest and to protect confidentiality, how can we explain decisions that are based on confidential information? Without an explanation, the prospective client is likely to feel personally rejected. Probably the best one can do is to say, "I'm very sorry to introduce a sudden complication, but I've realized as we talked that I have some personal connections I can't disclose that make it a bad idea for me to take you as a patient. I'm really sorry; I think I would enjoy working with you. Let me think about who might not have this conflict who would be a good match for you."

A special case of threats to clinical privacy and the principle of the patient's inviolability concerns requests for information from parties outside the treatment. While I respect the reasons that insurance companies or disability evaluators or adoption agencies or police or attorneys may want access to privileged information, the therapist's job is to protect the client's privacy as scrupulously as possible within the law and to insist that the *means* used by these professionals to achieve their ends are compatible with the protection of the therapy.[2] Wherever possible, the therapist should decline such requests, even in the face of being urged by the client to cooperate. Although there are too many conceivable scenarios of intrusion to cover in an introductory book, I want to make one critical point: When asked by outsiders—even by licensing boards or professional bodies—for confidential information, before doing anything else, the therapist should consult with an attorney experienced in mental health law, an increasingly complex specialization (see Chapter 12). State associations in the various professions usually have lists of lawyers with this expertise. Because there are often legitimate ways to protect one's patients and oneself that therapists have no reason to know about until they are in a potentially compromising situation, a legal consult is well worth the expense.

I should say a few words, however, about a common demand on therapists *from* attorneys. Lawyers are like therapists in that to whatever extent is legally possible, they put their clients' interests above everything else. Hence, they frequently ask clinicians to testify on behalf of their clients in disability proceedings and other legal evaluations. To an attorney, it is a simple matter: Who could know the person better, and more sympathetically, than the therapist? From the viewpoint of legal counsel, using the client's therapist also requires less time and expense than hiring an outside expert. But when one testifies on a patient's behalf, one corrupts the treatment. Leaving the role of professional trying to understand and convey understanding for the role of advocate or rescuer can have numerous grave, unintended consequences. For American psychologists, it may be effective to inform an insistent attorney, in a tone of regret, that the ethics code of the American Psychological Association stipulates that one may not perform the dual roles of therapist and witness.

As stated previously, clients who know that the therapist will be making a report on them cannot be expected to speak perfectly freely; they will consciously or unconsciously show their best side and often minimize the very issues the therapist was originally employed to address.[3] Most practitioners intuitively sense this and shrink from the prospect of writing statements or appearing in court on their clients' behalf, but it can be hard to resist an attorney's pressure. In such situations, experienced therapists have learned to take advantage of the fact that legally, there is no such thing as partial confidentiality; any decision to waive confidential privilege requires the therapist to write honest reports and to respond candidly to *all* queries from judges and opposing counsel. Persistent attorneys can usually be dissuaded by comments such as:

> "You don't want me to do that. I not only know a lot of positive, exculpating things about our mutual client, but I also have some clinical information that will cast a pretty unflattering light on him [or her]. If I testify [or write a statement], I will have to say things that, believe me, you don't want in the legal record. I recommend that you hire a forensic psychologist or psychiatrist to do an independent evaluation. The court will regard the testimony of a personal therapist as biased and therefore suspect anyway."

The fact that such testimony will wreck the psychotherapy is not something of particular salience to an attorney, nor is the fact that the ethical codes of most psychotherapy professions prohibit forensic activities by practitioners untrained in forensics. But the fact that the psychotherapist's participation might reduce the chances of a positive legal outcome will get a lawyer's attention.

To the client, who may be pleading for the therapist to go to bat in this way, one has to insist that any involvement with agendas other than trying to understand and help in strictly psychological ways will compromise the therapy. One can also point out to the client that evaluating bodies tend to regard a devoted, personally hired professional as biased and therefore will discount or discredit the clinician's contribution; hence, the therapist is in a less influential position than a presumably neutral professional (a reality that may surprise patients with idealizing transferences, who ascribe indiscriminate power to the therapist). Such a stance leaves the therapist free to assist the patient with feelings and fantasies about being evaluated psychologically for legal purposes by a stranger. In my own experience, after the client has expressed anger over the frustration of the normal wish to be rescued, he or she frequently becomes aware of contrasting feelings of relief and gratitude that the therapist is protecting the boundaries of the treatment.

One final recommendation: For the therapist confronted with a request to release confidential records on a client or to become involved in a legal matter, it is politic to treat the inquiring entity as well-intentioned, and then to temporize. It may protect both the patient and the tenor of the treatment to put the onus of not cooperating on someone else. Bryant Welch (2003) advises being warm and cordial while saying something along the lines of "I'd love to be of help, but let me check this out in terms of my state law and professional ethics first; I may have a conflict of interest here." Buying time to get one's own legal consult or advice from officials of one's local professional association can be crucial in these situations.

Time

The convention in analytic psychotherapy has been for the "hour" to be forty-five or fifty minutes long, so that the therapist can use the remaining ten or fifteen minutes to write some notes, stretch, use the bathroom, return phone calls, and make the emotional transition from the previous patient to the next one (see Greenson, 1974). Adequate space between sessions also reduces the probability that clients will run into each other coming and going, an experience that many find awkward or disturbing. Although the forty-five- or fifty-minute session works quite well, there is nothing sacred about it. Some experienced therapists (e.g., Hammer, 1990) have suggested that longer sessions—a full hour or an hour and a quarter—are better for people with obsessional defenses, because such patients take a long time to get into their feelings. Others (e.g., Putnam, 1989) have suggested that for abreactive sessions with dissociative and traumatized patients, an hour and a half or more might be scheduled to accommodate the processes of approaching the traumatic material, experiencing the feelings, and reflecting on what happened. Some therapists who work with couples like to see them for a double-length session so that each partner feels there is enough individual air time and so that the therapist has sufficient opportunity to feel out the dynamic between the two in addition to noting their individual psychological operations.

I ordinarily see individual people for forty-five-minute sessions. I used to see some patients, especially those who commuted a long way to get to me, for a double session: an hour and a half. According to the clients involved, it worked satisfactorily, though I noticed that psychotherapy proceeds to some degree according to Parkinson's Law (work expands to fill the time available). It seems that if one has an hour, the important material tends to appear in the last ten minutes, and if one has two hours, it also tends to appear in the last ten minutes. In Russia, professionals who want to get psychoanalytic training despite the dearth of analysts in their country have been allowed by the International Psychoanalytic Association to have "shuttle analysis," whereby instead of going to a local person four times a week, they fly once a month to a foreign city for an extended weekend and see their analyst three or four hours a day for three or four days in a row.

Interestingly, some patients regularly come five or ten or twenty minutes late no matter when the session is scheduled, how long it is set up to go, or how earnestly and accurately the clinician tries to make sense of this behavior. It is as if they are trying to titrate the amount of exposure to the therapist and keep it to a tolerable level. I find that interpretations, even if accepted, do nothing for this phenomenon; the only thing that influences it is the long, slow assimilation of the experience of the therapist's trustworthiness.

The intended moral of these observations is that highly motivated people can adapt to many different time arrangements, and people who are frightened of therapy will find ways to resist whatever accommodations are made. It follows that practitioners with control over their time should set their schedules up with primary concern for their own convenience. When my children were nursing infants, I scheduled forty-five-minute appointments back to back instead of with fifteen-minute intermissions and then took at least an hour-long break after three sessions in a row. Thus I could be gone from the baby for two and a quarter hours rather than three. (Three, as they each unambiguously let me know, comprised more time than they were willing to go without a meal.)

The same softheartedness that impels many therapists to make other exceptions for their clients affects their scheduling. Many of us end up extending ourselves too much, seeing clients on weekends or at some ungodly early-morning hour or too late in the evening. And when someone asks for an extra session, it is all too common for therapists to stretch themselves as far as possible to fit the patient in. It is my impression that this tendency is found in women more than in men (probably because of dynamics that are also at play in women's greater willingness to work for lower fees; see Liss-Levinson, 1990). My colleague Elinor Bashe (1989) did a doctoral dissertation on pregnancy in the therapist, in which she conducted intensive interviews with ten women who had gone through at least one pregnancy while treating patients. One of her serendipitous findings was that almost all of her subjects volunteered that once they were doing so for the baby rather than for their own "selfish" purposes, they found it much easier to set limits on the times they were willing to be available. And, more important, they learned that their patients simply adapted to their limitations. "I wish I'd known that ten years earlier," was a common refrain. Considering that control over one's time is one of the most attractive aspects of being a therapist, it is a shame to let our patients' predilections control us more than necessary—to our own disadvantage and not to their ultimate benefit.

Therapists also differ on how promptly they terminate a session. Some people are so aware of their need for the free interval, and hence so resentful of running overtime, that they end each meeting like clockwork. I have never been comfortable being that rigid about time; one of the reasons I work a forty-five-minute rather than a fifty-minute hour is that it gives me a bit of latitude in bringing the session to a close. When I have an initial interview with a prospective patient, I explain that I schedule forty-five-minute sessions and will usually end them right on time, but I add that sometimes, if we are in the middle of something compelling, we may find ourselves going a couple of minutes overtime. Patients seem to appreciate this, and I feel more natural in handling the end of each meeting that way. Still, I have to think about it when I notice that I am running over a lot with a particular patient; there is typically some very interesting dynamic that the person and I are enacting that needs to be converted into words and addressed directly.

I occasionally have a client who likes to keep track of the time and end the meeting before I announce that the session is over. Some like to have a clock in view; others deliberately avoid watching the time because they want to sink into a sense of timelessness as they free associate. Whatever people's responses to the time arrangements, it is always valuable to investigate their reactions to them. Again, in situations in which there is no prevailing institutional rule, the professional judgment and personal preferences of the therapist should dictate time conventions, because most clients will manage in their individual ways with whatever parameters are set, either accepting them graciously or resenting them no matter how generous they are.

I should say a few words about getting the client out the door, something I have observed to be quite an art, and one not typically taught in training programs. Everyone who has practiced for any length of time has encountered patients who seem to hate to separate, at least not at the initiative of another person, at the end of the session. Some pick the last five minutes to drop an informational bomb or break suddenly into emotion so intense and moving that the therapist feels like a boor even to imagine interrupting the outpouring. Some wait until the clinician announces the end of the session and only then remember that they have to talk about a scheduling problem or a friend who needs a referral. Others take an inordinate amount of time looking for their checkbook, then searching for their pen, then trying to remember the date, then ploddingly writing out a check, while the therapist stands around awkwardly waiting for the money and hoping to get to the bathroom.

As soon as a pattern of procrastination becomes evident, it is important for the therapist to enforce the time boundary. There are some relatively graceful ways of doing this. With the emotionally undone patient, I have learned to say, "I'm very sorry to interrupt you while you're in the middle of so many powerful feelings, but we do have to end. If you'd like to sit for a while in the waiting room composing yourself, so that you don't have to leave here feeling ragged, please take as much time as you need." With the person who laboriously writes the check while I shift awkwardly from one foot to the other, I have become good at saying, "I've noticed it takes some extra time for you to write out a check here, and I often have a few things to do between sessions. I don't want to stop our work earlier to make time for it, so how about making it out before you come?" I have also learned that with patients who tend to cling at the end of the session, it helps for me to stand up, walk to the door, and open it for them, while saying something in a warm tone about the next session—for example, "That felt like a heavy session today. I'll look forward to talking more on Tuesday."

If, despite these efforts at tact and consideration, someone insists on seeing me as rude and insensitive, there has probably been a rude, insensitive authority in that person's life for whom I need to be used as a surrogate in the service of the patient's growth. In other words, the worst that can happen is that the client will have the therapeutic opportunity to tell me off. Expressing anger at limits can be a highly therapeutic experience for someone whose earlier caregivers could not receive criticism without counterattacking or withdrawing. On the plus side, most patients eventually appreciate the chance to identify with someone who takes care of business in a kind but self-regarding way. "Something I've learned from you," one of my clients remarked after several years of analysis, "is that you just get things done. You take care of yourself. I'm trying to be more like that."

With limit-setting interventions, sometimes the patient simply defers to the therapist's wishes, and sometimes he or she has a reaction that illuminates important and previously invisible dynamics. Some people are insensitive to boundaries such as time for relatively straightforward reasons—for instance, because no one has ever asked them to observe them, or because their previous therapist was casual about limits, or because in their ethnic group it is polite to linger and show reluctance to part. Others manifest a resistance to the ending of the session that is pregnant with emotional meaning, often including shame about dependent feelings, or anger about having to submit to someone else's authority, or even—in the case of dissociative patients who lose time—genuine surprise that the session is over. Typically, one has to enforce a limit before the behavior that prompted the limit can be examined. It is a common mistake of newer therapists to hope that some interpretation will influence the patient to be more cooperative without the need to set an explicit limit. My clinical experience has consistently supported the original Freudian notion that people act out what they cannot remember or what they cannot allow themselves to feel. It follows that as long as people are able to enact a dynamic (in this case, most frequently a disavowed dependency or a compulsion to be in control), they do not have to think about why they persistently behave in a particular way. When there are no negative consequences for their behavior, interpretations just roll off them.

Money

Therapists who shift from an agency setting to one in which they set and collect the fee are often unprepared for the multitude of issues around money that arise in both themselves and their patients. People who can talk with no embarrassment about their kinkiest sexual practices are often completely tongue-tied when it comes to negotiating financial matters. One of Freud's more astute observations was that it is helpful for patients when their therapists treat money as a realistic aspect of life rather than a dirty secret (see also Dimen, 1994). Again, the depressive tendencies characteristic of many therapists may make it hard for them to be matter-of-fact about asking to be paid. Beginning therapists in particular often feel they have no right to charge a fee that gives what they see as the misleading impression that they know what they are doing. The first thing a newer therapist has to do with respect to the fee is to remember that psychotherapy is the way he or she makes a living, that it is an honorable and highly disciplined way to do so, that it requires extensive training, and that it is a lot more valuable than serving fast food—even if it initially feels like "just sitting there trying to understand." In contemporary Western cultures, respectful listening is rare enough to justify a decent remuneration; we tend to undervalue activities that are receptive rather than based on doing, producing, manufacturing, achieving, and so on.

As many practitioners have noted, money is a critical aspect of therapy. It is the means by which the two participants have a kind of moral equality, a genuine reciprocity. The therapist takes care of the patient emotionally; the patient takes care of the therapist financially. Because the therapist is getting paid by the patient, there is no other way in which the patient is expected to take care of the therapist. When the therapist accepts a given fee, the message is that this amount of money will be considered an even exchange for his or her professional services. Not collecting a fee damages this straightforward equivalence, creating an imbalance in the dyad whereby the patient is essentially being exploitive. Collecting anything in addition to a fee (stock tips, expensive gifts, special services) tips the scales of the relationship in the opposite direction: The therapist is being exploitive. Collecting goods or services instead of a fee has been found to create many problems that a simple monetary arrangement avoids; consequently, the American Psychological Association has considered barter arrangements to be questionably ethical.

Some years ago I read about research revealing that the fees of physicians are completely uncorrelated with their seniority or level of skill or professional reputation. I suspect the same thing is true for therapists' fees. Some people fresh out of training charge literally twice what I do, and some practitioners with more experience than I have charge a lower fee. Kernberg (1987) has judiciously recommended that one set the fee not at the highest level the market will bear, for that smacks of arrogance and greed and invites patients to believe the therapist can perform miracles, but that one also not set it at the low end of standard rates in one's community, a practice that many patients will interpret as meaning that the practitioner feels that what is being offered has little value. Realistically, one's colleagues will resent a therapist who sets a fee well above the prevailing scale, because they are affronted when others act as if they are worth such disproportionate amounts. At the same time, they will resent a practitioner who routinely charges much less than the going rate, because low fees contribute to the general devaluation of psychotherapy—an outcome that managed care companies do not need extra help to accomplish.

Also realistically, one's fee should adequately contribute to supporting one's family and should reflect something about one's expenses. The home office of a solo practitioner involves virtually no overhead, while a consulting room in the city's high-rent district, especially if secretarial help is part of the office package, is extremely costly. Patients to whom it matters to be seen by a Park Avenue therapist can expect to pay for the privilege. Clinicians without children will be able to have more flexibility about their fee than those who have three kids to put through college. Therapists typically have considerable ongoing expenses for continuing education, supervision, and personal therapy; their income must also compensate for their numerous unremunerated hours spent in activities such as keeping records and writing reports.

Having defended the practice of earning a decent wage, I would also like to affirm the value of seeing some clients at a lower fee. For many therapists, a large part of their identity as mental health professionals includes a wish to reach out to impoverished and underserved populations. These days, with mental health agencies grievously overburdened, sometimes the only option for real psychotherapy that a disadvantaged person has is a private practitioner with some low-fee time slots. One way to balance one's altruistic ideals with the need to earn a living is to find a way to earn good money in one role in order to underwrite the other role. Not only will this provide adequate financial resources and less reason for resentment, but in addition, poorer clients who know that their therapist has other sources of income may be spared unnecessary guilt. One of my former students, a Latino who grew up in a desperately indigent family, spends part of his week consulting for a hefty fee to a corporation about issues of diversity and the other part treating the urban poor for virtually nothing.

Many experienced therapists have asserted that offers of free treatment, at least by an individual practitioner, are unwise on many counts and can feel unconsciously demeaning to the patient. I once regarded this argument as a rationalization for greed, and it can certainly function as such, but I have also come to respect its validity. Some agencies, such as college counseling centers funded by tuition payments, provide "free" treatment without many problematic side effects, though even in such settings, staff members often complain of attitudes of entitlement that complicate their efforts to do effective psychotherapy. There is a dignity for the recipient of charitable services in making a reciprocal contribution, even if it is only a pittance. When I have seen clients for very little, I have found myself enjoying the extra few dollars and feeling less out of sorts during the rough spots in treatment than I would have if I were working *gratis*. It also enriched the therapy to involve money transactions, because a lot "goes on" around the fee. Just one memorable example: A male colleague of mine treating a woman who makes a marginal living as a lap dancer had a lot of material to work with when his client started paying him with crumpled, damp, one-dollar bills that she peeled one at a time off a large wad of paper money.

Another consideration concerns therapists with a strong desire to do analysis whenever possible, or at least to see clients more than once a week, a preference that characterizes most practitioners trained in analytic institutes. Joan Erle (1993) has written about how patients' grandiose fantasies of being "special"may be reinforced if they perceive a therapist as having given them a lower fee than is usually charged, and yet it is an important part of the identity and self-esteem of many psychodynamic therapists to want to do more intensive work. For that reason, they are often happy to charge less per hour to people who come multiple times a week. Erle recommends that such practitioners state their fee as a range, with the explanation that they prefer to work more intensively and expect to use the lower part of the range to accommodate people who want to come more than once weekly or who are good candidates for more intensive exploratory work. As early as 1955, Glover noted that analysts' legitimate economic motives are counterbalanced by a desire to practice psychoanalysis rather than psychotherapy. He recommended that a "guiding rule" with potential analysands should be "never to insist on a fee that is likely to be burdensome to the patient" (p. 22).

Experienced therapists would add, however, that care should be taken in adjusting the fee when the client already in treatment wants to increase the frequency of sessions. It is better, assuming that the patient is paying out of pocket or that any third-party coverage allows this, to keep the regular fee for the existing appointment and to charge a significantly reduced fee for the session being added. This practice applies especially to patients with borderline and narcissistic tendencies. Many clients have considerable unconscious ambivalence about greater intensity and may change their mind or act out, under the sway of the part of their personality that fears increased attachment. It happens quite frequently that someone whose fee has been reduced across the board to accommodate another weekly session decides to cut back again and assumes that he or she will keep the lower fee, leaving the therapist feeling cheated and struggling with a vague sense of awkwardness about raising the issue. If insurance arrangements do not permit different prices for different sessions, the best way to avoid this enactment is for the therapist to explain, when the patient wants more frequent meetings and asks for a break on the price, that he or she is willing to charge a set amount less per session for clients coming more than once a week, because it is more satisfying and productive to meet more often, but that if for any reason the person goes back to the lower frequency or begins missing the additional meeting, the fee will revert to the original amount.

When a client begins to be unreliable about payment and fails to bring the issue up, the therapist tends to feel uncomfortable and frustrated. When I was first practicing, I tried to find relevant, interpretable material in the associations of someone who had stopped paying, in the hope that the interpretation would open up the question of why this was happening and motivate the person to meet his or her financial obligation. I found that even when I made what I thought were brilliant connections that the patient acknowledged as accurate, there would seldom be a change in behavior. Again, Freud's insight applies: When something is being acted out, it is not analyzable; talking about its meaning does not foster insight and growth. As learning theorists would point out, as long as a behavior is being reinforced or is not costing anything, there is no incentive to behave differently. Stanley Moldawsky, my supervisor at the time of my earliest struggle with a deadbeat client, advised me to figure out my limit (in terms of either the length of time I was willing to wait after billing or the amount I was willing to carry as a debt) and state it. I was amazed that when I did, the patient, without comment, simply paid me. Only months later did we talk productively about what had been going on at that time. (I think his self-respect would have suffered if he had had to endure simultaneously both the disappointment of having to pay and the mortification of talking about it.) Since then, I have become better at saying, with a smile, "Hey. You haven't paid me lately, and I could use the money. When can I expect it?"

The depressive dynamics that impel so many therapists toward generosity can work against them financially. One of my colleagues says she always charges her full fee "because I might as well start there, since I always end up lowering it." The tendency for therapists to feel automatic credulity and sympathy when hearing another person's bad fortune can also make them victims of patients with notably ungenerous psychologies. I cannot count how many of my fellow therapists I have heard lamenting the financial concessions they made in response to an earnest description of penury, only to find later that the client has bought a Jaguar or is planning a vacation in Tahiti. Individuals who have trouble managing money—and lately, therapists seem to be seeing more and more people at all socioeconomic levels who are deeply in debt—will be glad to take advantage of a therapist's willingness to underwrite their self-defeating habits by reducing the fee or "carrying" them for a while. Not only is it not in the therapist's interest to promote this accommodation, it is not in the client's interest, either.

What about the question of raising one's rates? After working with someone for months or years, a therapist may notice that the charge per session has fallen below what is customarily charged locally. Or, after treating someone long enough to have a good sense of the client's finances, the therapist may realize that he or she is resenting having accepted a low fee based on the client's initial claim of poverty, which turns out to be questionable. Or, because of the success of the treatment, the patient's income and money management have improved enough to warrant paying a standard rate. When I have raised my fee, I have encountered the whole gamut of reactions, from "How can you be so greedy?!" to "Okay" to "Of course" to "I thought you'd never ask— I've been feeling guilty about paying you so little." It is always illuminating to explore the patient's experience of this critical aspect of the professional relationship.

Therapists differ as to how they handle asking for raises. Some simply announce an increase in their fee and let the chips fall. Some feel strongly that whatever charge was originally negotiated should remain the same throughout the treatment; to them, it is a matter of principle not to change the rules in the middle of the game. Some, taking seriously the fact that the client is their employer, present a rationale for a fee increase and ask their "boss" to consider giving them a raise. Of course, therapists who do it this way are taking their chances on a negative response, but if one is genuinely willing to be refused, this is probably the approach most consistent with the mutuality and reciprocity toward which we aim in psychoanalytic work. Ann Appelbaum (personal communication, January 3, 2002) tells me that she once said to a patient, "I'd like you to consider giving me a raise so I won't be embarrassed around my colleagues by having a fee that's so out of line with the going rate. I'd be grateful if you'd give it some thought and let me know if you're willing to do that." Somewhat to her surprise, the patient came back the next session with the announcement that she had decided against it; she did not think her employee deserved the raise. "Actually, I was delighted," Appelbaum told me, "because it represented extraordinary progress for her to be able to criticize me and assert herself like that."

I had a similar experience once with a patient who denied me permission to publish a description of her treatment. My disappointment in her refusal was more than compensated by my appreciation of the fact that growing up, she had always sacrificed her own needs to her father's narcissism, whereas now, she was insisting that her wishes take preference over the narcissistic agenda of an authority figure. I would have liked to use her material, but I liked even more seeing the evidence that she had made significant changes in her way of negotiating with others. Anecdotes like these illustrate another interesting feature of transactions around boundaries: Sometimes the limit setting goes in the opposite direction. When patients set reasonable limits on therapists, both parties can frequently see just how much progress has been made. Evidence of the identification of the client with the clinician's comfort in being clear about what is and is not okay can be so moving to the therapist that it trumps less powerful gratifications, such as getting a higher fee or writing about a fascinating case.

Finally, a tip for practitioners working in the United States with clients who use private insurance: Wherever possible, the therapist should insist that they pay up front, submit the bills themselves to the insurance company, and collect the reimbursements. For those who plead poverty and ask the therapist to accept a copayment with reimbursement later, their financial problem should be addressed in some other way (e.g., by suggesting that therapy begin once they have saved up enough to cover the first two months, after which reimbursements should come regularly). There can be serious negative consequences to accepting the copay and waiting for the rest of what is owed. For one thing, this arrangement contributes to unrealistic ideas about health care expenses by engendering in patients the habit of thinking that the therapy costs only the out-of-pocket amount. More relevant to the clinician's needs, if the patient is in charge of submitting, he or she can neglect to do so, especially in states of unconscious hostility, leaving the therapist in the unenviable position of nag. Even worse, most of us who have made such a deal have had at least one client who sent in the bills, received the reimbursement, and then spent it, evidently oblivious to the legal implications of committing insurance fraud or the interpersonal consequences of stealing from the therapist.

If the therapist is in charge of submitting, he or she may end up spending precious professional time dealing with all the errors and delays typical of third-party payors, who have an economic interest in stalling while their resources earn income, and who consequently have an extraordinary talent for losing bills, misplacing records, quibbling over technicalities of submission, and so on. Because the therapist's free time consists of short periods between sessions, being put on hold for fifteen minutes by an insurance company employee can make it impossible to resolve a problem over billing and reimbursement. I recommend that therapists say explicitly to clients that they prefer for the clients to deal with insurers because they dislike sacrificing professional time to fight with bureaucrats. I tell my patients, "Better you than me!"

Cancellations

Time is precious; it may be the only nonrenewable resource we have. Psychodynamic therapists have traditionally found ways to insist on the value of their time and to hold patients accountable for their own relationship to it. Respecting the finitude of time is consistent with psychoanalytic attention to other painful truths, such as mortality, the ubiquity of conflict, the limits of personal power, and the unattainability of perfection. Perhaps more salient at an emotional level, wasting time, losing productive hours, can cause resentment in a therapist that undermines his or her commitment to a patient. In addition to whatever justifications one has for a policy of making the client responsible for professional time lost, it is important to set up one's working arrangements such that one avoids the emotional burden of resentment. Having some kind of negative consequence for missing a session also exerts a counterforce to the resistances that some clients express by absenteeism.

Freud (1913) said he had learned to explain to patients that he was "leasing" them certain specific hours during the week, emphasizing that they were responsible to pay for them whether or not they came to every one—much as one would pay for all the classes in an academic course whether or not one cut some of them. This made sense in a time when an "analysis" lasted between a few weeks and a year. Many contemporary therapists find Freud's practice too rigid, preferring to ask their clients to give them at least twenty-four hours' notice if they find they must miss a session; with a day's advance knowledge, one can plan to use the free hour productively. Other practitioners have a policy of charging for a canceled session only when it cannot be rescheduled. Some of my colleagues charge half the fee for a missed appointment. In contrast, a few are even more exacting than Freud, insisting that their patients schedule vacations to coincide with their time off or else pay for the sessions they miss. This arrangement may be defensible for psychoanalysis proper, because an analysand seen four or five hours a week contributes a sizable portion of the analyst's income.[4]

Agencies often have no requirement that clients pay for missed sessions, an omission that may account for the high number of cancellations and no-shows in counseling centers and clinics, and an omission that also may significantly reduce a clinician's power to get patients to examine avoidant behavior. The absence of a cancellation policy in many institutions reflects the fact that third-party payors understandably balk at covering services not rendered. Most private therapists have explicit penalties for cancellations, however, especially last-minute ones (which may entail giving a client one bill to submit for insurance reimbursement and an additional one for canceled meetings). The fact that a client's insurance company will not pay for unused hours may provide additional motivation for the person to push past resistances and come to treatment.

Again, the details of such policies depend partly on the practitioner's specific situation. Because I have a home office, cancellations are not burdensome to me; I can always use the time constructively. And because my fees are adequate and my overhead is minimal, I can afford some flexibility about missed sessions. My policy, therefore, is that I do not typically charge for cancellations, though I try to reschedule if possible. On the other hand, I do charge when a patient simply does not show up, because in that situation I am sitting in the office, waiting, thinking about the patient, unable to use the time in another way. There are some clients with whom I am more demanding: When agreeing to work with someone with notable psychopathic tendencies, I insist from the beginning on payment for all sessions, whether the person comes or not (see *Psychoanalytic Diagnosis*, McWilliams, 1994, for the rationale). And irrespective of their individual psychologies, with clients who cancel so often that I feel the treatment is compromised, I engage the patient in a problem-solving discussion about the issue, and we negotiate together a specific policy that will promote the person's attendance.

One reason I deviated from the more common practice of requiring payment in the absence of adequate notice regardless of "extenuating circumstances" was that I slowly realized, when I did have such a cancellation policy, that I had "borrowed" it from supervisors without thinking through whether my heart was really in it. It worked for my mentors because it served their individual needs, but it was not serving mine. For one thing, I encountered a number of patients with whom haggling over whether my policy was fair did not seem to be advancing the therapeutic process. In this culture, many find this kind of rule self-serving and authoritarian.[5] For another, I met people who told me they had become estranged, overtly or in the privacy of their feelings, from a prior therapist because of having been charged for an appointment when they had been taken ill suddenly or were stuck in an unforeseeable traffic jam. They had experienced the enforcement of the policy as a vote of no confidence, an implied suspicion that they were not all that sick or were exaggerating the traffic problem. It did not feel worth it to me to hold to a principle at the price of damaging the working alliance. Now that I am comfortable with the policy I have, I implement it without conflict.

For the description of a similar professional evolution, consider the following comments by Kim Chernin (1995) about her own idiosyncratic cancellation policy:

> My clients and I devised a flexible policy of cancellations, with a certain number of uncharged cancellations (usually three in a year), easygoing substitutions, (whenever possible in the same week), paid cancellations (for more than three in a year, when these did not prove to be rearrangeable). There were also exceptions to these categories (emergencies, illness, traffic accidents), I leaving it to the client to determine into which category the cancellation fell. . . . No one, in the years since we evolved this policy, has taken advantage of this flexible arrangement, probably because it had been worked out with an articulate awareness of the clients' need not to pay for sessions they were unable to attend, [and of] my acknowledged need of regularity in the earning of my living. (p. 158)

I have gone into detail about my own solutions not to recommend them to others so much as to illustrate the diversity in business practices among professionals. A colleague who read the foregoing section called my attention to the fact that my attitude toward money is markedly more casual than my attitude about time, an observation that immediately rang true. I am not the only breadwinner in my family, and my practice income has always been supplemented by fees for teaching, two factors that have affected my cancellation policies. I should therefore stress that anger and resentment when one's expected salary is unexpectedly diminished is a natural reaction, and in itself a legitimate reason for enforcing an agreement that clients pay for sessions canceled without adequate notice. Especially when someone explains that his or her job demands conflict with a scheduled appointment, it is clear that one of the two therapy partners has to take a loss, and it is not the therapist who is instigating the rupture in the routine.

Availability

Like questions of money and time, the amount of personal availability a therapist may reasonably extend to a client depends on the specific needs of the patient and the personal preferences and circumstances of the therapist. In agency practice, there are often regulations protecting therapists from dealing with patients outside scheduled working hours; for example, it is against the rules of some organizations for an employee to give out his or her home phone number. In an emergency, a client is expected to call a designated service. As a consequence, just as with the issue of money, many practitioners do not face the question of the boundaries of their availability until they practice independently.

With some clients, a limit to the therapist's availability never needs to be specified because they naturally establish it themselves: They respect the professional's privacy and need for personal space and hence telephone or e-mail only around scheduling issues. Others can seem insatiable, calling whenever they are upset, asking for advice, treating the therapist as a bottomless source of emotional supplies. It can be hard to set limits on such patients, especially when their pain is palpable and they experience limits as an attack. Nonetheless, it is critical to do so. If the therapist has strong feelings of not wanting to be intruded on, he or she must say so and talk with the patient about what resources are available between sessions if the person becomes overwhelmed. For example, "I'm sorry to say that I feel very strongly about my free time, and I don't take professional phone calls at home. I fully understand, however, that you may need to reach out for help, so let's talk about what your options are." These options may include, among other things, calling hot-line or emergency-service numbers, writing things down to bring to the next appointment, talking with a friend, meditating, doing relaxation exercises, or even calling the therapist's voice mail. Many clients have told me that it grounds them in some unspecifiable but deeply comforting way to hear me on tape (perhaps this widely reported clinical phenomenon is related to the discovery [DeCasper & Fifer, 1980; DeCasper & Spence, 1986] that infants discriminate their mother's voice, and respond by calming, even *in utero*).

If the therapist feels some personal flexibility on the issue, a negotiation may be possible. For example, "I'm realizing that we're spending a lot of time on the phone together, and we need to figure out some plan to reduce that. I don't have a lot of extra time to give, and I'm not always available, either. Plus, we can't get much of value done in the few minutes I can typically spare. Let's talk about other ways you can try to get through the rough spots between sessions." Some of my colleagues allow patients to put long messages on their voice mail, some limit calls to a certain number per week for no more than a certain number of minutes, and some charge for phone time so that they will not feel exploited. Others permit unlimited e-mail contact because it is much less intrusive than phone calls. I have worked with some patients who used my e-mail address as a kind of transitional object (Winnicott, 1953); they did not require my immediate presence, but they wanted to feel they could "talk" to me in my absence, knowing I would get the message. Of course, if I were to feel that a client was "spamming" me to the point that I was dreading going on line, I would talk with the person about keeping the communications to some agreed-on number of e-mails between sessions. Many therapists establish that they are happy to receive e-mail but unwilling to answer it; others may send a short response.

Because there are many clients—seemingly an increasing number over past decades—who need to go through a developmental process in which they rail against limits, let me stress again that the therapist is not going to preempt this difficult process by being generous. Excessive liberality with such patients only insures that their demands will escalate until a limit is finally reached and the developmental struggle can happen. It is better if this occurs before the therapist is in a stew of rancor and self-criticism. Most overtly clingy, dependent patients have an equally strong covert need to express anger and oppositionality. It is thus preferable to set reasonable limits on availability than to infantilize them by an overly caretaking response. Limits provide such clients the pleasures of indignation and the consequent use of the angry energy to learn to meet their needs themselves, not to mention the lesson that the therapist sticks with them through their furious tirades, like parents who remain devoted after an adolescent rejects them in a rage.

THE ART OF SAYING NO

Setting limits is rarely pleasant, especially for therapists, who like to make others happy. It may also be harder than it used to be, when there was more of a "party line" about the rules of psychoanalytic treatment. One of the more challenging side effects of current movements toward more flexibility, individuality, and elaboration of different treatment styles for different clients is that therapists, when explaining their boundaries to their patients, can no longer hide behind the justification, "That's just how psychoanalytic therapy is done." We need rationales for what we do, and we usually have to give some account of these to our clients. Despite the fact that this process requires more thoughtfulness than knee-jerk appeals to orthodoxy, I think it is much better for both therapists and patients to talk out, and even struggle around, issues of the frame.

I have found that when I discuss limits, patients are much more willing to cooperate with my rules when I relate them to my own needs than when I make a speech about how the limit is really in their best interest. Most of us can remember how unsatisfied we were with parental explanations in the form of "This is for your own good," or "This hurts me more than it hurts you," even when such statements may have been at least partly true. And those clients who need the therapist's limits spelled out are usually individuals who did not experience their parents as having their best interests in mind. As a result, they are particularly skeptical that an authority, even one they have hired to help them, would do anything for the sake of another person's well-being. They regard "therapeutic" rationales for boundaries as self-serving rationalizations, and they are probably right that there is usually that element in the practitioner's position.

Given this skepticism, it is more persuasive to boundary-testing clients for the therapist to acknowledge the self-serving basis for a limit. Thus, even if it is a practitioner's actual clinical rationale, I do not recommend saying, "I'm refusing to lower the fee because it would only reinforce your feeling that you are not worth much." Far better to say, "I'm just not willing to work for less than what I've charged. If I did, I would find myself resenting you, and I doubt I could do you much good in a state of resentment." Or, "I'm sorry, but I can't become known as the practitioner who always subverts the fee scale that the organization has established to support its work." Or, "Much as I enjoy my fantasies of cheating HMOs, and even though it might make your life a lot easier, I'm not willing to commit insurance fraud. That could cost me my license." Explicitly self-serving explanations are much more believable somehow than altruistic ones.

There is also nothing wrong with apologizing for its negative effects at the same time one is stating a rule. For example, "I know it's really hard on you when you get into these horrible states of mind between sessions, and I know it would probably help if I could always be available to talk. But I can't reasonably do that, and if I tried to, I'm afraid I'd come to feel more burdened than is good for my relationship with you. I'm really sorry I can't stretch a bit further, but I have to be realistic." Or, "I'm truly sorry I can't see you for a lower fee. I appreciate how difficult your financial situation is, and I'd like not to make it any harder, but I can't ignore my own financial realities." One of my patients made an interesting point after I apologetically refused to do part of our session by phone as she threaded her way through unforeseen road construction that was making her late (I felt that, given the statistics on accidents and cell phones, to do so would be vaguely complicit with a self-destructive tendency she had). She told me, "I was angry that you wouldn't do that, but I could almost hear the gears in your mind clanking, asking yourself whether you'd resent it and deciding that you would. And it relieves me that, unlike my mother, you protect yourself against resentment. To be cared for resentfully is very shaming."

Finally, after having set a boundary, therapists should be alert for evidence of the client's negative reactions. Positive reactions may also be part of the picture, but no person should be put in the inherently shame-tainted position of being told that he or she is saying "Thanks, I needed that!" when a desire has been frustrated. If a clinician avoids rubbing it in that a given boundary has had positive effects, the client will often volunteer later that the limit was a good thing. It is a completely different experience to offer such an observation on one's own authority than to be told this by the person who thwarted one's requests. The aftermath of boundary setting provides precious opportunities in psychotherapy, opportunities that would be missed if the therapist tried to conciliate clients instead of being clear about what is acceptable and what is not.

Very often in the session after a limit has been set, the patient will come late, or will report feelings of not having wanted to come, or will have trouble talking. At this point the therapist can bring up the possibility that the client felt hurt and/or angry about the transaction. For example, "I wonder if I hurt your feelings when I ended the session right when you were in the middle of some very painful memories. It would be natural to resent that." When the therapist makes such a speculation, even if the client reacts to it with indifference, an important point is being made: In this therapy one is required to cooperate in certain ways, but one does not have to pretend to like cooperating. Actions and feelings are separate things; some actions may be unacceptable, but no feeling is beyond the pale.

CONCLUDING COMMENTS

Boundary issues can tax anyone's clinical ingenuity. They create issues for all therapists, not just those with a psychodynamic sensibility. In fact, because conventions about privacy, time, money, cancellations, and availability characterize most professional relationships, I am hoping that this chapter will be of use to beginning clinicians and counselors across a wide range of settings, orientations, and specializations. But questions about boundaries present perhaps the most difficult challenges to those who identify with the analytic tradition. First, a psychoanalytic attitude—including acknowledging the complexity of motivation, idealizing empathy, and appreciating radical differences in subjectivity—may complicate one's comfort with standing alone and diminish one's confidence in the reasonableness of rules that represent personal preferences. Second, by encouraging ongoing, powerful attachments, psychodynamic practitioners invite regressive wishes that can manifest themselves as incursions on boundaries or invitations to transgress them. This invitation may have a developmental purpose or

value but still challenges the professional balance. Third, the characterological tendencies that may accompany an attraction to psychoanalytic ideas and modes of working can militate against ease in setting
limits and tolerance of the negative reactions they inevitably produce.

In this chapter I have tried to honor the importance of the therapeutic frame without becoming dogmatic about its specific dimensions. I have looked mainly at aspects of the contract between client
and practitioner that present themselves early in treatment. Issues of
privacy, time, money, cancellation, and availability must be addressed
directly in the initial interview or as soon as they arise. Depending on
the client, they can be received as mundane, predictable requisites of a
professional relationship or as harrowing impingements that inflict humiliation or incite protest or inspire ingenious experiments in defiance. Whatever the response, these arrangements must be negotiated
in all therapies. Whereas in most parts of this book I attest to the probable trustworthiness of therapists' gut feelings and intuitions about
what is helpful, there is something about setting limits that is counterintuitive for many of us. Consequently, I have given that process special
attention. In Chapter 7 I discuss more client-specific boundary issues,
especially those that may develop as a therapy moves into deeper and
deeper territory with the patient's progressive disclosures and the therapist's affective responsiveness to them.

NOTES

1. My friend Kerry Gordon finds these generalizations, which may not apply
to therapists whose personalities are not depressively organized, much too
sweeping. A significant minority of therapists have, as I noted in passing in
Chapter 1, a schizoid character style, and hence may have an opposite attitude toward boundary issues. And, of course, the therapeutic community,
like any large conglomeration, contains people of widely different temperamental sensibilities and character types, and the different disciplines from
which psychotherapists may come (psychiatry, psychology, social work, nursing, education, religion, and others) may attract and nourish discipline-
specific sensibilities. Some psychiatrist colleagues have commented that
they do not identify with the depressive dynamics I describe. "One of the
things you learn to do as a doctor is to inflict pain without feeling guilty,"
one of them told me. A participant in a conference for pastoral counselors
at which I spoke commented that I had "nailed about eighty percent of the
audience" with my elaboration of schizoid dynamics. I continue to think
that the depressively inclined therapist is modal, but the reader can be the
judge of the aptness of the comments in this section.
2. I am personally a radical about confidentiality. Ever since the 1976 *Tarasoff*

decision, in which a California court held that a therapist should have
warned the intended victim of potential harm by his patient (in fact, the psychologist in question had tried to get the man hospitalized and was
thwarted in the attempt by a supervising psychiatrist who did not agree that
he was dangerous), there has been a disturbing erosion of patients' safety to
say everything they think and feel to a therapist. Without this freedom, therapy with many clients is not really possible (see Bollas & Sundelson, 1995;
Szasz, 2003). For individuals without problems controlling their impulses,
legal limitations on therapeutic privacy pose minimal problems, but for
others—often those who need professional help most—the "duty to warn"
laws deter them from seeking or staying in treatment.

I know of many cases in which a therapist's dutiful report of abuse or intended harm to others helped no one and in fact damaged the possibility of
help. The patient who is reported after confessing harmful actions or intentions, even if he or she has signed a consent form specifying the limits of
confidentiality, typically feels betrayed and enraged and leaves treatment.
Ironically, state authorities frequently respond to a clinician's report by investigating and concluding that the parent or family needs therapy—therapy
that is now essentially impossible because the reported party is thoroughly
disillusioned with treatment. Although I believe we need laws requiring citizens in general to report child abuse, I think it causes more problems than it
solves for therapists to have to report statements made by patients in a privileged relationship. When a client confesses abusive acts or intentions, we
can use all the clout in the therapy relationship to get the person to control
the behavior, including threatening to stop the treatment if it goes on, but if
we become instruments of the state's control, we destroy the trust on which
the therapeutic relationship is based. Although we must obey the current reporting laws, I regard the rationales for them as naive and the implementation of them as deeply problematic.

3. In a comparably oblivious policy, many psychoanalytic institutes once required, as a condition of graduating, that a candidate's training analyst report on his or her psychological suitability to practice as a psychoanalyst.
   You can imagine how effective those analyses were. For obvious reasons,
   such rules have disappeared, but while they were in force, the conventional
   wisdom in such institutes was that after one finished the "didactic analysis,"
   then one could undertake a "real" or "therapeutic" analysis with a person of
   one's choice.

4. Still, I do not recommend this. Clients experience it as a shameless justification of greed. For individuals whose job requires an irregular schedule,
   such a policy is particularly problematic. A woman with a stellar acting career told me she had been seeing a therapist in Los Angeles productively,
   for several months, three times a week, when she told him she would be
   spending July and August out of state. He stated that unless she paid him
   for three sessions a week throughout the summer to "hold her place," he
   could not guarantee he would have room for her in his practice in the fall.
   Not surprisingly, she declined his terms and left treatment. I have heard
   many stories like this.

5. Interestingly, Bader (1997) reports that in Norway, in the context of a social-ized health care system and less cynical assumptions about individual moti-vation, such rules are treated as reasonable and realistic rather than as man-ifestations of selfishness; hence, Norwegian clients do not see paying for missed sessions as an act of humiliating submission. Another observation on cultural context comes from Jan Resnick (personal communication, March 11, 2003):

> In West Australia, we find a very casual, easy-going, informal culture where such rules may be experienced as a persecuting attack or, alternatively, as the revelation of such avaricious, professionally sanctioned greed—to extort money for doing nothing—that [the cancellation policy] is taken as proof that the therapist is out for themselves and has no genuine care for the cli-ent. (I have experienced both.)
>
> So, I have found success in making clear the rule right from the start and applying it with a good deal of gentle flexibility in an attempt to profes-sionalize the public in the respect of learning to value time that is reserved for them.

Chapter 6

Basic Therapy Processes

> [Psychotherapists] hold no brief for the greatness of their
> hearts—they are among the least of those who work
> beyond themselves—but to some extent they lessen the
> man-made misery of man. They stand by. Hatred they
> endure, and do not turn away. Love comes their way, and
> they are not seduced. They are the listeners, but they
> listen with unwavering intent, and their silence is not
> cold.
>
> —ALLEN WHEELIS (1958, p. 246)

Analytic therapy requires one person to talk freely and the other to listen receptively, neither of which is easy to do. There are many different technical approaches in psychoanalytic work, depending on the client, the clinician, and the context, but all of them involve the joint effort of therapist and patient to appreciate the themes and meanings in the patient's self-expression. People who are pleased with their psychotherapy experience seldom report that it was a practitioner's dazzling verbal interventions that brought about significant changes. Rather, our satisfied customers mention the quality of our presence and the sense that we care. Most of our copious literature on technique represents efforts of different writers to specify ways we can facilitate a natural process of self-understanding and psychological maturation.

D. W. Winnicott (1958), a pediatrician who became a psychoanalyst, emphasized how critical it is to the development of a sense of identity and agency for an infant to experience the sense of "being alone in the presence of the mother." For the psychotherapy patient there is, ideally, an analogous sense of being alone in the presence of the therapist. The practice of taking oneself seriously and listening to oneself respectfully is often a new accomplishment for individuals adapting to the role of client, an experience for which they may need considerable support. Helping individuals to embrace the goal of the examined life may take considerable tact, patience, and technical flexibility.

Psychotherapy is a conversation, a back-and-forth collaboration in which listening and talking alternate on both sides of the therapeutic partnership. As such, it is represented rather artificially in sections on listening and talking, respectively, as if those processes were separable, but for purposes of organization, I describe aspects of that conversation under these headings. Then I share some observations about various influences on therapeutic style and speak briefly about combining psychoanalytic work with other therapeutic approaches. Finally, I consider the respective roles of power and of love in the psychotherapy process.

LISTENING

Psychotherapy technique has more to do with how one listens than with how one talks. Most ordinary conversation depends on assumptions that a psychodynamic practitioner takes pains not to make, such as that the person talking feels friendly toward the listener. Social dialogue includes a lot of extraneous "noise" created by the fact that both parties to a conversation have needs for both self-expression and acknowledgment from the other. Friends may interrupt, talk over each other, and change the subject at whim. In contrast, listening in a professional capacity is a disciplined, meditative, and emotionally receptive activity in which the therapist's needs for self-expression and self-acknowledgment are subordinated to the psychological needs of the client. The condition of therapeutic receptiveness shares with hypnotic states the combination of deep relaxation and an enhanced capacity for concentration (Casement, 1985; Freud, 1912b; Ogden, 1997). It is also ultimately exhausting (see Chapter 11).

It is not uncommon to hear people characterizing psychoanalytic therapists as "being paid just to sit there." They should only know how hard it can be just to sit there! When it is done well, "just" sitting there encourages clients to get brave enough to confide something painful, to figure out their own solutions, to find their sense of agency in the presence of a person who welcomes their increasing confidence and competence. The therapist is deprived of the illusion that it is his or her clever formulations that created that change, a frustration that it takes a good deal of training to be able to give up. We do not let our clients struggle along without any responsiveness from us, but we also do not rush to tell them that we understand or that we have a solution. We are keenly aware of the fact that full understanding of another person's psychology is impossible, and that a coping strategy that might work for ourselves could be disastrous for someone else.

Psychodynamic therapists vary how much they interact verbally, depending on the specific needs of each person—with some clients we may sound almost chatty, but we try to do so in a state of mindfulness of therapeutic goals. Bertram Karon (personal communication, January 25, 2003) described to me a young, relatively unsophisticated woman who went, on his recommendation, to a psychodynamic therapist after having been treated on and off since age eleven with psychoactive drugs and short-term cognitive-behavioral interventions. She came back to thank him after a therapy experience that had been deeply healing, saying, "I know now how to tell you've got a psychoanalytic person for a therapist. They're the ones that when you talk, they hear you."

Preliminary Considerations

In psychotherapy, listening is more important than talking. In fact, most of the ways that therapists talk during the clinical hour are intended to demonstrate that they are listening. We live in an age and civilization in which emphasis tends to be on doing rather than being, in which prevailing conceptions of science emphasize prediction and control rather than disciplined naturalistic observation, in which pop gurus counsel people about how to have various effects on others rather than about how to let others become comfortable being themselves. The idea that listening should be privileged over talking comes up against a strong Western cultural bias. Still, most of us can probably remember transformative instances when we felt the effect of someone's thoughtful attention, or when we were touched by someone's understanding, or when we were struck by an insight that entered our consciousness in a moment of repose.

Bion (1970, p. 57) counseled therapists to listen to each session "without memory or desire." By this impossible advice I understand him to mean that we need to clear our heads and try to take the patient's thoughts and feelings in without preconception. He emphasized the therapist's role as a "container" of images and feelings too toxic for the patient to tolerate. Winnicott's (1955) emphasis on the "holding" function of the psychotherapist and his (1971) and later Ogden's (1985, 1986) stress on "potential space" are similar: We have to create a space in which it is possible for the person to tell the truth of his or her experience. This can be much harder than it sounds. As Charles (in press) commented about her effort to be a container for a deeply unhappy, angry, and demanding client, "*My* work, during this arduous first year, consisted of containing my own distress sufficiently that I could provide an environment in which Ruth could continue to tell her story" (p. 32).

The therapeutic effects of being carefully listened to are substantial. Many patients, especially those from families that had depressed, distracted, or overworked caregivers, are amazed to learn that the therapist actually remembers what they say. Later, they tell us how much that meant to them. I often comment, toward the beginning of a course of therapy, "I'm going to be pretty quiet for a while, just trying to get a better sense of you and the problems you came to work on. As I start to feel I understand something, I'll let you know what I'm thinking, and you can tell me whether that feels right or whether I'm off in some way." With patients who have considerable background in disciplined introspection, including those with previous analytic therapy, I may comment that for a while they will know a lot more about themselves than I know about them and that I will appreciate their tolerating a period during which I am catching up with what they have already figured out about themselves. It is rare that someone responds to statements such as these with irritation and impatience; rather, clients seem relieved that I will not be trying to impose on them my prepackaged understandings and pet recommendations.

Early in treatment, it is unwise to let silences extend or accumulate. Silence can sometimes be profoundly meaningful to patients—as in occasions in which they feel deeply and wordlessly understood, or sincerely respected by the therapist's willingness not to hurry them, or warmly appreciative of a reticence to impinge upon their moments of silent contemplation. But they are unlikely to have anything other than an unproductively anxious reaction to early silences. When clients have trouble talking, it is better to address the problem and work out a temporary solution. One option is to ask what the therapist might say or do to make it easier for them to talk. Another possibility is to engage in mutual problem solving, exploring what the effect would be of different responses, such as the therapist's attempting to draw them out versus the therapist's waiting quietly. Silence is tolerated much better if the patient understands it as respectful and has participated in the decision not to rush to fill the air space.

The primary aim of the psychoanalytic therapist is to encourage free expression. An effect of our doing so is that we give patients the experience of having a relationship in which honesty is possible. The appropriateness of any intervention or therapeutic stance should be judged by the criterion of whether it increases the patient's ability to confide, to explore more and more painful self-states, and to expand access to more intense and more discriminated emotional experience—

in other words, to elaborate the self. The classical analyst's reserve has this aim (Greenson, 1967), but so does the empathic mirroring of the self psychologist, the patient- and analyst-centered interpretations of the Kleinian (Steiner, 1993), the here-and-now/you-and-me confrontation of the transference-focused therapist with the borderline patient (Clarkin et al., 1999), and the countertransference disclosure of the relational therapist (Aron, 1996). All the psychoanalytic approaches to technique are designed to facilitate this ongoing, deepening, ultimately self-righting process of self-exploration and self-expression. They apply more and less well, respectively, to different patients, different stages in the clinical process, and the personalities of different therapists.

I mentioned in Chapter 4 the empirically derived work of Joseph Weiss and Harold Sampson and their colleagues (Weiss, 1999; Weiss et al., 1986), who have concluded that patients know at some level what they need from treatment and have an unconscious "plan" for therapy. Then they test the therapist to see if he or she can cooperate with that plan. This fits my clinical experience. With most clients, I become impressed with the power, notwithstanding all the anxieties about change that impress the analytic therapist as resistance, of their wish to take in new experience and grow. If we listen carefully, they will try to tell us (usually in the first session) what they need from us in order to do so. Although they may subsequently behave in ways that evoke responses from us that are opposite to the ones they said they needed, I think Sampson and Weiss are right that such experiences constitute tests, and that our therapeutic role is to try to stay supportive of the client's original plan.

For example, some clients will tell a therapist—either in words or in actions—that they cannot stand too much warmth, that they need to be challenged and confronted, that they are allergic to motherly concern. They experience caring as a soul-threatening seduction, or they worry that the longing it evokes for what they lacked in childhood will pull them into a malignant regression. Or they know that their self-esteem will be traumatically shattered by the evocation of their dependent wishes. Consequently, despite the therapeutic effect of warmth on most clients, such individuals will regard a therapist's effort to offer empathic resonance as tantalizing, entrapping, and consuming, a threat to their continued existence as separate individuals. This dynamic is frequently found in people with trauma histories, toward whom it may be hard *not* to express sympathy. They typically find ways to demonstrate their preference for our keeping a certain respectful distance, but then, unconsciously to test us, they may behave in ways that invite us to rescue them with our love. The therapist who listens carefully and develops a tentative psychodynamic formulation of each person as a unique individual (see McWilliams, 1999; Peebles-Kleiger, 2002) will do much better with such stresses than the therapist who applies a favored theory to everyone.

Styles of Listening

As therapists, we essentially use each patient as a consultant, learning from him or her what style of listening and responding is most helpful (Casement, 1985, 2002; Charles, in press). There is usually a fair amount of bumbling along, especially at the beginning of any treatment. During this bumbling, the main thing for a therapist to keep in mind is the importance of helping the client to talk freely, to expose as much inner life as possible. Asking periodically, "Are you feeling comfortable talking with me? Is there any way I could make it any easier for you to be frank and open?" can help both client and therapist with their adaptation to each other. Even in short-term, structured psychodynamic treatments, there should be an effort in the first couple of sessions to be sure that the client has been put sufficiently at ease to tell his or her story with the least possible interference by inhibition of any sort.

The therapist thus tries to convey an attitude that will prevent or reduce feelings of shame and humiliation about whatever is revealed. Throughout treatment, but especially in the beginning, whenever shame emerges, addressing and reducing it are high-priority matters. I have known several individuals who have learned a lot about their dynamics in psychotherapy but who seem to remain deeply ashamed of them. Self-knowledge is one goal of psychoanalytic treatment, but a more profound goal is self-acceptance. The more one accepts aspects of the self that have been seen as shameful, the less one is controlled by them. Psychoanalysis as a field has tried to name one after another propensity that comes with the territory of being human, including all the seven deadly sins, with the assumption that acknowledging these tendencies allows us to find better ways to deal with them.

One way to communicate acceptance and to dissolve shame is by what I think of as the "Yeah . . . so?" response, either verbally or nonverbally. In other words, we take in whatever the patient has confessed with a tone or a look of unsurprised matter-of-fact-ness, implying that we are not quite sure why this is such a big deal. Sometimes we make a quick connection that allows us to make a casual comment to the effect that given what the person has said about his or her family of origin, the disclosure is hardly surprising. Or we mutter a comment such as "Well, naturally," or adopt a puzzled tone and ask, "So what's so terrible about that?" when a patient seems to be drowning in shame while disclosing some crime of the heart. Sometimes it is helpful to ask, "Do you have a sense of why this seems to involve a lot of shame for you?" conveying that it is not self-evident why someone would be mortified by confiding something human beings inevitably feel.

It is also important throughout the therapy to try to keep one's own temptations toward narcissistic display under control. What I mean by this is that it is natural to want to demonstrate our competence, to show our patients that we have something to offer. This inclination can get in the way of maintaining enough reserve to let people make their own discoveries and come up with their own solutions to the problems in their lives. Therapists must be careful not to one-up their clients. A tone of "So you've finally figured out what I've known all along" can poison the process. The temptation to do this is especially strong with patients who are devaluing and challenging. Better to comment wryly, "Sounds like you can't imagine how a bonehead like me could be of help" than to try to demonstrate one's clinical brilliance.

The much-parodied verbal tic of the analytic therapist ("Hmm" or "Mm-hmm") is an effort to convey our "there-ness" without interrupting the client. Greenson (1954) noted that the sound "mm" is predominant in words used for "mother" in a great number of languages and may also express delight at something tasting good. Perhaps with this locution we are nonverbally signaling to clients that we are as open to their hunger and aggression as a nursing mother. I find myself making a number of facilitating grunts and nods intended to give messages such as "I'm listening," "Keep talking," "That's interesting," "That surprises me," "That must have been painful," "I'm not sure what you mean," and "I get it."

Lawrence Hedges (1983) delineates four different listening perspectives, for patients with a neurotic personality organization, narcissistic personality organization, borderline personality organization, and "organizing" personality, respectively. His last category refers to those clients whom others have called primitive, understructured, and psychotic-level, who probably correlate highly with the disorganized attachment style described in the empirical literature (see Coates & Moore, 1997; Fonagy et al., 1996; Main & Solomon, 1991). He recommends listening for Freudian themes (drive motivations, structural conflict, and defense) with neurotic-level clients, self-psychological themes (self-cohesion and fragmentation in relation to selfobjects) with narcissistically organized clients, object-relational themes (merger vs. abandonment, affect differentiation, separation, and individuation) with borderline clients, and Kleinian themes (greed, envy, hatred, the paranoid–schizoid position) with personalities trying to organize themselves. Hedges's recommendations, made in the context of an erudite exploration of relevant philosophical and psychoanalytic literature, are generally consistent with those that I summarized in *Psychoanalytic Diagnosis* (McWilliams, 1994) with respect to different orientations toward patients with differing levels of personality organization. They are consistent also with the assumptions underlying Kernberg's "structural interview" (1984).

TALKING

How one talks in the role of therapist expresses a unique combination of one's theoretical orientation, understanding of the client's psychology, and individual personality and conversational style. The intellectual effort to formulate one's comments according to the rules of some expert can interfere drastically with the receptive sensibility that moves treatment along. Although there was a rather perfectionistic era in psychoanalytic history (roughly coinciding with the years when American analysts were trying to define psychoanalysis as a specifiable medical procedure), when analytic practitioners idealized the concept of the "accurate" as opposed to "inexact" interpretation (Glover, 1931), contemporary psychodynamic therapists tend to follow Spence (1982) and Schafer (1983)[1] in regarding the therapist's communications as efforts to promote the development of mutual understandings that account for the patient's experience.

In addition to having rejected its former perfectionism, the analytic community has, for the most part, outgrown its early, naive confidence in the capacity of a therapist to "uncover" the truth of a person's history in the way an archeologist can excavate ruins or a detective can solve a mystery; instead, we regard the project of psychotherapy as a joint effort to develop a narrative that makes sense of a person's subjective experience and personal problems. Most of us view truth claims (especially those made in a tone of undiluted certainty) as suspect, both because validation for clinical hypotheses and historical reconstructions are hard to come by and because both therapist and patient have unconscious reasons to ignore or distort phenomena that make them anxious. The upside of this change toward embracing not-knowing is that there is much less pressure on beginning therapists to craft their interventions along the lines of some rigid model of interpretive precision.

Facilitating the Therapeutic Process

As I argued in the previous two chapters, the earliest comments of the therapist should be oriented toward establishing safety, communicating a wish to understand, explaining relevant aspects of the process of therapy, clarifying the frame, and identifying any issues that might get in the way of the person's willingness to collaborate or the therapist's capacity to help. Next, I recommend that therapists devote a session to taking a comprehensive history, during which they may develop and find a way to share a tentative dynamic formulation of the individual's problems.[2] After this, the therapist's activity should be oriented toward increasing the client's capacity to speak freely and with full emotional engagement. Interventions such as "Can you say more about that?," or "Sounds like there's a lot of feeling there," or "That must have been difficult," or "Have you been in similar situations?," or "What comes to your mind as you think about that?," or "Does that remind you of anything?," or "How are you feeling as you tell me this?" are common ways of doing this.

Each clinician must find words that feel personally genuine in the situation; otherwise, he or she will sound mechanical and insincere. In advising therapists about the tone that should inform psychodynamic treatment, Schafer (1974) has urged that we not bracket ourselves off patriarchally from the therapeutic conversation by speaking in stilted versions of professional speech. Instead, he reminds us that psychotherapy is an "I–Thou type of exploratory dialogue." He gives the following examples of natural, more egalitarian styles of speech as opposed to stiffer locutions:

> "I am wondering what that could be about" as against persistently remaining thoughtfully silent. "Congratulations!" as against "You must be very proud of yourself." "I don't feel at ease somehow and I have a hunch you are trying to get me to feel that way" as against "You are trying to make me feel ill at ease." "That's a helluva way to live" as against "Your life does not seem very satisfying or easy." And "I'm not surprised" as against "That might have been expected." (pp. 512–513)

Sometimes, when the phrase of a patient has seemed pregnant with unspoken feeling, a therapist will simply echo it in slower or softer tones than the patient used, hoping to elicit the affect behind it. Many psychoanalytic therapists, including me, bring up the subject of dreams early in treatment, inquiring about recurrent dreams, memorable childhood dreams, and recent dreams in order to expand the client's sense of the topics that are welcome in the therapy room. Asking about fantasies, or explaining that it will be valuable to think about the client's fantasy life together, is also helpful.

If the patient is talking freely without the therapist's facilitative comments and educative inquiries, there is no reason to speak until toward the end of a session, when the client may reasonably expect some verbal response. This response may come in the form of a question about the way the client has been interpreting the incidents that have been recounted (i.e., a request for clarification), or a statement of encouragement to continue talking about the material so that the two parties can get more understanding of it (a reinforcement of the therapeutic alliance), or an exploration of how the patient is feeling having made these disclosures to the therapist (a preliminary examination of transference reactions), or a comment on ways in which the person seems to be keeping the material at an emotional distance (analysis of defense), or a summary of a theme that the therapist has been hearing between the lines (a tentative interpretation), among many other possibilities. Again, the most important feature of any intervention early in treatment is the communication that the therapist has been listening.

Addressing Resistances to Self-Expression

Because we want our patients to speak from the heart, we gently try to reduce any verbal defensiveness that interferes with or mutes that process. With tact, we call attention to the ways they seem to keep the full intensity of their experience at arm's length. Common defenses against frank verbalization include such mannerisms as talking in the second person (e.g., in response to "How did you feel?", "Well, you know, you feel bad when that happens"), talking in the third person ("I guess it's natural for people to feel bad in that situation"), dramatizing or demonstrating things that could be simply expressed ("I was SOOOOO angry!" with an exaggerated eye-roll that slightly ridicules the feeling it portrays), trying to bring the therapist into the experience ("Can you believe the bastard did that to me?"), avoiding the naming of affects and substituting a vague term ("How did you feel?," "Kinda weird, I guess"), changing the subject when feelings get too close, talking in baby talk or some other affected way about more intimate topics, and many other unconscious strategies to keep pain and shame at a distance.

There is a vast clinical literature—not just in psychoanalysis but in the other humanistic therapies such as Gestalt, client-centered, and existential approaches—on helping people become more connected with their feelings and more comfortable expressing themselves directly. Therapists who work with couples often find it valuable to give both parties the direct instruction: "Speak to each other in 'I' statements and say what you feel" (and then often, they have to go on to explain that the locution "I feel that you're insensitive" is not exactly what they meant). When partners can move from describing what is bad in the other to what is experienced in the self ("I feel hurt when you ignore me"), a giant step has been taken toward improvement in the relationship. Individual therapists usually take a less didactic stance than professionals trying to improve the communications skills of two partners, but the aim is similar: to encourage clients to speak nondefensively and in the first-person voice about their emotional experience.

Many analysts (e.g., Fine, 1971; Greenson, 1967) who write about ways to increase the therapeutic power in the clinical conversation have urged their colleagues to use straightforward, ordinary language, including for experiences as intimate as sex (e.g., "You went down on him" rather than "You engaged in fellatio"). Greenson (1950) has noted how advantageous it is for clients brought up in other cultures if the clinician is familiar with the language of their childhood. Schafer (1976) recommended that therapists use, and encourage clients to use, "action language"—that is, emphasizing verbs rather than nouns, especially abstract ones ("You're feeling pretty guilty" rather than "You're suffering pangs of conscience" or "Your superego is attacking you"). Levenson (1988) advised "the pursuit of the particular," that is, asking for the details of experiences when the client makes a general statement ("What exactly did you say when you 'asserted yourself'?"). Learning a client's personal metaphors and developing vivid metaphors together can further this process of greater expressiveness as well.[3]

Every therapist–patient dyad evolves its distinctive rhythms of speech and silence, self-elaboration and reflection, talking and listening. Some patients hardly let the therapist get a word in edgewise, while others sit there helplessly waiting for the professional to steer the conversation. One of the reasons psychoanalytic therapists are so fond of the literature on infant–caregiver relationships, even though we are quite cognizant of the fact that the adult in treatment is not reducible to a fixated infant, is that the process of synchronizing oneself with a patient's idiosyncratic style feels strikingly similar to descriptions of parents' efforts to adapt to the temperament and rhythms unique to their baby (Brazelton & Als, 1979; Escalona & Corman, 1974; D. N. Stern, 1995).

INFLUENCES ON THERAPEUTIC STYLE

Many disparate and converging factors influence the style and tone (prosody) adopted by the clinician in any given therapy session. Among them are the characteristics of the patient, the stage of the treatment, and the personality of the therapist. In addition, there is the matter of the practitioner's theoretical orientation or choice of a particular type of dynamic therapy that suits the circumstances (e.g., a short-term model such as that of Mann, 1973, or Luborsky & Crits-Christoph, 1990, that prescribes a particular focus). I confine myself in the next section to a discussion of the first variables, as the explication of different psychoanalytic models is beyond my scope here.

Patient Characteristics

How we talk with people depends on the situation they are in when they come to us and on our understanding of their personality structure. Obviously, people in crisis require an immediately responsive, problem-solving kind of attention. Those who come for more gradual or general problems need to develop a relationship in which those problems can be elaborated and examined in depth. For individuals who seem to have considerable ego strength, who readily make a friendly connection with the therapist, and who have a lot of self-observing capacity, less is more. That is, the more we can get them talking, and intervene only when they seem to get stuck, the better. The most typical mistake that beginning therapists make with mature, high-functioning people is to say too much or speak too often. Unfortunately, such clients are much rarer in the practices of most beginning therapists—and probably also more seasoned ones—than much more disturbed and difficult individuals.

For patients who are more terrified, who struggle with psychotic-level anxieties, who feel unable to regulate their emotions, containment is the main function that the therapist's style of interaction must provide. Clarity about boundaries and tolerance of their intense and often negative reactions to the therapist's limits are critical. Closeness is often a much more terrifying condition than abandonment for them, but they are also exquisitely reactive to separations and consequently cause therapists to struggle with guilt over time off. Clear boundaries are also critical for clients in the borderline range who have profound difficulties with affect regulation, as is the exploration of the stark good-versus-bad polarities in which they see the world. People with borderline dynamics also respond well to therapists who do not try to hide their own affective reactions in the name of trying to be professional or neutral (Maroda, 1999; Holmqvist, 2000).

There is a continuum from predominantly supportive (in the technical sense—all therapy is of course supportive) to predominantly exploratory psychotherapy (Rockland, 1992). Where we work on that continuum with any client correlates reasonably well with Kernberg's (1984) levels of severity of psychopathology: For those in the neurotic range, we can keep opening up questions and inviting exploration; for those in the borderline range, we expect a dyadic struggle that requires us to be active, limit setting, interpretive of primitive dynamics, and focused on the here-and-now relationship; with those in the psychotic range, we need to be educative, normalizing, and explicitly supportive of the patient's capacities. Prosody varies also depending on the patient's personality type: the tough tone that comforts a paranoid person (at any level of severity) is quite different from the sympathetic attitude that comforts a depressive person, irrespective of the severity of any depressive symptoms or the level of personality organization (McWilliams, 1994). No matter how well read we are, most of us adapt our tone to the patient on the basis of intuition and experience.

In a 1991 article I argued that devotion and integrity, which can be understood as the preeminent values expressed in good mothering and good fathering, respectively, must both be present in psychotherapy. I had become impressed with empirical research that was documenting infants' needs for both soothing and stimulation (e.g., Brazelton, 1982; Yogman, 1981) and the apparently universal tendency for babies and young children to associate soothing with mothers and stimulation with fathers, irrespective of the personalities or roles of their caregivers (Lamb, 1977; Clarke-Stewart, 1978; Belsky, 1979). It struck me that different psychoanalytic theorists have tended to emphasize either more soothing-maternal or more stimulating-paternal styles of therapy. For example, Freud was more paternal in style and tone, while his colleague Ferenczi advocated a more maternal sensibility. Over the course of psychoanalytic history, there have been many highly publicized controversies between a more paternal theorist or school of thought and a more maternal one, both of whom were competing for status as the favored paradigm (e.g., Fenichel vs. Reik, Melanie Klein vs. Anna Freud, Brenner vs. Stone, Kernberg vs. Kohut, the classicists vs. the relational analysts).

Like most therapists (e.g., Pine, 1998), I find such debates rather arid. As many clinicians have argued, different kinds of patients need different kinds of responsiveness. The balance of maternal and paternal tone differs for different clients, and usually practitioners figure out what is helpful by trial and error. For example, most of us find ourselves behaving in more Kohutian, maternal ways with people with more empty, depleted narcissistic dynamics (McWilliams, 1994), who tend to experience interpretation as attack. But we learn to interpret in the more paternal, confronting tone of Kernberg when trying to deal with the more arrogant, entitled version of narcissistic pathology, because such patients tend not to respect anyone who fails to stand up to them. Most patients need both tones, and the capacity to shift grace-fully from one mode to another is central to the art of psychotherapy.

Research on attachment suggests that therapists adapt their man-ner to the specific attachment style of each patient (see Cassidy & Shaver, 2002; Cortina & Marrone, 2003; Fonagy, 2000). Individuals with secure attachment patterns respond well to interpretation of inter-nal conflict, whereas those who have an anxious attachment style may require more soothing. Therapists may have to tolerate an oscillation between fears of engulfment and fears of abandonment in clients with an ambivalent attachment style (cf. Masterson, 1976). I have mentioned previously several problems that arise when one works with people whose attachment paradigm is disorganized and disoriented.

Eventually, we will know a lot more about differences in the brain that make one person long for a straight-talking, tell-it-like-it-is style of intervention while another responds to the therapist as traumatically interfering whenever he or she introduces the most gentle of questions. The work of neuropsychoanalytic scholars such as Mark Solms, Joseph LeDoux, Allen Schore, Antonio Damasio, and Bessel van der Kolk is al-ready giving us a whole new language for understanding the nuances of interpersonal experience, including that of psychotherapy. But hav-ing new paradigms, including respectably scientific ones, will not obvi-ate the need for therapists to rely on their right brain and to go through an intuitively informed, sometimes painful trial-and-error pro-cess with each client.

Phase of Therapy

What any given person needs from a therapist may change over the course of the work. I learned this originally from the narcissistically devastated woman I took on as my first long-term client. At that point in my professional development, I was palpitating to do the classical psychoanalytic work that had been so helpful to me, and this woman wanted to come three times a week. I knew that she was too regressed to be a candidate for the couch, but I wanted to try to be as orthodox as possible otherwise. When she would ask me, with the intention of talk-ing about some relevant issue, whether I had seen a certain movie or read a certain novel, I tried responding with "I wonder why that is com-ing to your mind now." After two or three unproductive exposures to the rage reaction that this response provoked, I decided it was more conducive to her self-exploration for me to say yes or no and wait for her to continue. Then at some point in our third year of therapy, she made such an inquiry, and I opened my mouth to reply. "DON'T ANSWER!" she exclaimed. "Don't you realize that when you answer, you cut off my ability to fantasize about what the answer is?!" Thus, once I had finally learned to work like Heinz Kohut, this patient had moved on to wanting Charles Brenner for her therapist.

Therapists are always having to strike a balance between more ostensibly passive and more obviously active interventions (often construed as empathy and interpretation, holding/containing and confronting, provision of experience and enhancement of knowledge). These two kinds of activity are perhaps always both present, but one usually predominates with a particular patient or in a particular phase of treatment. Several theorists (e.g., Josephs, 1995; Seinfeld, 1993; Stark, 1999) have explored the coexistence and oscillation of these two therapeutic processes. Seinfeld (1993), who also (independently) explored maternal and paternal metaphors for therapeutic style, suggests that the more maternal voice is a better fit with psychologies of developmental arrest or deficiency, whereas the more interpretive, paternal tone is better suited to the treatment of problems caused by unconscious conflict. Like many writers, he notes the artificiality of contrasting these activities as if they were mutually exclusive or even qualitatively different (see, e.g., Moses, 1988; D. B. Stern, 1984, 1988): A good interpretation is taken in as deeply empathic, and the therapist's empathic attitude can be received as an interpretation—for example, as a nonverbal way of saying, "Despite your feelings of shame, it is possible to accept you as you are."

Seinfeld goes on to note that the psychologies of most of us contain both deficit and conflict. It follows that at different points in treatment, anyone in therapy tends to be working in one or the other place predominantly. Thus, many patients whose backgrounds contain serious deprivation need a fairly long period of experiencing the therapist as a noncritical, available, and supportive other before they are able to tolerate more focused attention on an area of internal conflict. They may need to take in the more maternal aspects of the relationship before they feel "held" enough internally to deal with an interpretive style that would have overwhelmed their previously more fragile sense of security and self-esteem. There are other patients—for example, virtually all markedly psychopathic individuals, some people with schizoid dynamics, and most people with paranoid psychologies, narcissism of the entitled sort, or significant hypomania—who are so suspicious of or frightened by maternal acceptance that they cannot take it in as supportive until they have established that the therapist is separate enough, strong enough, and tough-minded enough to "get" the way they see the world and survive their toxicity.

In the case of a person who needs a long period of a reassuring maternal presence before being able to take in anything more stimulating, a movement from deficit to conflict may be signaled by a change in the therapist's countertransference. The first time this happened to me, I thought I was losing my empathy. A man I had been working with patiently and supportively for months began ridiculing himself in familiar ways, a tendency I saw as related to his growing up with six siblings. In his family, the only way he could get attention from his beleaguered mother was by playing the helpless fool. But suddenly one session, instead of thinking "Poor guy, given his history these masochistic reactions are inevitable," I found myself wanting to smack him. I was irritated, impatient, and barely in control of the impulse to unload my hostility in an interpretation.

Instead, I ran to supervision, full of shame about my countertransference (an interesting parallel process [Ekstein & Wallerstein, 1958], by the way, to the client's self-hating attitude). My supervisor and I figured out that over the course of our work, this man had been quietly moving toward more capacity for self-assertion. Now when he debased himself, he was no longer behaving in the only way he knew to relate to others (in therapy, he had slowly learned a different way to relate); instead, he was defending against the fears that would have attended his behaving with self-respect. He was not stuck at this point in a state of deficit. Rather, he had a conflict about whether or not to change his behavior, and because he was frightened of change, he was choosing the regressive option. This behavior irritated me now, as it had not before, because I knew he could do better. As long as I had felt that change was not possible yet, I could be genuinely accepting of his symptomatology, but when I began to feel he was selling his capabilities short, I smoldered. Having understood this, I found a way to challenge his behavior that did not feel like unloading on him. Interestingly, my countertransference irritation was more genuinely empathic to his state of mind—that is, to both his capacity and his fear to change—than an effort to condole with him for his self-hatred would have been.

The Therapist's Personality

Years ago, in the context of working intensively with two excellent supervisors who had markedly contrasting therapeutic styles, I became fascinated with the interaction between a practitioner's personality and his or her therapeutic style and theory of healing. One of my mentors, a reserved and somewhat socially awkward man who described himself as schizoid, put considerable emphasis on being spontaneous, warm, real, alive, and flexible. The other, an affectionate, demonstrative, sociable person who joked about his hysterical and exhibitionistic tendencies, would go on at length about restraint, discipline, reserve, and the most judicious use of "parameters." I gradually realized that what each of my supervisors was most concerned to pass on to me was an orientation that corrected for the disadvantages of his own temperament. It was also the attitude that each one seemed to feel would have been most healing to him as a patient.

Around the same time, I began noticing that some theorists recommended a particular therapeutic attitude that they not only believed would have been helpful to them as clients but that also normalized and generalized their own dynamics. Heinz Kohut might be a convenient exemplar of this tendency. Strozier's (2001) biography depicts a man who thrived on the experience of being idealized by others. Kohut's urging the analytic community to accept idealizations from admiring patients, rather than trying to resolve idealizing transferences by interpretation, was consistent with his personal *modus vivendi* and was the stance that he clearly believed, given the autobiographical nature of his most famous case (Kohut, 1979—see Note 1, Chapter 11, here) would have been more healing to him than the standard analytic interpretation of defense. Another irresistible example is Melanie Klein, who was frequently experienced by others as forceful and opinionated (Grosskurth, 1986). Klein urged analysts to name children's presumed dynamics with confidence and to interpret them authoritatively, a therapeutic version of her own interpersonal style.

I have concluded over the years that when clinicians talk most passionately about an attitude or process that is "at the center of" or that is "the essence of" the healing process, they often prescribe a stance that either normalizes their own dispositions or compensates for the limitations of their character type. In either case, they seem to be trying to heal themselves. Generalizing about what is helpful in therapy on the basis of one's own psychology is frequently useful, because we are all much more similar than we are different as human beings. There are times, however, that to be a good therapist for a particular patient we must find and draw on specific qualities in our personalities that, if evident in our therapist, would *not* have facilitated our own treatment. For example, if the therapist of an individual with marked antisocial tendencies is unable to connect with the more ruthless, power-oriented parts of his or her own personality and thereby set an authentically skeptical, no-nonsense, tough-guy tone, he or she cannot expect to develop any semblance of a working alliance.

As I observed in the previous chapter, many therapists have depressive dynamics and as a result emphasize availability, the holding environment, noncritical acceptance, and similar attitudes that are healing to those of us with this psychology. The work of Donald Winnicott, who certainly had a powerful depressive side, is often cited by therapists for whom depressive themes are personally resonant. I notice that my own metaphors for psychotherapy tend to have a maternal-availability-as-healing tinge, and not surprisingly, Winnicott's writings have always appealed to me. There is evidence, however, that as a therapist, Winnicott had trouble tolerating his own aggression and thus had difficulty setting limits. His inability to do so may have been rationalized by his belief that very troubled patients need to regress to a state of primary dependence (see Rodman, 2003). His painfully public failure with Masud Khan (see below) and his probable mistakes with Margaret Little have been widely regarded as evidence for this limitation (Flournoy, 1992; Hopkins, 1998; Rodman, 2003).

Again, one of the reasons for therapists to have personal therapy is that we all need to find parts of our personalities that can be accessed for work with people whose dynamics are different from our own central themes and variations. Such explorations in the nether regions of our psyches help us to stretch as therapists. And yet because there are limits to everyone's flexibility, some patients will not be a good fit with a particular therapist's range of authentic treatment styles. I would not recommend that any practitioner, novice or otherwise, try to adopt a tone that feels either false or too distant from his or her most temperamentally congruent inclinations.

INTEGRATING PSYCHOANALYTIC THERAPY WITH OTHER APPROACHES

Unlike theorists and researchers, who understandably prefer their categories to be uncontaminated, most therapists want to do whatever helps their patients most and fastest. They readily combine psychoanalytic treatment with nonpsychoanalytic efforts to reduce suffering, including cognitive-behavioral therapy, twelve-step programs, eye movement desensitization and reprocessing, hypnosis, relaxation training, support groups, Gestalt exercises, meditation, and other interventions. Evolving out of the pioneering work of writers such as Wachtel, Messer, and Arkowitz (e.g., Arkowitz & Messer, 1984; Wachtel, 1997), there is now an international organization concerned with the integration of different models of psychotherapy: the Society for the Exploration of Psychotherapy Integration. It has grown rapidly and has attracted considerable clinical enthusiasm.

Recent articles in psychoanalytic journals (e.g., Conners, 2001; Frank, 1992) have described circumstances in which analysts should consider supplementing their usual work with cognitive-behavioral interventions. Some of us do the collateral therapy work ourselves, and some refer to other practitioners, either because they have better training in a given technique or because it would complicate the transference unduly for us to be in two rather different roles. To us, this is no big deal. Working therapists are rarely purists, a fact that may come as a surprise to people who assume that analytic clinicians are ideologues. Interestingly, Freud was the first therapist to advocate moving beyond the customary interpretive stance into an "active" problem-solving approach. In 1919, noting that standard analytic technique arose from work with hysteria and must be adapted flexibly to the treatment of other problems, he recommended an early version of exposure therapy:

> One can hardly master a phobia if one waits till the patient lets the analysis influence him to give it up. He will never in that case bring into the analysis the material indispensable for a convincing resolution. . . . One succeeds only when one can induce [people with agoraphobia] by the influence of the analysis . . . to go into the street and to struggle with their anxiety while they make the attempt. (p. 166)

POWER AND LOVE

Both the virtues and the dangers of psychoanalytic therapy lie in the fact that the therapist is in a position of substantial emotional power. Power is morally neutral: It can be applied to good or evil ends. It can turn a therapist's unthinking act of ordinary thoughtfulness into a revolutionary therapeutic moment, and it can convert a minor lapse into a full-scale calamity. Appreciating the extent of one's power is critical to the lifelong process of trying to maximize good and minimize harm with which conscientious therapists struggle every day. Psychoanalytic therapy also generates love between practitioner and client; in fact, I believe it is love that endows the therapist with the emotional power to foster change and love that gives the patient the courage to pursue it. It is not the only therapeutic factor, but love may be the one that allows the other curative processes to do their work.

Power in the Role of Therapist

Much of the power in any kind of therapy derives simply from the therapist's role. Anyone who has been promoted from an institutional position of equality to that of a higher-up has learned the emotionally startling lesson that one's former colleagues immediately begin to act with a special circumspection, deference, or hostility, no matter how relaxed

they were formerly. Role and status are potent realities. In secular Western society, being a therapist is probably psychologically comparable to
being in the sacred status accorded in other cultures to gurus, religious
leaders, teachers, healers, prophets, shamans, elders, oracles, and other
tribal authorities (cf. Frank & Frank, 1991). Whatever the therapist's
theoretical orientation, the situation in which one person has a need
and the other has expertise to address it tilts the power relationship
heavily in the therapist's direction. In the psychoanalytic literature,
Phyllis Greenacre (1959) was perhaps the first to elaborate insightfully
on the "tilted" nature of therapeutic collaboration. The therapist may
take an egalitarian tone, but the playing field is not level (see I.
Hoffman, 1998, for a more recent exploration of this topic).

An additional source of power specific to therapy inheres in the
fact that the client is asked to reveal sensitive information, while the
therapist discloses little of a personal nature. Again, this imbalance applies to all types of treatment. In psychoanalytic work, this aspect of the
power imbalance is magnified by the fact that the therapist may ask
about dreams, fantasies, sexual practices, and other intensely intimate
domains of experience. Even the most shame-free, self-confident client
feels the asymmetricality of the analytic collaboration; not surprisingly,
most people are conscious of being more than a little frustrated by it.
Patients may seek to rectify the power differential in numerous ways: by
seizing on small indications of a therapist's personality and commenting on them, by reading articles that the therapist has written, by looking up information on the Internet, by asking personal questions, by
behaving seductively, by bringing gifts or giving advice that sends the
message that the client, too, has something to offer to the other person
in the relationship. Novelists and other writers portraying a treatment
on the couch have depicted how carefully patients listen for the pencil
scratching away behind them, as they try to discern something about
the therapist's interests from figuring out which topics seem to inspire
the note taking ("scribble, scribble, scribble," one of my analysands
teased).

Once someone is perceived as in a powerful position, it is virtually
impossible for him or her to counteract the perception of power by being voluntarily out of role. I once sat on a board of education where
members would sometimes feel aggrieved if they had tried to speak
with a teacher "just as a parent, not as a school board member!" only to
find the teacher unable to talk nondefensively to a person who, whatever the board member's current self-definition, was the teacher's employer. Bill Clinton (Renshon, 1998) reportedly could not comprehend
why anybody cared about his sexual indiscretions or why Monica
Lewinsky might have found it hard to refrain from telling her friends

that she was having oral sex with the President of the United States. He seems to have wanted to believe he could be perceived by the public and by his girlfriend the way he perhaps perceived himself: as a somewhat overweight and insecure guy who finds sexual fidelity difficult. He may be at some level just that, but his role made the perception by others of that self-representation out of the question.

Thus, the one kind of power we do not have in an authoritative role is the ability to suspend our power. We cannot just redefine a situation that by its nature evokes in others the universal primary experience of being dependent on people considerably more powerful than they are (i.e., that elicits transferences). As Freud learned when he tried to talk his earliest patients out of their insistence on projecting parental qualities on to him, transferences cannot be unilaterally suspended. Along the same lines, the first analysts, including Freud, overestimated the extent to which a transference could be "worked through" in a short period. Later psychoanalytic writing on transference (e.g., Bergmann, 1988) assumes that once people are in a powerful role, especially that of analyst, they are never likely to be seen as just another human being struggling along in life. Changes in the ethics codes of various psychotherapy professions in the direction of prohibiting sexual contact between client and treater for a considerable time after therapy has ended reflect the accumulated experience of individuals who have suffered because the psychological power differential does not go away even after a treatment is over.

Psychoanalytic Listening and Therapeutic Power

In psychoanalysis and psychoanalytic therapy there is an additional power problem that goes beyond role. It is a morally challenging issue that may say a lot about the widespread animosity toward the psychoanalytic tradition even as it accounts for the effectiveness of many analytic treatments. That is, in psychoanalytic work, therapists draw power to themselves. By attending repeatedly to the reactions that a client has toward him or her, a therapist selectively reinforces the patient's attention to and preoccupation with the therapeutic relationship. My understanding of the reason we cultivate the client's transference in traditional analytic work is that if we are to modify the very powerful, unconscious, pathogenic voices that haunt the people who come to us, we must accrue a degree of power comparable to that of their internalized early objects.

If change were easy, psychotherapists would be out of a job. People do not come to therapy if their own sense of agency or the experienced power of the authorities in their current life is great enough to bring

about solutions to their problems. Sometimes the nontherapeutic resources a person has are powerful enough: Good advice, emotional
support, and even insightful interpretation of disavowed motives by
friends and acquaintances can sometimes set off chain reactions of increasingly healthier behavior. The salutary effect on the forger Frank
Abagnale by FBI agent Carl Hanratty portrayed in Spielberg's film
Catch Me If You Can is a poignant case in point. In that movie, Abnagale
became less desctructively psychopathic as a result of Hanratty's influence. People seek psychotherapy, however, when ordinary resources
are not sufficient to foster the kind of adaptation they need to make. It
is not uncommon for an individual coming to treatment to have exhausted friends, relatives, teachers, doctors, and spiritual counselors in
an effort to solve some intractable psychological problem. And often,
these failed sources of help have behaved with impeccable intelligence
and concern, only to confront ultimate exasperation in the face of
someone's incomprehensible resistance to change. Schlesinger (2003)
astutely compares trying to make serious changes in someone's personality organization with trying to make significant reforms in an entrenched bureaucracy.

Even authorities in a very powerful position, including therapists,
do not have adequate clout *via their role alone* to counteract the effects
of many messages from childhood that rattle around in less accessible
areas of the brain. A friend of mine who had been raised by sexually repressive parents in a strict Boston Irish Catholic subculture struggled to
develop her stifled erotic potential; in particular, she felt a formidable
internal prohibition on masturbation. Intellectually, as an adult, she
found her inhibitions absurd. She wanted to be able to enjoy her body,
but every time she even thought about touching her genitals, she became either unbearably anxious or physically anesthetic. A priest to
whom she confessed her problem explained to her that most authorities in the contemporary Church do not consider masturbation a sin—
in fact, they regard it as preferable to forms of sexual expression that
exploit or misuse other human beings. He encouraged her to enjoy
God's gift of her capacity for self-arousal. She went home exhilarated,
expecting that this authoritative permission would liberate her. And
yet when she tried to masturbate, she was still overcome by guilt, and
her physical responsiveness shut down completely. Subsequently she
saw a sex therapist, but when she found she could not bear to do the
carefully graduated homework exercises she was assigned, she dropped
out of treatment.

In contrast to this experience, she described to me how later, in
analysis, her transference had slowly reached an emotional peak. With
the invitation to explore her emotional life in the safety of her analyst's

office, she started to experience herself as more and more like a child in the presence of her prudish, intimidating mother. As the analyst's ordinary boundaries began to feel like arbitrary and irrational restrictions on her freedom, she slowly found the courage to express her anger and resentment without censorship. After weeks of attacking her therapist for what she was experiencing as his oppressive "rules," she was able to take in the fact that he was actually on the side of her capacity to enjoy her sexuality. At that point the masturbation taboo began to dissipate. Once the analyst had become, in her subjective world, as emotionally powerful as the repressive mother of her girlhood, his "permission" carried much more clout than that of either her sensitive priest or her competent sex therapist.

This story is both illuminating and cautionary. It has a happy ending because the analyst could tolerate the emotional storms that were unleashed by his cultivation of the transference and because despite the siege on his boundaries, he was unfailingly clear about keeping them. He was appreciative of the power he had and did not misuse it. Other, more ominous endings would have been written if the analyst had acted in a way that made his patient feel humiliated about either her inhibition or the intense feelings that surfaced as she tried to address it, or if he had prematurely tried to "reason" with her, or if he had defensively explained away her rage at being constricted by insisting that these feelings belonged to her mother rather than to him (this could have easily been rationalized as "interpreting the transference")—not to mention the disaster that would have ensued if he had been narcissistic enough to decide that what his patient needed from him was not emotional availability and professional discipline but sexual stimulation.

A quarter of a century ago, Hans Strupp and his colleagues published a book aptly titled *Psychotherapy for Better or Worse* (Strupp, Hadley, & Gomez-Schwartz, 1977), written partly in response to claims that psychotherapy is ineffectual. Some psychologists had concluded from outcome studies that therapy (presumably psychodynamic treatment, as that was the major kind available at the time) is no more effective than spending an equivalent amount of time on a clinic waiting list. Strupp and his colleagues noted that when one carefully examines the data, therapy appears to have been *either* beneficial *or* damaging for the patients studied. A reasonable inference is therefore not that therapy does not matter but that it matters for good or ill—not exactly a comforting finding for clinicians, but at least not a shocking one to those of us who make our living trying to help people, who see again and again the unmistakable positive and negative consequences of our work and that of our colleagues. The problem of "negative effects" still troubles the field and is the flip side of the phenomenon of the therapist's power.

Resistances to Appreciating One's Power as a Therapist

When I first began doing psychodynamic therapy, despite all my training I found myself shocked by the fact that my patients took my interventions seriously, developed powerful transferences to me, and got better. I remember thinking, "It makes sense that I would react to *my* therapist that way—after all, he's a very powerful person. But I'm only me." We all carry around as a primary identity the sense of being a child, of being the one dependent on the power of others, perhaps even of being an innocent. For many people with significant power, it never ceases to be a bit surprising that others defer. Unless a defensive grandiosity has silenced the weak child within, most powerful people harbor some fears of being found out as an ordinary human being. Inadequate appreciation of the far-reaching implications of their power is not uncommon.

I doubt that most clinicians fully appreciate the nature and extent of their power. By temperament and calling, most therapists identify automatically with the weak and relatively powerless. Not only do we all have the residue of our childhood belief that it is the other people who are really in charge, we also have recurrent experiences that remind us how slow and incremental our work is. Especially in contrast to the compensatory childhood fantasies that may have attracted us to this way of earning our living, we must repeatedly acknowledge how little capacity we have to instigate the dramatic rescues we may have once imagined. It can consequently be a rude awakening every time some casual or even carefully empathic remark precipitates a devastated reaction in a client. It is not surprising that therapists have a reputation for carefully weighing their words, even outside the clinical situation. It is a hard habit to break.

On the other hand, there are aspects of the therapy situation that insidiously reinforce grandiosity and buttress the attractive assumption that one's words are *intrinsically* powerful, not just powerful because of one's role and activity in that role. A psychotherapist seeking support for unconscious fantasies of omnipotence does not have to be clinically effective or interpretively brilliant or even competent. On any given day, a therapist sees one person after another for whom he or she, by virtue of a particular ritual and role, has become a highly significant figure in that person's current life. Even when a client conveys hostility and devaluation, a sensitive clinician can feel how much preoccupation and emotional energy those feelings contain. Clients put us at the cen-

ter of their affective experience, supervisees look for someone to idealize, and only the most courageous students readily take issue with mentors who are in a position to influence their careers. After a while, it
becomes easy for those of us with clinical authority and narcissistic vulnerability to believe we are pretty special.

Anyone who wants to see the worst-case illustration of this dynamic should read Linda Hopkins's (1998) chilling reflections on the
personal and professional fortunes of Masud Khan, the brilliant but
characterologically flawed *enfant terrible* of midcentury British psychoanalytic circles. My friend Arnold Lazarus, who delights in providing
me with examples of the most appalling aspects of psychoanalytic history, recently forwarded an article on Khan to me, evidently having
concluded that psychoanalysis has been irredeemably corrupted by omnipotent misbehavior of this sort by everyone from Freud on down. I
have seen enough integrity in analysts and enough malfeasance in deni-
zens of other therapeutic communities to suspect that the problem is
not so much with analysis as with human nature and the seductions of
power. But it is incontestable that psychoanalytic therapy provides fertile territory for misusing one's role.

Empowering the Patient

In the course of psychotherapies that are going well, clients gradually
feel more realistically powerful and less dependent on their therapist's
power, more emotionally equal and less inferior in their role. Many of
the standard features of psychoanalytic practice represent the effort to
help patients find, embrace, and expand their power. For example, by
withholding advice and overt personal influence, therapists implicitly
express their confidence that patients can discover or craft their own
answers once they understand themselves better. By waiting for the client to choose the topics discussed in any session, we try to convey a
sense of trust that some inner dynamism in the patient "knows" how to
get to the problem area. By surviving the intensity of their negative
feelings, we demonstrate that their power is not necessarily destructive.
Even when we work with people whose psychology requires us to be
more active and advisory, we take pains to respect their potential autonomy as far as this is possible and safe.

By the phrase "realistically powerful" in the previous paragraph, I
allude to the fact that there are clients who begin treatment with a
sense of omnipotence (sometimes of psychotic proportions) and thus
feel anything but weak. Some of these clients are miserable because
they feel their power is evil and dangerous; others complain that despite their obvious power, there seems to be something wrong with

their capacity to enjoy life. For such individuals, the sense of power is defensive: Their grandiosity protects against feelings of terror, rage, envy, humiliation, or unbearable grief. It is also ultimately illusory. It contrasts stunningly with the realistic power expressed in a growing sense of authentic competence, perception of options and choice, willingness to take risks, and confidence in one's ability to handle problems—in other words, those capacities that arise in therapy out of repeated experiences of unpunished self-expression and mutually examined efforts to alter self-defeating patterns.

Under ideal circumstances, by the end of a successful course of therapy the patient feels grateful for the therapist's professional competence but not awe-struck at the therapist's wisdom, goodness, or power. Some degree of idealization may work in favor of the therapy process, but as termination approaches, idealizing feelings should have shrunk to normal appreciation, by both parties, for a job well done. The patient feels empowered to leave and also to choose to come back if problems arise in the future. By this time, there is typically a warm, egalitarian feeling between client and clinician. (Therapists joke among themselves that the job is a masochist's paradise: Just as we come to feel that a patient is easy to be with, pleasant to listen to, someone we would enjoy having as a friend, we have to let him or her go and greet the next miserable malcontent.)

The foregoing description may not apply to patients with severe psychopathology—some of whom have to hire and fire several therapists before they can settle in with one they dare to try to trust. It also does not fit the circumstances of practitioners who work in settings where the length of therapy is not under the patient's control. Under conditions of forced termination, the best a therapist can do is to try to maximize his or her power during the main portion of the treatment and then take care toward the end to try to "return" it to the patient. A common way of doing this when the work has gone well is to congratulate the client for the progress and to make explicit statements about how whatever was accomplished reflects not just the therapist's skill but the patient's talent and hard work. Residual idealization is probably more common after short-term than long-term work.

Love

The psychotherapy situation naturally elicits love from clients. In fact, it does so in such a reliable way that Martin Bergmann (1987, p. 213) has observed, "For centuries men and women have searched for mandrake roots and other substances from which a love potion could be brewed. And then . . . a Jewish Viennese physician uncovered love's se-

cret." The secret is to listen carefully, to be genuinely interested in the
other person, to react in an accepting and nonshaming way to his or
her disclosures, and to make no demands that the other party meet
one's emotional needs—defining aspects of the psychoanalytic arrangement.

It has long been known that many patients fall in love with or
come to love their therapists. It has been less highly publicized that
therapists love many of their patients, though there is a certain amount
of fantasy about this that can be inferred from some movie versions of
psychotherapy. Matter-of-fact acknowledgments in the psychoanalytic
literature that we love our clients are rare, and even rarer are suggestions that it is our love that is the main therapeutic agent (see, however,
Ferenczi, 1932; Gitelson, 1962; Hirsch, 1994; I. Hoffman, 1998; Lear,
1990; Little, 1951; Loewald, 1960; Nacht, 1962; Pine, 1985; Searles,
1959; Steingart, 1993). In fact, there has been a certain amount of disdain in some psychoanalytic quarters for the idea that love cures.
Kohut's theories were more than once critiqued on the grounds that
his ideas were reducible to trying to heal patients via the analyst's love
and hence were *ipso facto* suspect.

But there are signs that the L-word is coming out of the closet. In
the year I was getting this book ready for publication, there appeared
two ground-breaking articles on the role of love in therapy, both from
analysts who assume intersubjectivity and mutuality in the psychotherapy process. Joseph Natterson (2003) suggests that we view psychotherapy as a "mutually loving process" in which the therapist's "subordinated subjectivity" fosters an actualization of love along with an
actualization of self in patients, through a natural progression of desire, belief, and hope. Daniel Shaw (2003), after noting the skittishness
with which psychoanalytic writers have addressed the question of their
love for their patients, concludes that "analytic love," which he differentiates from romantic, sexual, and countertransferential love, can be a
critical element in healing. Shaw raises an interesting question:

> Psychoanalysis provides a ritualized setting for a process that encour-
> ages the development of the analysand's intimate awareness of him-
> self. In the process, analyst and analysand inevitably and necessarily
> become intimately involved with each other, intellectually and emo-
> tionally. At the heart of this endeavor . . . is a search for love, for the
> sense of being lovable, for the remobilization of thwarted capacities
> to give love and to receive love. This may seem a more fitting descrip-
> tion of the analysand than the analyst, but consider our choice of
> profession. Is it not likely that we chose our work, at least in part,
> because it affords us the means of realizing the aim of being especially
> important to—especially loved and valued by—our analysands? (pp.
> 252–253)

I would add that being a therapist offers us the opportunity to experience ourselves *as loving*, a state of mind that is inherently rewarding and good for the self-esteem. And as Racker (1968) noted, the loving attitude inherent in conducting therapy also assuages guilt by symbolically making reparation to early love objects whom we unconsciously believe we have damaged.

It is increasingly clear from empirical studies of psychotherapy that it is the relationship that heals. But "the relationship" is a bit of an abstraction. What happens between two people when one enters the relationship suffering and leaves it feeling less symptomatic, more alive, more agentic, more genuine? Neuropsychological studies are revealing that objectively, when we remain in intimate emotional contact with another person, changes take place in our respective brains (see Chapter 11). But subjectively, it certainly seems that love has been generated in the dyad and has been taken in by the client with therapeutic effects. I think Bergmann (1987) is right (and this was Freud's meaning as well, in his comment to Jung that psychoanalysis is a cure through love) that what initially inspires the patient's love for the therapist is the sense that the therapist is both similar to (by being in a caregiving role) and different from the childhood caregivers. After the alliance is established, it is often the ways the therapist differs from the parents that touch clients most powerfully.

But at some point (early with more borderline and psychotic clients and later with neurotic-level people), the therapist is experienced as just like the pathogenic early love objects. With each new patient I become awed once more by the emergence of transference and transferential reenactments. The recurrence in the therapeutic relationship of the main emotional currents in the client's history is a wondrous phenomenon. What makes it especially fascinating is that both parties to therapy start out earnestly resolving that what happened to the client earlier *will not happen* this time around. The patient is looking to undo the prior damage and thus tries to choose a therapist who offers a contrasting experience to the one internalized in childhood; the therapist longs not to fail the patient as the early caregivers did. And yet with stunning inevitability, both parties find themselves caught up in repetition: Patients who are convinced that all authorities are critical elicit the critical part of the therapist, those who presume that all men are narcissistic somehow evoke the narcissism of a male clinician, and so forth. If our hopes that we can love someone into health via understanding and good intentions are doomed, if instead we replicate the pain of the past, where does the love come in?

I think the therapist's love is experienced mainly in processing the repetitions. The client may feel hurt in ways excruciatingly like his or her childhood suffering, and yet the therapist, unlike the early love objects, tolerates the client's pain, knows that the interaction feels horribly familiar, and by empathy and interpretation contributes to the client's capacity to distinguish what has happened now from what happened in the past. The patient's activity in recreating the situation is examined nonjudgmentally, leading ultimately to an increase in the sense of agency. The affects attending the repetition are accepted and processed as they were not the first time around. And frequently, the therapist's remorse about having participated in replicating a painful early experience is evident to the client, who feels the loving repair that is inherent in apology. It can be deeply touching to patients to realize that the therapist's narcissistic wishes to be perfect or to be seen as innocent take second place to his or her honesty and wish to restore the therapeutic connection.

Winnicott (1947) was doubtless right that hatred is as inevitable and important as love, and that many patients need to evoke the therapist's sincere hate before they can tolerate his or her love. And Ferenczi (1932, cited in Shaw, 2003) seems intuitively accurate in bemoaning the fact that one cannot just decide to love a patient; the feeling must be genuine to be therapeutic. Those clinical populations that are most damaged in their capacity to love, namely, antisocial and narcissistically organized individuals, are also the most notoriously difficult to help. Could that be because their incapacity to love makes it hard for therapists to feel genuinely loving toward them?

I have worked with people it took me literally years to love. I had to endure a lot of hostile, defensive posturing that was very off-putting before I felt I had made contact with the hurt and lovable person under all the layers of self-protection. It troubles me when I cannot find something to love in a person who comes to me for help, and I suspect that this feeling is not uncommon among therapists. With the patient I mentioned in Chapter 3, whose passive hostility sparked the unsatisfying interchange with my would-be Rogerian supervisor, I was not able to feel any genuine compassion toward her until I serendipitously caught a stomach flu. My gastrointestinal symptoms were strikingly similar to those of the psychosomatically implicated ailments about which she interminably complained, and they were miserable. When I "got" viscerally the kind of pain and nausea she coped with every day, discomforts I had to bear for only a day or two, my heart finally went out to her. In a similar vein, my friend Nicole Moore, a psychiatrist in the U.S. Air Force, confided (personal communication, August 20, 2003):

> I don't like *myself* when I can't find something to love in a patient. I *look* for it. Often I can find something in the person's history that stirs my genuine compassion; I can love the child who went through that and

hold an image of that child in my heart. I think when patients see the love reflected back at them, they start to believe they are lovable after all, and they start to get better.

I want to make it clear that psychoanalytic love includes respect and is anything but infantilizing. It is not incompatible with all the negative feelings toward patients that get stirred up in therapy, nor is it incompatible with setting limits, interpreting defenses, confronting self-destructiveness, and inflicting inevitable pain—both by accurate observations that are hard on a patient's self-esteem and by inaccurate ones that disappoint because the therapist has again demonstrated fallibility. Like any kind of love worth the name, it is not based on distortion; that is, therapists do not idealize clients in order to feel loving toward them. We try to love them as they are and have faith that they can grow in the ways they need to grow.

I doubt that anyone can feel truly loved unless he or she has been truly recognized as a combination of positive and negative qualities, good and evil. Here I return to the theme of honesty: In supporting the effort to pursue and name what feels true, no matter how unattractive, the therapist creates the conditions under which clients can feel loved for who they really are. In the context of this love, they can begin to expand, to experiment, to hope, to change. As Shaw (2003) concluded:

> Analytic love is indeed complicated and dangerous, and like all loving, carries the potential for devastating disappointment. This knowledge, rather than leading us to ignore, omit, or cancel our love, seems instead a call to persist in loving, as authentically, deeply, respectfully, and responsibly as we can. (p. 275)

NOTES

1. Although Spence and Schafer take their observation in radically different directions, they have both pointed out that clinical narrations cannot be assumed to be historical "facts." Schafer has recently commented, "Donald Spence ... a confirmed empiricist ... criticizes psychoanalysis for not amassing hard historical facts through scientific research that would satisfy hard-nosed experimentalists. I view Spence as my polar opposite. For me, clinical narrations are versions of a life that are as close to true versions as one can hope to get through analysis" (1999, pp. 348–349).
2. I have made the argument for formal and comprehensive history-taking in Chapter 1 of *Psychoanalytic Diagnosis* (McWilliams, 1994). I have discussed

the process of developing and sharing a dynamic formulation in Chapter 2 of *Psychoanalytic Case Formulation* (McWilliams, 1999).

3. For an interesting use of this principle within a classical psychoanalytic treatment, see Volkan (1984). In more recent psychoanalytic writing on helping therapists to help patients to speak with feeling, Martha Stark's (1994) explication of her distinctive interpretive style, Stephen Appelbaum's (2000) book on "evocativeness," and Karen Maroda's intended book on technique from a relational perspective document different ways of furthering authentic expression.

Chapter 7

Boundaries II: Quandaries

What other occupation requires of its practitioners that
they be the objects of people's excoriations, threats and
rejections, or be subjected to tantalizing offerings that
plead "touch me," yet may not be touched? What other
occupation has built into it the frustration of feeling
helpless, stupid and lost as a necessary part of the work?
And what other occupation puts its practitioners in the
position of being an onlooker or midwife to the
fulfillment of others' destinies?
—EMMANUEL GHENT (1990, p. 133)

Most of this chapter concerns issues that might be labeled
"Things they didn't tell me in my training program." Recently, in preparation for a lecture I had agreed to give on that general topic to a convention of therapists, I asked members of one of my consultation
groups to associate freely and out loud about common clinical quanda-
ries for which their formal professional training had not prepared
them. It was a fascinating meeting, punctuated by the laughter of mutual recognition and the eye-rolling of reciprocal condolence. It also
raised important questions about the lacunae in our literature on psychotherapy, the inadequacy of academic psychology and descriptive
psychiatry to give us insight into some very common but unresearched
phenomena, and the inevitable insufficiencies of our ethics codes.

Therapists often begin their professional life having been told
(or having inferred) that they must accept the client as is, and that
their own needs and feelings must be subordinated to the task of
empathic understanding, regardless of what the patient presents. This
well-intentioned position can be taken too far. A colleague of mine
describes how she was asked, when interning in a mental hospital, to
do psychological testing with a man whose problems included com-

163

pulsive masturbation. He was brought to her office in a bathrobe, and as she began the evaluation procedure, he opened it and began playing with his penis. Because no one had ever emphasized that she had a right to define her own professional boundaries, she did not feel comfortable insisting that he wear street clothes and control his behavior during the testing. It must have been an awkward couple of hours.

I have arbitrarily divided the topic at hand into accidental or unpreventable boundary problems and unconsciously orchestrated enactments. Admittedly, many of the most troublesome interactions between therapists and clients have aspects of both conscious innocence and unconscious premeditation. In addition, seemingly similar incidents can have substantially different dynamics or radically different meanings to the participants. Nevertheless, it makes a difference to a therapist whether one is confronting a situation unforseen by both parties or whether one has been presented with a dilemma that the client, often with the therapist's unconscious participation, crafted in order to stage and work over some internal conflict.

In a separate section, I deal with the question of the therapist's self-disclosure. During the past couple of decades, this topic has inspired a vast literature, especially by analysts in the relational movement. In that literature as well as in case conferences and workshops, analytic practitioners have been increasingly forthcoming about the fact that their behavior with clients often deviates from the idealized "classical" model with which many of them were originally inculcated, a model that took literally Freud's injunction to the analyst to "be opaque to his patients and, like a mirror, . . . show them nothing but what is shown to him" (1912b, p. 118). I cannot do justice to all the nuances of self-disclosure issues in a short space, but I can at least give readers a sense of the landscape and its main features.

Finally, I take up the multifaceted question of touch in psychotherapy. That topic is so complex, so redolent of deep emotional memories, so dependent on context for its meaning, and so culturally various in its expressions that it requires its own treatment. Every experienced psychoanalytic therapist I know has had patients who have requested or demanded a hug, or who have suddenly grabbed the therapist in an embrace. And yet all of them also say that their training in psychotherapy did not prepare them for how to deal with these situations. Beyond their teachers' exhortations not to have sexual contact with a client, there is a vast expanse in which beginning therapists often find themselves at sea. In what follows, I hope to make it a little easier for them to navigate those waters.

ACCIDENTS AND MORE OR LESS
INNOCENT EVENTS

Chance Encounters

One of the most burdensome side effects of being a therapist is that
when one runs into a patient unexpectedly, all kinds of problems may
arise. This is true to some extent for members of any profession with
emotional power—many people find themselves self-conscious and
hypersensitive when they have out-of-role interactions with their gyne-
cologist or their child's teacher or any kind of celebrity—but the question of how to handle unexpected encounters is particularly problematic for psychoanalytic therapists and their patients. Practitioners in
Manhattan tell me that chance meetings happen often enough even
in large, urban environments; in small, rural communities, managing
out-of-office interactions with patients is a chronic fact of professional life. Among pastoral counselors, interactions with their clients
within their communities of faith are commonplace. In university settings, running into patients is virtually unavoidable. When one of my
clinical psychology graduate students decided to round out her life
by doing something utterly unrelated to psychotherapy training, she
arrived in her leotard for the first meeting of a small dance class,
only to have a client show up for the same instruction. Another colleague encountered a client at a four-person meeting for academics
interested in Buddhism.

Handling intrusions into what one expected to be private space is a
source of significant unacknowledged stress for therapists. The fact that
one has to exert a constant discipline *inside* the consulting room is an expected demand of the therapeutic role, but it can come as a painful shock
that a comparable degree of discipline is often required in one's free
time. Moreover, many therapists have fantasies about the dangers of personal exposure that rival the nightmares of their most paranoid clients.
Suggesting that therapists do not talk enough among themselves about
the dynamics of their own dread of being found out in some horrifying
way, Jonathan Slavin (2002) recently quipped to an appreciative audience
of psychoanalysts that unexpected run-ins with patients are frequently
described with the affect appropriate to a "near-death experience."

Beyond our neurotic reasons for discomfort with unplanned encounters, there are some perfectly realistic professional problems that
they raise, mainly because the emotional context is complicated. People who are unexpectedly confronted with the off-duty presence of
their therapist tend to be conflicted in their reactions, and individual
patients differ about which side of the conflict they express. On one

hand, the asymmetrical nature of psychoanalytic relationships (the fact that therapists know intimate details of their clients' lives, whereas clients know comparatively little about the lives of their therapists) can make the real-life existence of the therapist a matter of intense fascination to clients. On the other, the fact that therapists hear people's most shame-filled secrets gives some patients more than enough motivation to hope they will never encounter their therapist anywhere but in the office. Some individuals are so secretive about even being in therapy—never mind the content of their revelations—that they do not want us to admit to knowing them, while others feel terribly wounded if they bump into us socially and are treated as invisible. Some are thrilled to find that the therapist is "just another human being," while others are distressed that their idealized image of the therapist has been tainted. It is important here, as in most other areas, to follow the patient's lead, but it is not always easy to figure out what that is.

What boundaries are appropriate for these "extratherapeutic" contacts? This question is more complicated than policies about money and time, because less of the issue is under the therapist's control. Moreover, at the beginning of treatment, it makes little sense to talk about a policy for out-of-office encounters, because unless the client has had previous psychotherapy, he or she has no experiential basis for expecting that it will be a big deal to run into the therapist out of role. Still, if the two parties have reason to expect that their paths will cross, they should at least discuss whether they will say hello or whether the patient prefers to act as if the therapist is a stranger. If they have significant overlapping social connections and there are other resources available, for the sake of both therapist and patient they should rethink whether it is a good idea to work together. If they live and work in a small community with limited therapeutic resources, there may be no choice but to contract for treatment knowing that they will encounter each other repeatedly. An early conversation about this fact of life may be critical to the success of therapy.

As with every aspect of clinical decision-making, much depends on the patient and the nature of the therapeutic contract. It is relatively easy to sound out a higher-functioning patient about how he or she prefers the therapist to behave at chance meetings (i.e., whether the therapist should acknowledge the client, whether the client would want to introduce the therapist to family members or friends, what signal the client could give when not wanting to be approached), and then to respect the person's wishes. In the special case where the patient is also a therapist or where the two parties are unavoidably in the same religious or political group, therapist and patient can expect to find themselves together at meetings, conferences, and social events. Typically, the therapeutic partners greet one another with a little cordial small talk and then keep a respectful distance.

Yet even with clients in the neurotic-to-healthy ranges, once strong transference feelings have developed, out-of-office encounters can create very troublesome situations for both parties. It is a frustrating fact of psychodynamic life that patients who are immersed in powerful transferences may assume that seeing the therapist out of role equates to seeing the "real" therapist. In other words, they may insist on the validity of their transference-driven perceptions because at this sighting, the clinician is not behaving with the reserve and discipline typical of his or her office behavior, and patients can find evidence, in this less inhibited version of their therapist, that everything they fear (or wish) is true.

An analysand of mine, a woman whose mother had wanted her to be a boy, was certain that I prefer males to females. One day she came to her session crushed, because she had seen me at a conference luncheon, where I had chosen to sit next to a man. In this instance, I happened to remember and so called to her attention the fact that the person on my other side was a woman. Her selective perception became obvious enough to her that she was able to entertain a small challenge to her conviction that, like her mother, I disdain people of her gender. Unfortunately, one does not always have such evidence available. I could just as easily have been sitting between two men, or between two women by whom I seemed bored. Or I could have been talking only to the man when my patient happened to be watching. It is much harder to analyze the client's contribution to a perception that is bolstered by evidence from outside the office, and when that evidence is interpreted in support of hurtful early beliefs, it is painful to both therapist and client.

With more troubled or emotionally vulnerable patients, extra-therapeutic contacts are frequently quite disturbing. Some narcissistic individuals cannot tolerate the damage to their idealization when they run into their usually elegant therapist at the mall, in jeans, looking harried and herding a preschool brood where they do not want to go. Clients with a paranoid streak have been known to fire their therapist because of seeing a politically unacceptable bumper sticker on the clinician's car. People with histories of sexual abuse can be terrified if they perceive evidence of their therapist's sexuality or seductiveness in social situations. Of course, it is critical to talk with patients immediately after any such encounter and to try to process their reactions, but occasionally they are too distressed to do so and bolt precipitously from treatment, leaving the therapist with an irrational but intense guilt. I once lost a paranoid client with whom I had worked productively for two years because he saw me at a restaurant, having lunch with a person he despised. Especially given the inevitability of unplanned encounters and the importance of therapists' having satisfying involvements outside their professional role, I do not know of any way to deal with these severe, therapy-destroying reactions other than with a philosophical attitude: Shit happens.

Some patients, especially when under the sway of an intense transference, actively seek out extratherapeutic interactions. They may also go to great lengths to find out information about their therapists; the Internet offers endless possibilities for intrusiveness. In individuals with serious psychopathology, especially borderline clients with any tendency toward erotomania, interest in learning about the therapist's "real" self can become intense and obsessive. A patient of one of my colleagues announced that she had joined her therapist's gym in hopes of seeing her naked. More than one practitioner I know has been stalked by a borderline patient. It is crucial for a clinician to make clear to such a person what behavior will not be tolerated, and what will be the consequences if the therapist's boundaries are ignored (e.g., a break from treatment for several days or weeks). With patients who invade their privacy, therapists must set reasonable self-protective limits and insist on compliance, even if that means reporting the client's harassment to law enforcement officials. In the absence of utterly consistent boundaries, efforts to interpret or to convey understanding of the client's driven behavior will only reinforce the invasive actions and the primitive fantasies they express (see Blum, 1973; Meloy, 1998).

As I stressed in the previous chapter, it is important for psychoanalytic practitioners to appreciate that to their patients, they are never really "out of role." The power in the role affects clients sufficiently that the therapist cannot voluntarily exit from a consequential place in their emotional experience. It can be tempting for many reasons to try to dissolve or ignore boundaries created by role and relate "just as one person to another," but the interaction is rarely received that way. In my community, a man who sat on the town council once created a local political disaster by criticizing an elected official in colorful terms to a neighbor. "But I wasn't speaking as a councilman," he protested; "I was just speaking as a friend." It was hard for him to assimilate the fact that he was not the one in control of how his remarks were received. Similarly, therapists must accept the reality that they are involved in something that has its own dynamic, a dynamic that is frustratingly unresponsive to a clinician's acts of will.

Innocent Invitations

Some of our customers arrive at our doorstep already knowing that it is conventional to keep the therapist–patient relationship uncontaminated by coexisting connections in the world beyond the consulting room. Others make the perfectly reasonable assumption that the therapist is like most other professionals—teachers, dentists, veterinarians, attorneys, accountants, clergy, doctors, people one might get to know in a social setting after the professional business is transacted. These clients may invite the practitioner to dinner or to a party or fund-raising event in the same way that they would invite any professional they got to know to such a function. Even when such invitations are full of unconscious wishes and fantasies, they may be extended with an innocent ignorance of their potentially problematic nature. In the early years of the psychoanalytic movement, before we fully appreciated the implications of the phenomenon of transference, analysts were similarly naive; they assumed it was natural to be in multiple roles with patients, just as they would have been had they been someone's family doctor. Freud used to introduce his analysands to his wife and children. He also took his friends, colleagues, and even his daughter into treatment. He meddled in his patients' love lives. Sometimes an analyst and analysand in the same professional community would go on vacations together and continue the analysis. Instances of what would now be considered boundary transgressions sometimes worked out reasonably well, but the more egregious examples had negative and even disastrous consequences (Gabbard, 1995).

Innocent invitations for out-of-office interaction tend to be extended early in therapy, before the transference heats up and the patient naturally comes to see the awkwardness of combining a therapeutic relationship with social interactions. The clinician's response to such an invitation should be something along the lines of "thanks very much. I appreciate the invitation, but I've learned over time that it's better in a psychotherapy relationship to try to avoid contact outside the therapy hour. It can get really difficult and uncomfortable, when you're exposing all kinds of intimate thoughts and feelings here, for us to interact in a matter-of-fact social way. It can feel oddly false, and although I'm sorry to miss out on what you're offering, I'm going to decline, based on my overall sense that it's better for you and me to keep our relationship uncomplicated by interactions outside our work here."

If the client persists and/or seems wounded, one has to clarify the message and reinforce it without acting out one's natural irritation at being put in the painful position of disappointing a person one cares about. One can say, for example, "Maybe I'm being too rigid, but I've found I just can't be in two different roles with people I work with as a therapist. It's one of those limitations I have that you and I will just have to live with." In subsequent sessions, it is important to be alert for evidence of the client's reaction, which may include a painful sense of having been rejected, a belief that the therapist is critical of the person for having asked, and fantasies that the "real" reason for the refusal is the therapist's distaste for the patient. Occasionally, there may also be some awareness of the relief that comes with learning that the therapist will preserve the boundaries even when given attractive invitations to transgress them.

Cultural and subcultural norms may complicate this issue (Foster, Moskowitz, & Javier, 1996; Sue & Sue, 1990). In some ethnic groups, parents, grandparents, or other family authorities may insist on meeting a family member's therapist before supporting the person's decision to go into treatment. I have known several practitioners working in ethnically distinctive communities who routinely accept dinner invitations from the families of prospective clients, knowing that in the subculture in which they practice, psychotherapy is not going to happen without the family's approval of the practitioner. While teaching in New Zealand, I learned that in Maori subcultures, families observe a ritual at the beginning of a member's therapy, in which the therapist symbolically becomes part of the family. At the end of treatment, there is a ceremony of leave taking from the family. Sometimes one has to become known to some extent as a "real person" outside the office before one can take a patient into treatment and slowly socialize him or her into the role conventions that govern psychodynamic therapy.

ENACTMENTS

Over the past several decades, analytic therapists have noted changes in the kinds of clients who come to them for help. The rigid, moralistic, inhibited patient of the Freudian era is not unknown, but much more common now is the person who repeatedly acts in driven, highly destructive, entitled, or self-harming ways. Suicidal and parasuicidal gestures, abusive behavior, sexual risk taking, self-mutilation, eating disorders, and addictions of various kinds seem to be the order of our day. We are seeing more clients diagnosed as borderline, personality-disordered, and posttraumatic. Whether or not societal changes have brought about a significant shift in psychopathologies (as many therapists believe), more individuals with serious problems controlling their behavior are seeking psychotherapy. Such patients typically com-

municate with their therapists more by enactment than by verbalization.

Relational analysts have persuasively argued that even the treatments of cooperative, verbally adept individuals are better understood
in terms of the progressive clarification and exploration of mutual enactments than by reference to the analyst's dispassionate interpretation
of free associations (see Hirsch, 1998). A consensus seems to be evolving (J. Greenberg, 1991; I. Hoffman, 1996; Jacobs, 1986; Mitchell,
1988; Renik, 1996; Slavin & Kriegman, 1998; Stolorow & Atwood,
1997) to the effect that it is not possible to avoid being pulled into the
dramas that are central in the patient's psychology (cf. Levenson,
1972). Nevertheless, there is a marked difference between the subtle
inductions into repetition that characterize the analyses of high-
functioning individuals and the stark pressures for special concessions
made by more troubled patients. My remarks in this section pertain
mostly to the less self-observing, more regressed and demanding clients who desperately need therapy yet repeatedly put the treatment in
jeopardy. There follows a discussion of some provocations and potential boundary infringements with which therapists often cope.

Attacks on Professionalism

Some clients behave toward the therapist in ways that broadcast a refusal to respect the clinician's professionalism. Often, a person is
overtly cooperative and friendly while being covertly devaluing. Young-
looking therapists and those the client knows to be in training are particularly vulnerable to this indirect yet palpably hostile depreciation.
Examples include the patient who immediately uses the therapist's first
name in a tone more appropriate to a teenage pal, the patient who in-
terrupts a discussion of serious issues to exclaim, "Nice earrings!
Where did you get them?," the patient who repeatedly touches the therapist's arm or shoulder with the familiarity of a buddy, and the patient
who flirts or tells jokes or tries to seduce the therapist into an alliance
against the other sex or some third party, as if the practitioner's appropriate role is to gossip about the perfidy of men or the exasperating
habits of mothers-in-law.

It is hard to respond in a professional manner to these incursions.
The client's behavior invites a kind of chumminess, yet if the therapist
accepts it at face value, an important resistance to authentic participation in treatment will be collusively ignored. On the other hand, a therapist who addresses the devaluation directly risks sounding as prim and
judgmental as a high school librarian enforcing a no-talking rule—thus
providing new ammunition for the client's campaign to avoid acknowl-

edging the therapist's position of responsibility and to escape the invitation to rely on it. The best way I know out of this dilemma is via one's sense of humor. Ideally, the therapist can find a way to enjoy the playfulness in the client's provocation (much as one would enjoy a three-year-old child who experiments with calling her mother "Emily"), and can make a light, slightly teasing, matter-of-fact quip that does not require a thoughtful response from the client. For example, "I see you enjoy being on a first-name basis," or "You'd rather talk about my earrings than about your problems?," or "If I didn't know you had come here because you're suffering, I'd think you were trying to pick me up!," or "Once we agree about everything that's wrong with men, maybe we can get into how particular men have disappointed you."

In carrying off comments like these, it helps for the therapist to have a kind demeanor and an unflustered tone. If the clinician seems too irritated, the client can feel devastatingly exposed (as a hostile provocateur) and/or privately triumphant (for successfully getting the authority off balance), and neither attitude is particularly conducive to the progressive self-revelation that therapy requires. If the therapist's annoyance does leak out and the patient picks it up, one can simply admit that it is hard to remain nondefensive when one feels subtly attacked. The therapist can follow up such a remark with some comment that shows that he or she has not lost a sense of humor. Even if the clinician's intervention is empathic and adroit, the patient is likely to feel a pang of humiliation; consequently, some processing of the interaction may be necessary.

Newer therapists are often flummoxed by disarmingly provocative clients. They may find themselves absorbing a lot of hostility before figuring out how to address the relentless devaluation to which an ambivalent patient is subjecting them. Taking one's time to find a nonpunitive, self-respecting stance in the face of a covert assault is certainly warranted, given how disastrous it can be to the treatment for the therapist to come off as either impotent and self-devaluing or defensive and heavy-handed. It may help to practice delivering a casual and slightly self-mocking line such as "So you're afraid I'm a rank beginner who doesn't know the first thing about helping you," or "You seem to be trying to tell me that at my tender age I couldn't possibly know enough to be of any value to you." Fortunately, one's skill in responding quickly and gracefully to such provocations increases over time.

Loaded Invitations

Sometimes a client's invitations are not so innocent as those I discussed earlier; that is, they are extended in the context of at least some awareness that an acceptance of them would constitute a departure from conventional professional norms. Such solicitations often express the client's natural wish for evidence that he or she is in some way "special" to the therapist. Sometimes the dominant emotional tone in an invitation is gratitude. More than one client has invited me to her wedding, explaining that she experiences me as a loving parental figure who simply "belongs" at such an important rite of passage. Sometimes an invitation strikes the therapist as full of aggression, conscious or unconscious, as if the client is trying to corrupt the therapeutic process or daring the clinician to enter a conspiracy to "break the rules." It is my impression that many treatments include at least one occasion when the practitioner feels put on the spot by a patient who consciously intends, by asking the therapist to a special event, to honor the powerful attachment between the two parties. It can be difficult to decide how to respond therapeutically to such invitations, or even how to think about them. One has to consider whether it might be reasonable to accept, and, if not, how to decline without injuring the patient.

When one is given an invitation by a client, it is often wise to stall: One can reasonably ask the patient for time to consider the implications together. The parties need to think about the meanings in this particular context of both acceptance and rejection and to explore the inevitably complex motives behind the proposal. Occasionally, there is a good therapeutic reason to accept a patient's invitation. It is arguable, for example, that a practitioner's understanding of a musician or actor or athlete will be increased by attendance at one of the person's concerts or plays or games. Even if appearing at a client's performance does not significantly increase the therapist's understanding, it may be a critical gesture from the viewpoint of a client who needs to feel known by the practitioner not only as the embodiment of psychopathology but also as an effective adult in the world outside the consulting room.

If the therapist decides there is justification for accepting an invitation, he or she should consider doing so on the condition that social interactions will be minimal. The therapist's comfort in the situation is not a trivial issue. Even if the patient is proud of being in therapy, it is awkward to be introduced as someone's shrink; it makes other people uncomfortable, and it tends to leave the therapist feeling vaguely inappropriate, like a person who wore a business suit to a picnic. Being identified as the patient's "friend" or "colleague," on the other hand, feels discordant with the overall commitment to honesty that sustains analytic psychotherapy. Subtle issues of confidentiality may arise. Thus, agreeing to see a performance but declining to go backstage and meet the client's cohorts, or agreeing to be present at a wedding but not at the reception may sometimes resolve the tension between honoring the client's wishes and keeping the treatment free of unnecessary complications.

If, as is more frequently the case, the therapist feels that accepting an invitation would not be in the best interest of the treatment—or if the therapist simply does not want to attend for personal reasons—there is no way to avoid some hurt feelings. With higher-functioning clients, the resulting sense of rejection can be useful grist for the therapeutic mill, but with more fragile people, it can feel devastating and can shut down the therapeutic process. In fact, it is usually an appreciation of the tenuousness of a client's self-esteem that inclines therapists to accept invitations that might be more wisely declined. As with more innocent invitations, injury may be mitigated if the therapist demurs not on the basis of "this is for your own good" but by reference to personal needs and feelings. "I'm sorry, but I just wouldn't feel comfortable," or "I appreciate your inviting me, but I don't like being in social situations with people I'm working with in therapy. It can feel too strange and false to be in this very intimate professional role and simultaneously acting more like a social acquaintance." Or even, "I'd love to go, but I wouldn't want to get in trouble for seeming to violate the ethical standards of my profession, which are very strict about therapists staying in their role." If the therapist speaks calmly and with self-assurance—that is, without guilt or equivocation—clients are more likely to accept the limit and not to keep pressing, whatever their emotional reactions to being turned down.

It remains a possibility, however, that the reason for a professional limit has nothing to do with the clinician's comfort and everything to do with what is for the patient's "own good." I have sometimes wanted to accept a client's appealing invitation yet had to respect the quiet, insistent internal voice telling me it would not be a good idea. Even with unappealing requests for dubious favors, I have been tempted to yield to earnest, persistent entreaties just to placate a client or to try to show how generous I am. In such cases, especially when a client is winningly imploring the therapist to make an exception, or is hurt and angry about the therapist's refusal, the best one can do is to say something such as "I may be wrong, but 1 don't think what you want is really in your interest. As your therapist I have to stand for what makes sense to me."

The more there is an unconsciously hostile dimension to the invitation, the more the processing of what has happened can feel miserable to both parties. The therapist's refusal can be taken by the unconsciously guilty client as a kind of "gotcha!"—an accusation that the client is engaging in a covert act of aggression. Unless the therapist's initial reaction to the loaded invitation is free of insinuation that the client is behaving inappropriately in extending it, it is unlikely that the patient will be able to acknowledge without humiliation that there was a thorn in the bouquet that he or she offered. Many of the most painful interactions in therapy are endured in the context of enactments involving invitations, as well as in the related question of gifts.

Gifts

Like invitations, gifts may be fairly innocent or may be loaded with meaning. Some clients send fruit baskets at Christmas to all the important professionals in their lives and see no reason to exclude their therapist from the list. Modest offerings of this sort are not much of a problem: The therapist simply says thank you. If the patient's train of thought suggests, after this matter-of-fact communication, that there is a larger unconscious issue in tendering the gift, the therapist or the patient can find a way to bring that up. One of my clients memorably announced that she had noticed she brought me flowers when she was having murderous fantasies about me. If it is the therapist who introduces commentary on the patient's less friendly motives, it is important to avoid any implication that the unconscious motives cancel out the positive, conscious ones, and instead to convey a matter-of-fact attitude that most transactions contain some emotional ambivalence and ambiguity. As with every intervention, it is critical that the client not experience the therapist's statements as reductive and shaming, as if the message is, "You may have *thought* you felt X, but you *really* felt Y!" Instead, the therapist's comments should communicate "We knew you felt X, but now we can see that you *also* felt Y."

Small gifts that would not be easily construed as indicating the therapist's exploitation of the patient's resources (e.g., a box of cookies, a poem, or an inexpensive book or CD of significance to the client) are often accepted by therapists because rejecting them can cause undue hurt. The original psychoanalytic rationale (e.g., Eissler, 1953) for not accepting client's gifts, even small ones, was that gift giving is an expression of something that should be understood rather than acted out. By accepting a gift, many ego psychologists argued, the therapist would be colluding in a communication that bypasses words and, in so doing, would be foreclosing an opportunity to look at an important dynamic. Eventually, especially in the context of Heinz Kohut's writings (e.g., 1977) about the preeminence of empathy over other aspects of therapeutic communication, clinicians began to note that sometimes the refusal of a gift not only does not generate important psychological material but actually can reduce the possibilities for doing so. Many began noting that the acceptance of a small present from the patient can increase rather than decrease the possibilities for understanding the transaction; that is, the patient who feels that his or her gift is accepted appreciatively is not put on the defensive and can therefore get nondefensively interested in the deeper meanings of the gesture.

Sometimes, however, the interaction is conspicuously devoid of elements of sincere (even if ambivalent) benevolence. One of my colleagues has a patient who has repeatedly tried to shower him with lavish gifts, despite his unambiguous refusal to accept even small items. Gift giving is a compulsive feature of this woman's life outside the therapy and seems to embody a great deal of power and domination and very little generosity. The client admits that her friends and relatives complain that they feel criticized and controlled by her relentless offerings, all of which seem to contain some hidden criticism (e.g., an expensive curling iron for a daughter-in-law whose hair style she dislikes). Recently, in the face of the therapist's patient refusals to accept the presents she brought to the office, she began ordering items from the Internet and sending them to him anonymously. He has not signed for the deliveries of these packages and has taken the position that he is not willing to work with her until this behavior stops. The clinical grounds for his position is that if there is to be any possibility of change, this determination to be the one in the role of giver must be talked about rather than acted out. There is a risk-management issue here also; by accepting expensive gifts, he would be vulnerable to the charge of exploiting his patients for extratherapeutic services. Patients who engage in these sorts of power struggles seem to be particularly inclined to make complaints to authorities when they do not succeed in getting what they (consciously) want.

Requests for Other Treatments

Very often when clients begin to feel impatient with psychotherapy and critical of the therapist, they ask about getting a more concrete or directive treatment, such as medication or hypnosis or eye movement desensitization and reprocessing (EMDR). Or they may go to Internet sites about particular disorders and come back with the impression that cognitive-behavioral treatments are the only effective therapies for their problem. Such requests may express a realistic, self-respecting interest in trying another approach, but they may also be a way to express negative feelings about the therapist and therapy without doing so directly. Therapists can usually tell by their countertransference reactions whether such a question reflects mostly a sincere interest in another modality or whether it is mainly a way of communicating hostility. If such a query is predominantly hostile, the therapist will feel irritated and defensive. Whatever the flavor of the inquiry, clients deserve an eventual response to their manifest question (such as the admission that the therapist is not trained in EMDR or regards it as inappropriate for the patient's problem, or the comment that most controlled research has established that hypnosis is not a reliable means of recovering early memories, or the statement that the therapist would be glad to refer the client for adjunctive EMDR or cognitive-behavioral therapy or medication).

If the inquiry seems a vehicle for hostility, it is also important for the therapist to find a way to help the client become more comfortable and direct with the negative messages. Very often, an awareness of the feeling of irritation that the therapy is not helping faster or more magically provides the first chance a patient has to acknowledge a normal, expectable, emotionally alive hostile feeling in the context of a supportive relationship—the first opportunity to tolerate simultaneous hatred and love for the same person. Experiencing and even enjoying one's angry, demanding side often liberates a wide range of other affects, positive as well as negative. One of my clients commented that it was as if her fear of the consequences of her anger was the stopper in a bottle that, once uncorked, turned out to contain all her tender and loving feelings. A sense of humor and a disposition not to take provocations personally are assets for therapists in such interactions. "I guess you're trying to tell me in a polite way that I'm not helping you fast enough," or "You've had enough of this what-comes-to-mind-about-that stuff and want me to get on with it and tell you how to feel better, right?"

Sometimes when powerful negative affects and enactments engulf both parties, there is nothing to do but endure it. As Winnicott (1955) originally observed, the fact that the analyst survives the patient's repeated emotional onslaughts is a central factor in healing. Over many generations now, different analytic writers (e.g., Brunswick, 1928; Fiscalini, 1988; Grotjahn, 1954; Lipin, 1963; Searl, 1936; Shane & Shane, 1996) have noted that in addition to the Freudian ideal of "working through" the person's unfolding relational difficulties, there is a lot of simply "living through" that we do with our clients. Even patently crazy demands can, in the empathic atmosphere of psychotherapy, have a kind of logic that defies easy interpretation.

I remember Otto Kernberg once talking about a woman he had treated who insisted that the only condition under which she would ever believe that he cared about her was if he would kill her. Her rationale was that if he were to murder her, he would finally be verifying that her pain was in fact so unbearable that the only humane option was to put her out of her misery—and on top of the obvious love in that action, he would be demonstrably elevating her needs above his own wishes to avoid criticism and stay out of jail. When he told this story, the audience of therapists murmured in a tone of polite sympathy for his clinical challenge, but they were much more deeply and delightedly engaged a couple of moments later when he added, "And you know, for a while, I couldn't figure out what was wrong with her argument!" Sometimes we get drenched by the storm the client brings into the consulting room and can only wait it out, insisting on enforcing safety precautions that make sense to us, until we find some way to redefine the turbulence so that it can be seen as offering new possibilities (cf. Benjamin, 1995).

A Cautionary Tale

A few years ago I was brought up on ethics charges by a disgruntled relative of a patient. Because I did not believe I had behaved unethically and was therefore not carrying a lot of guilt or shame, I was not particularly reluctant to talk to other therapists about being in this situation. Fortunately, I was eventually exonerated. Since then, the fact that most of my colleagues know that this happened to me has prompted many of them to call me when they have been the object of a complaint or investigation, or when they run into other situations with legal ramifications, such as being stalked or threatened by a client. It has been eye-opening to learn how many very competent, conscientious, and highly ethical therapists have been through something like this. Having a window on my colleagues' confidential and diverse experiences over several years has given me a sense of what are the professional scenarios that most commonly spell trouble.

Any litigator familiar with mental health law in the United States will confirm the fact that the most dangerous situations for therapists involve child custody issues. Consequently, there has come to be a fairly helpful risk-management literature (e.g., Haas & Malouf, 2002; Hedges, 2000; Koocher & Keith-Spiegel, 1998) on how to avoid some of the minefields in that territory. But another scenario has come to my attention repeatedly, usually unrelated to concerns over children. This story line involves a patient who begins to regress and make heavier demands on the therapist. The therapist, identifying with the hungry, needy part of the client (but not the raging, entitled, sadistic part) starts to try to give more. Soon there are extra sessions, special meetings, exceptions to regular practice designed to give the patient the message that the therapist really cares (and the therapist really *does* care). Eventually, the client, who has been needing to discharge an unbearable amount of negative affect, develops a psychotic transference in which the therapist is wholeheartedly believed to be a bad object.

The therapist, who cannot tolerate being distorted in this way, steps up the effort to demonstrate goodness. He or she sees the patient late at night or agrees to hug the patient or goes to the patient's home or talks about personal things in a frantic effort to reveal the caring human being that the patient is now seeing as a persecutor. These efforts only inflame the patient, who then complains to a regulatory board or ethics committee, citing as evidence of malfeasance all the therapist's deviations from the frame. The investigating body looks at the evidence of the therapist's disregard of ordinary professional boundaries, senses the therapist's feeling of guilt about the patient's regression, and rules in favor of the patient (who is sincerely convinced of the therapist's badness and who does not look or sound crazy anywhere but with the therapist).

Dear reader: Do not let this happen to you. Get enough therapy yourself to know what your own dynamics are and to distinguish them from those of your patients. Learn to listen to the small rumblings of irritation and anxiety in yourself that suggest that the client's request for special treatment contains hostility and terror as well as desperation and need. Set an example of a person who can insist on working under reasonable conditions, who collects a living wage, whose time is valuable, whose ground rules demand respect. This is how you would want your client to conduct his or her life. When the client rages, do not get defensive, but do not acquiesce. Many patients are so terrified of emotional intimacy that they are driven over and over again to provoke crises that allow them to distance with impunity (see Hedges, 2000). They may be unable to tolerate evidence of the therapist's charitable nature—they cannot find this in themselves, they envy it in others, and they consequently seek to destroy it or expose it as fraudulent (cf. Klein, 1957). It does them no service for a therapist to keep tormenting them with generosity. Instead, one must be prepared for a long period of limit testing, provocation, and the slow, painful effort to make sense of the rage within. Putting out crackers and cheese is reasonable when visitors show up with wine, but not when they arrive with cyanide.

Notwithstanding all these warnings, sometimes there is a good therapeutic reason for doing something relatively unconventional. Ideally, if a therapist comes to think that a deviation from standard boundaries is clinically warranted, he or she should seek the opinion of an experienced colleague and, if the colleague supports the clinician's judgment, go ahead with what seems called for clinically, keeping a record of the consultation and the rationale for the clinical decision. Sometimes, however, one does not have the luxury of time; clients may put practitioners on the spot either with deliberate (albeit sometimes unconscious) provocation or because of their ignorance of standard therapy rules. One of my patients, for example, used to send me a flower arrangement at Christmas; another would occasionally bake her special bran muffins for me. In both instances, I felt it would be injurious to the person's self-esteem to reject the gift and insist on exploring the motives involved. (In fact, as I mentioned previously, it was easier to analyze the complex motives for the gift when I did accept it, because the person then did not feel criticized and was not on the defensive.) When therapists have to make split-second decisions to behave in a way that might be critiqued by an unsympathetic and literalistic outsider, however, they are well advised to record their clinical rationales for doing so.

DISCLOSURE

The burgeoning literature on self-disclosure of the last two decades has been a breath of fresh air to those therapists who had previously felt strangled by orthodoxy. Relational theorists have made scholarly and thoughtful arguments to the effect that in the intense atmosphere of a therapy session, explicit disclosure of aspects of the self can be preferable to the pretense that one is, or can be perceived as, a "blank screen" (e.g., Maroda, 1999; Renik, 1995). Such reasoning has relieved practitioners, who, if they had any self-awareness, had to know they were not all that inscrutable, even when they were assiduously trying to keep their personal feelings and attitudes invisible. In the sections that follow, I discuss self-disclosures over which one has no choice, disclosure of personal information because it is vital to the patient, disclosure of conscious countertransference reactions, and disclosure of biographical information about the therapist. This is not an exhaustive set of categories, but I hope it covers the main territory in which beginning therapists find themselves.

Inevitable Disclosure

As many writers have pointed out (e.g., Aron, 1991; Greenson, 1967; Levenson, 1996), therapists reveal a great deal about themselves via such factors as their style of dress, office decor, physical appearance, and personal demeanor. Most patients observe whether or not the clinician wears a wedding ring. They make note of what kind of car the therapist drives and what shape it is in. If the treatment is conducted in a home office, patients may glimpse members of the family, service people, and other features of the practitioner's life outside the consulting room. If the therapist has written professionally, clients can read the publications. They can get to know people in the therapist's circles and ask questions. In recent years, the Internet has provided ample information for any person curious enough to do a little on-line research. And over time, patients certainly become aware of their therapist's "real" personality and of aspects of the therapist's self that are theoretically private (Crastnopol, 1997; C. Thompson, 1956).

Patients may also be confronted serendipitously with information about the therapist's private life. A few years ago my colleague Albert Shire was the victim of a freak accident: He was walking with his wife to a local movie theater on a Friday night when a building collapsed on them. He awoke in the hospital to learn that although he had sustained only minor injuries, his wife was dead. *The New York Times* carried the story, and before a day had gone by, all his patients knew about it. When he went back to work a couple of weeks later, in addition to dealing with his grief, he had to contend with clients who felt guilty about taking up any of his emotional energy. Understandably, they wanted to take care of him and not add to his pain, but their consequent inhibitions against talking about their own problems were also functioning as a resistance to the therapy work. Eventually, he said to those who were particularly tongue-tied, "Want to take care of me? Let me do my job."

Clients inevitably learn a great deal about their therapist's personality, conflicts, and narcissistic needs by making conscious and unconscious inferences from the clinician's body language, facial expressions, and choices of intervention. Greenson (1967) tells the story of a patient who figured out his political preferences because "whenever he said anything favorable about a Republican politician, I always asked for associations. On the other hand, whenever he said anything hostile about a Republican, I remained silent, as though in agreement" (p. 273). Greenson had been completely unaware of this pattern. Jennifer Melfi (to take one of the few media portrayals of a psychodynamic therapist that approaches believability—see Gabbard, 2002) broadcasts a "keep your distance but come closer" conflict via the combination of sitting quite far away from her patients yet wearing short skirts and crossing her legs appealingly, and it is pretty clear that Tony Soprano perceives that conflict. (I recommend sitting closer and not showing so much leg.) Patients can read their therapists' psychologies from vocal tone; answering-machine messages; policies about time, money, availability, and cancellation; and other expressions of the treater's professional individuality. A man I know who had had a less than satisfying experience with a therapist he saw for a couple of years remarked, "I stayed too long with him. I should've left when I realized that the interesting fish he had in his office tank was a piranha."

It can make a beginning therapist excruciatingly self-conscious to

be watched so carefully, but one gets used to it over time, and to whatever extent it is possible to relax and just accept the fact of being scrutinized, it will make the job of listening and helping easier. If one tries to
be virtually invisible, the result will be either to behave so stiffly that
the patient's comfort will suffer, or to lie to ourselves about what is possible, or both. We simply do not have total control over what we reveal.
Theodor Reik, referring to therapists as well as patients, represents
Freud as believing "that mortals are not made to keep a secret and that
self-betrayal oozes from all their pores" (1948, p. 23). There is a lot of
evidence supporting this prejudice. Hence, my only recommendation
about one's attitude toward inevitable self-disclosure is to get used to it.
It may help to remind oneself that what we know empirically about
therapeutic effectiveness is that outcome is much more highly correlated with an attachment to a vivid individual person than with the application of any specific techniques (Luborsky et al., 2002).

Disclosure of Information Vital to the Patient

Patients have the right, as consumers of our services, to know things
that will have a significant effect on them and their therapy. Some of
these matters should be conveyed in the initial session. For example,
clients should be told at the beginning of treatment about such things
as the legal limits of confidentiality. It has become standard practice in
the litigation-crazy United States to ask prospective patients to sign a
consent to treatment form that spells out such conditions. Karen
Maroda (personal communication, January 4, 2000) tells me that she
states at the start of each treatment she undertakes that she will be raising her fee every year in accordance with inflation. Physicians in training or graduate students in psychology or counseling who expect to
leave for a residency or internship should let their clients know of those
plans at the outset, even if the move is three years in the future and
even if the client is asking for a short-term therapy (clients often change
their minds when they get comfortable). Clinicians who decide that
they are going to retire or move out of the area, even if the event is a
few years hence, should tell new patients of their plans. In fact, any limits to the length of the therapy that are known in advance should be
shared, lest the patient feel betrayed later, when his or her assumption
of control over how long the treatment can last is traumatically refuted.

    When one plans a vacation, patients should be given the dates well
before the separation, both for practical reasons (so that they can plan
their schedule and finances accordingly) and for therapeutic ones (so
that they have ample opportunity to process their reactions to the
planned interruption of the therapy). If the therapist becomes preg-

nant, around the time this becomes evident she should let her clients know her plans for taking time off, and the two parties should discuss how they will proceed if the pregnancy becomes medically complicated or if she goes into early labor. If a clinician has to cancel one or two sessions abruptly because of illness or emergency, it is not so important to tell the patient the details; one can simply say, "I'm sorry, I've come down with something and have to cancel tomorrow," or "I'm sorry but there was an unexpected and pressing personal matter I had to attend to." In these instances, it is important to examine the person's fantasies about what happened, but occasional calamities requiring a couple of days off are understood by most people as part of life and hence require no disclosure. Many contemporary therapists will, however, disclose something specific ("I had to have my dog put to sleep" or "I threw my back out"), out of a combination of motives: They feel the patient deserves some explanation for a rupture in consistency, and they expect that the patient's responses to the information will be richer and more clinically useful than their reactions to a lack of information.

Most gay, lesbian, bisexual, transgendered, and intersexed patients need to know something about the therapist's attitude toward their sexuality or toward the political positions they have taken about sexual or genital diversity. Prospective patients in sexual minorities may insist on knowing the therapist's sexual or at least political orientation, and although I believe that therapists have a right not to disclose aspects of their sexuality to patients, they should understand that lack of disclosure may be an insurmountable barrier to the person's working with them. Some individuals have a strong preference to go to a professional of their own sexual orientation. Therapists who want to work with such patients need to be willing to announce their similar orientation or to talk frankly about not meeting the qualifications set by the patient. Efforts to change the client's mind about the importance of this factor would only add insult to the injuries such individuals have already sustained by being in a sexual minority. (See the section on "Disclosure of Personal and Biographical Information," however, with respect to the complexity of divulging sexual orientation to some patients.) A similar consideration applies to patients in any minority (ethnic, racial, religious) who want to be seen by someone of their "own kind."

Some prospective patients need to know something about the therapist's spiritual orientation, or at least that the therapist is not contemptuous of the client's religious concerns. People whose occupations or avocations involve political positions or activities—union organizers or newspaper columnists, for example—may need to know that the therapist is not contemptuous of their politics. These various examples of requests for revelations that the therapist may be better off address-ing directly (rather than deferring and exploring) all illustrate the fact that for many patients, understanding something about who the thera-pist is as a person is vital to the attainment of a working alliance (see McWilliams, 1999, Ch. 2, for more elaboration).

More problematically, it seems to me that patients have the right to know at any point in treatment if the therapist is seriously or termi-nally ill (see Abend, 1982; Dewald, 1982; A. L. Morrison, 1997; Phillip, 1993; and B. Pizer, 1997, for disparate views on this topic). It is unfair, to say the least, to drop dead on someone whose attachment you have cultivated, when there was a possibility of talking about the impending loss together. Inquiries into how therapists deal with the question of their approaching death (e.g., Fieldsteel, 1989) have revealed that de-nial seems to be the defense of choice for afflicted practitioners. I have known several people whose therapist was visibly wasting away while hiding behind the notion of neutrality and insisting that the therapy go on as if the perceptions of the therapist's ill health were all in the mind of the client. The analytic requirement to be honest with oneself is no less stringent for therapists than for patients, and no matter how pain-ful it is to acknowledge one's looming demise, it is a professional re-sponsibility. It is also important to keep a list of practitioners that cli-ents might consult after one's death and to be sure that at least one other person knows where it is.

There are also instances in which a patient will ask point-blank about something that may require a disclosure because the alternative (simply exploring the question) is too unsupportive of the person's sense of reality. A few years ago I was diagnosed with breast cancer. Be-cause the tumor had been removed in the surgical biopsy, I was told I could postpone further treatment for a while; my options were a mas-tectomy or a wider excision plus radiation. I decided on a mastectomy and scheduled it for the Friday before a holiday weekend three months away so that I could take an extra day off that weekend and otherwise keep working as usual. I was managing considerable anxiety, because I knew that until a pathologist had looked at the excised breast, I could not be completely sure it was free of other tumors that may have eluded mammography. I felt fine physically, however, and continued to see clients without a break.

Of all my patients, who at that time included two therapists who prided themselves on their keen sense of my emotional state, only one person suspected that something was bothering me—a shy, sensitive woman with no psychological training. As she was growing up, her mother had repeatedly told her she was "hypersensitive" or "overreacting" or "making a mountain out of a molehill." At the end of a session she tentatively raised a question: "I don't want to invade your privacy, but is anything wrong? You seemed a little preoccupied lately." I was not about to duplicate her mother's defensive reactions to her perceptiveness, and so I responded, "Yes, there *is* something I'm bothered about. It's medical, and to the best of my knowledge, I'll be fine. But I will tell you if I find out it's more dire, and I'll know within a few weeks." Because I thought it would be validating to her growing confidence in her acuity, I went on to say, with admiration, that she was the only one of my clients who had noticed.[1] I think that this kind of disclosure can advance the therapeutic process and, more compellingly, that its absence can retard it.

Disclosure of Countertransference Reactions

There is a huge literature, including some serious controversies, about whether and under what circumstances one should acknowledge to clients the emotional reactions that one feels in their presence. Divulging a countertransference is usually a powerful communication, provoking intense and complex responses. The question is burdened by the fact that one can never make full disclosure because so much of any state of mind is not in consciousness (cf. Aron, 1997). The guidelines I have developed for myself in this vexed area are to admit to feelings that are obvious to the client anyway, to try to respond honestly to direct questions about my feelings whether or not I explicitly disclose, to bring up my emotional state when I am pretty certain it will further rather than complicate the client's work, and, when I do reveal my feelings, to do so in ways that run the least risk of making the patient feel either blamed for my reactions or impelled to take care of me.

It seems to me that it is subtly dishonest to act as if one is "blank" when one in fact is full of feeling, and that a more candid reaction than putative neutrality often deepens the work. For example, when a chronically self-destructive woman reports that she has again put herself in harm's way, despite weeks of work on understanding why she does that, I am likely to feel rage, and my best poker face is not good enough to hide this. If she then asks if I'm angry, it feels evasive to say something like, "What's your fantasy about that?," or "What comes to mind about your question?" I would rather say, "Well, it doesn't thrill me to hear that you've had unprotected sex again with a stranger. If you want to get a therapist upset, one of the best ways to do it is to keep demonstrating that her efforts to make you less self-destructive are in vain. What's your reaction to having gotten this reaction from me?"

Then I might go on to explore whether she has run into irritated reactions from other people, what she had been expecting from me, whether there was a test in her communication, what she imagines will be the consequences of my anger, and so forth. I might also wonder with her whether she feels hostility toward me and is expressing it via self-destructiveness rather than with a direct statement about her feelings. Because many people associate expressions of negative feelings with punishment or rejection, it can be valuable for the therapist to acknowledge anger without any punitiveness attached. It teaches that anger is just a feeling like any other and can often be felt safely and expressed safely.

Ever since Racker's (1968) seminal argument that strong feelings in a therapist usually mirror either the same feelings in the patient (concordant countertransference) or the feelings that important others have had toward the patient (complementary countertransference), analysts have felt they have more options about using the information that they get via their less intellectual faculties. Sometimes it moves things along for the therapist to acknowledge what is emotionally obvious. For example, "I'm getting this powerful feeling that nothing I do is going to be right by you. Is that a feeling that you've had yourself?" Or, "I'm noticing that I feel confused. Do you get that reaction from other people? Do you feel confused yourself?" Or, "I'm noticing that I'm feeling a deep sadness as you talk. Are you in touch with any feelings like that?"

Probably the most difficult countertransference to manage in the clinical situation is sexual attraction. I feel strongly, along with Benjamin (1997), Gabbard (1998), Maroda (2002), and others, that confessing sexual attraction to a patient is virtually never therapeutic; it is too close to actual seductiveness to be discriminated from it. As my colleague Seth Warren once observed, "Sometimes talking about sex *is* sex." It might not be destructive to make a comment such as, "Are you feeling that there's a subtle flirtation going on between you and me? I'm sensing some seductive vibes in the atmosphere," but in a situation with such an emotional power imbalance, admitting sexual desire can be disastrous. Again, if evidence of the therapist's sexual responsiveness is inescapable (as in the time I wrote a bill for an attractive male patient and wrote "sex" instead of "six" sessions), the patient's reaction can be explored via a question like, "Well, what's your response to this eruption from my unconscious?" Readers who are interested in psychoanalytic reflections on this topic may enjoy a series of articles in *Psychoanalytic Dialogues* inspired by Davies's (1994) thoughtfully written article about a session in which she disclosed her attraction to a patient.

Disclosure of Personal or Biographical Information

There is much less in the analytic literature about whether and when to share with a patient some fact about the therapist that is not directly relevant to the well-being of the person in treatment. But it is my impression that even therapists who self-define as classical or orthodox find ways to let their clients know personal information that signals that they might understand what the patient is going through. For example, with a music-loving patient, a therapist can find ways to communicate the information that he or she is familiar with the musical works about which the patient is talking. A therapist whose politics are similar to those of a patient can smile knowingly when the patient criticizes a mutually disliked public figure. Sometimes when therapists are working with individuals having problems related to a parental role, they find excuses to tell a story that reveals that they are parents, too, and that they appreciate the difficulties of the job. With people in the psychotic range, who frequently need their experiences normalized, and with those who are constrained from coming longer than a few sessions, self-disclosure of this sort is very common and valuable. Good therapists working in supportive modes have talked about themselves to patients in disciplined ways for decades.

The inclination to make comments that let the client know of some area of similarity between therapist and client seems to be fairly widespread. I assume such statements are often made in an effort to strengthen the working alliance. My student Craig Callan, who is writing his doctoral dissertation on this topic, is finding that many of the analysts he has interviewed, when invited to talk about a clinical encounter in which they revealed some biographical information to a client, readily thought of such an instance. I have heard from numerous friends and colleagues that such a disclosure from a therapist was a therapeutic watershed for them, and I experienced a few memorable moments like this in my own analysis. I suspect that when we want our patients to know something about ourselves and yet suffer from internalized prohibitions about self-revelation, we unconsciously find ways to let the information slip out. The analytic ethos of honesty suggests that it is better, to whatever extent one can, to be conscious of what one is doing and why, and to substitute a more conscious choice for a less conscious, less agentic disclosure.

There is a substantial literature at this point about whether or not to disclose one's sexual orientation (see, e.g., Isay's groundbreaking article, 1991). For therapists who identify as heterosexual this is usually a nonproblem. For those working in practices serving gay, lesbian, bisexual, and transgendered clients, disclosure is also less of a hot issue be-

cause people coming to such facilities assume therapists' intimate familiarity with sexual diversity. But for clinicians in sexual minorities
who treat a general clientele, to tell or not to tell can be a paralyzing
quandary. It is intrusive to burden the client with a disclosure that has
not been asked for, yet the alternative may be to feel vaguely and un-
comfortably dishonest. This quandary is particularly vexing when one
works with heterosexual or sexually conflicted patients who talk about
sex on the assumption that the therapist identifies as straight. With
conflicted patients, a sexual-minority therapist is in an especially agonizing dilemma: The patient may need a model of comfort with minority status, yet disclosure can provoke upset and even rejection because
of the unconscious homophobia creating the conflict. I have no easy
answer here other than for therapists in this bind to read the relevant
literature, consult with a sensitive supervisor, and make the best call on
the basis of knowledge of the client's psychology.

My general suggestion to beginning therapists is to be very conservative about biographical self-revelation, except during the initial session, when clients deserve answers to questions that for them are pre-
requisites to hiring a particular mental health professional. Even
granting the relational point that neutrality and anonymity are not possible, there are good reasons to be careful with revealing personal information. First, the toothpaste cannot be put back in the tube. If what
was shared in an effort to enhance the connection has the opposite effect, the revelation cannot be undone. Once when I told a client I knew
what she was going through because I had suffered a similar experience, she reacted with dismay. She felt I would not be objective enough
to help her, and although she stayed in treatment, she continually
threw up to me afterwards her belief that she could not trust what I had
to say in certain areas because I was obviously biased. I suppose a dismissive transference would have emerged in any case, but because her
minimization of my open-mindedness was bolstered by the "reality" of
my disclosure, it was hard to explore the transferential aspects of her
attitude.

Second, sometimes patients experience such disclosures as a
frightening role reversal, as if the therapist is confiding in the patient
with the hope of being comforted. Individuals who had a significantly
depressed parent or who were "parentified" as children are particularly
prone to this reaction, as are people with significant narcissistic tendencies. Devaluation, rather than the grateful feeling of being understood, may greet the therapist's well-intentioned divulgence. More than
one person has told me that he or she left a therapist because the practitioner "started telling me about his [or her] *own* problems!" It is painful to learn that interventions made in a spirit of trying to normalize or
comfort are experienced as being made with a very different intention,

but this is one of the areas in which such misunderstandings can be spectacularly evident.

Finally and perhaps most important, such information will not ordinarily have a lot of therapeutic power unless it comes after a long period in which the patient realizes how deeply convinced he or she is that the therapist cannot possibly understand—in fact, any potential therapeutic power in such a revelation can be lost if it is made too soon. As a patient in the late 1960s, I kept worrying that my analyst (whose background was in social work and who ran a settlement house on the Lower East Side of New York) was a right-wing ideologue like my father. Intellectually, I knew this was improbable in the extreme, but I kept finding myself in a severe state of anxiety when I talked about my leftish involvements. Eventually, after I had explored for months many different aspects of my gut-level conviction of my therapist's rigid conservatism and found myself stuck going further in describing my activities, he told me that he was politically rather liberal. This revelation, which hit me at the emotional rather than the cerebral level, touched me deeply, dissipated my resistance, and provided a corrective experience of talking about politics to a male authority who did not pathologize me for my convictions. But if he had told me that about himself at the beginning of treatment, I would never have understood the power of transferential fears. This is a good example of the general principle that deviating from the frame is only powerful when the frame has become reliable (I. Hoffman, 1998).

TOUCH

Holding, in the psychological sense, is a *sine qua non* of psychotherapy (Slochower, 1997; Winnicott, 1963). It should not be surprising that many clients want a more concrete expression of the sense of being held by a caring professional. Similarly, being in psychotherapy involves letting oneself be touched emotionally. Whether therapists should ever hold or touch the client physically has been the subject of considerable controversy (see Casement, 1985; Toronto, 2001). Recently an entire issue of *Psychoanalytic Inquiry* was devoted to the topic (Shane & Shane, 2000), and very little common ground was reached.

Physical Holding

Every psychoanalytic therapist I know has been entreated by a patient to be hugged. My own experience is that requests or demands to be held come from many people with borderline features, most people with histories of trauma (especially sexual trauma), and many less damaged clients who allow themselves to regress in an intensive psychoanalytic process. Unhappily for the therapist's comfort, they do not bring it up in an intellectualized, hypothetical way; instead, the request comes on the heels of their being mired in grief or flooded with painful memories or armed with the entitled determination of the person who will not be denied. These clients can fill the therapist with dread that a refusal will devastate or retraumatize them or provoke a flight from therapy. As I noted at the beginning of this chapter, being on the receiving end of a person's earnest rationale for needing physical touch is one of the most common clinical situations we encounter, and yet very few textbooks talk about the issue beyond discouraging the therapist from gratifying the patient's wish. If only a simple rule could help us to deal sensitively with the clinical challenge!

Classically, one frustrates the demand, subjects the wish to therapeutic scrutiny, and manages not to humiliate the patient. But I find that when I am in the situation, I can do only the first and, with luck, the last. Analyzing the meaning of the wish or demand usually comes a lot later, and preferably at the initiative of the patient: As I stressed in Chapter 5, there is less shame for people in raising touchy issues themselves than in having the issues brought up by a therapist. When clients feel the overwhelming wish to be held, the yearning may be sincere, but they are also frequently trying to avoid some negative feelings. By misunderstanding the patient as *needing* to be held, as if physical comfort is developmentally required in the treatment, a therapist would be implicitly accepting the patient's preference to be seen as a needy child rather than as a conflicted adult. Many of us, perhaps especially women, are more comfortable with our dependent longings than with affects such as hostility, envy, and hatred, and when those feelings start to surface in the therapeutic relationship, we want to be reassured that we are embraced, as it were, despite our aggression.

A therapist who holds a patient may enjoy being seen as the omnipotent parent who can fix things with a hug. Realistically, however, we are not parental or omnipotent, and to hug someone feeds the fantasy that we, rather than the patient, are ultimately responsible for coming up with sources of comfort. It is infantilizing to accept uncritically a client's version of the self as *defined* by a small child needing physical comfort rather than as *including* the sense of being that small child. In addition, physical contact of this sort collapses the "space" (Winnicott, 1971; Ogden, 1985) between the two parties—the area of symbolization, play, and "as-if" relating—that has been so carefully constructed over the course of the therapeutic work. Such a collapse reduces to a concrete physical act the complex metaphorical meanings of the longing to be held, and it creates unconscious anxiety that other strivings—ones that are not so attractive (such as the wish to attack physically or exploit sexually)—may also be acted out.

Here are some possible things to say:

> "I can feel how deeply you want to be held, and I agree that you weren't held nearly enough as a child. But I'm not comfortable acting on your wishes. I can be with you as you grieve for what you didn't have, but I don't feel right taking on the role of the person who can make it better."

> "I've never integrated physical touch into the way I do therapy. It's just not something I could do naturally in the context of my role, and if I tried to do anything that went against the grain of my role as I understand it, it wouldn't be the kind of hug you want anyway."

> "I'm very touched that you can tell me what you want, and I wish I could offer it, but all I can offer in my role as your therapist is the opportunity to understand what you want right now and to work through the anger and grief that go with not getting it."

> "I'm sorry. In my role as therapist, I'm just not a hugger."

These examples constitute efforts to implement the principle I talked about earlier, that it is better to set boundaries based on one's own limitations than on the basis of "what's good for you."

There are some situations in which most therapists do hug patients. As hugging is becoming a more common form of greeting and leave taking in American culture, it is not unusual for a course of therapy to end with a hug. Most of us have been hugged spontaneously by a patient and have felt it would not be right to stiffen up in the moment and invoke "the rules," though we may have gently raised a question about the meaning of the patient's gesture in a subsequent session. One man I worked with, who carefully cultivated a tough-guy exterior, grabbed me for a hug at the end of a session in which he had broken down in tears about having just been diagnosed with a terminal illness. I was not about to peel him off me. I have been known to touch a grieving person on the shoulder or arm as he or she leaves the session, usually while saying something like "Hang in there" or "Good luck coping with all of this."

But somehow a spontaneous expression of sympathy that has a physical dimension feels utterly different to me from a situation in which the patient makes a direct request in the context of an intense transference. Interestingly, I often have fantasies of touching or holding patients when they are not asking for physical comfort, whereas my countertransference when someone makes a point of asking has never been to want immediately to hold that person. Instead, I feel vaguely aware that there is more going on here than unadulterated love, I feel bothered by being put in a difficult position, and I find myself curious about the less conscious piece of the patient's experience. Although I have emphasized how moving and therapeutic it can be to deviate in a spontaneous way from an established therapeutic pattern, it is my strong impression that the time to break the frame is not when the patient is imploring one to do so. Usually in such situations, people need to be angry and then to grieve.

One of my patients, a woman whose childhood deprivation of physical comfort was extreme, asked me to hold her at a point in her analysis when she was beginning to feel more empowered and was noticing that often, when she made her wishes explicit to her family and friends, they were willing to grant them. She realized that she had never taken the risk of asking me for a hug, having simply assumed that physical contact was out of bounds. So she made such a request in the context of her pleasure and pride in having learned that when one asks, sometimes one gets what one wants. It was particularly painful for me to say no in this situation, and it was even more painful for her to have her proposal rejected. Still, both she and I noticed that shortly after her witnessing my clarity about a difficult boundary, she was able to set a long-overdue and very effective limit on some family members who had been taking advantage of her.

Cultural and situational differences affect decisions about touch. In South America, it is not uncommon for a therapist to greet a client with a kiss on each cheek. Freud used to shake hands warmly with patients at the beginning and end of every appointment. One of my students told me about a transformative session she had had with an HIV-positive man who was deeply moved by the fact that she shook his hand warmly on meeting him, demonstrating, as he saw it, her feeling that he was not a lesser being or a source of contamination. Most therapists learn to trust their instincts about when touch is contextually warranted—that is, when it furthers the relationship and its goals—and when it is a resistance, a way of avoiding what needs to be understood together.

Sex

To my knowledge, no one has yet come up with a credible, generalizable rationale for having sex with a patient or ex-patient.[2] In the 1970s, when all kinds of conventional limits were under widespread attack, one occasionally heard the argument that it would be "good for" a particular patient if the therapist were to engage in sex with her. (It was usually a her. The maverick practitioner was usually a he.) In the few instances I knew of in which such a therapeutic regimen had been carried out, I had the strong impression that it was only the younger, more conventionally attractive patients of a given clinician that this prescription was considered "good for." I would have given more credence to the alleged therapeutic impulse here if the therapist had also offered his sexual tutelage to his older and less attractive clients. As to whether sexual enactments can be harmless or even beneficial, after considerable anecdotal, clinical, and empirical attention to the fate of both clients and therapists who have entered into a sexual relationship (Gabbard, 1989; Pope, 1986), the evidence has come in soundly on the side of abstention. The stories of patients who became sexually involved with therapists or ex-therapists are almost always sad ones, and only the most psychopathic of sexualizing practitioners look back on their actions without pain (Gabbard, Peltz, & COPE Study Group, 2002). Consequently, at least in the United States, the legal and professional rules have become unambiguous. As Welch (1999, p. 4) pithily put it in a risk-management bulletin for therapists, "The only safe course is 'don't' and 'never.' "

But beyond the practical question of the therapist's self-protection, or the protection of the patient, or the repudiation of the dishonesty inherent in rationalizing one's sexual experiments as in the service of a client's growth, there is the issue of understanding what is going on when there is a compelling sexual undercurrent in therapy. We are all subject to the power and energy of sexuality—I suspect that Freud got it right in putting desire at the center of his theory—and the clearer it is that we will not act them out, the safer we tend to be with our pervasive sexual feelings. Erotic images and fantasies are common in psychotherapy. They energize and enrich the process, but they become problematic when one or both therapy partners gets stuck in an implicit or explicit sexualized state. Clear ethical standards are useful but not sufficient to help clinicians with this difficulty.

A therapist who, when confronted with a seductive or sexually mesmerizing patient, construes the issue as about sexual expression may be seriously misunderstanding the psychological forces in play. While sexualized transference–countertransference situations may have many different meanings (see Gabbard, 1994), I think it is safe to say that overall, clients' attempts at seduction rarely express love and sexual attraction as much as they express primal fears and the wish to gain compensatory power in a struggle that the patient needs to lose in order to learn that not all authority is corruptible and not all relationship is about exploitation. Before one can explore the dynamics of sexualization, the boundary must be clear.

As straightforward as the no-sex position appears, it can be difficult for clinicians to find ways to say a resolute "no" to a client who is
persistently seductive—and not just because of their own sexuality and
susceptibility to the flattery of being desired. Even people who feel no
strong erotic temptation struggle to handle this delicate situation therapeutically. Very often, the therapist rightly intuits that the client's self-
esteem is directly attached to the capacity to seduce, and that a sexual
rejection will therefore be humiliating. Rejecting someone's sexual invitation without making that individual feel rejected as a person is not
easy—as anyone who has had to do this in his or her personal life
knows. Some women I know have been told by their therapist, in an apparent effort to soften the "no," that they are attractive and in another
situation could have been a sexual partner. I think this is too seductive.
It also invites the patient to cut the treatment short so that the two parties can be in "another situation." It is much cleaner and probably more
honest to say, "I'm sorry. I don't do that." Or, "I'm sorry. I don't have
sex with clients." If the person pressing for a love affair has a psychopathic streak (as is not uncommon) and therefore cannot imagine the
personal code of conduct that impels the "no," it may be more effective
to say, "I'm sorry. No matter how persuasive you are, I'm not going to
jeopardize my career by doing something I could lose my license for.
End of story."

If the therapist does feel a distracting degree of sexual attraction
to a patient, whether reciprocated or not, the best course of action is to
consult with trusted colleagues and to bring it up in one's own therapy.
I have found in consultation groups for professionals that when one
participant exposes a strong erotic countertransference, the other
group members usually pick up on all the other dynamics involving
narcissism, idealization, power, and grief that are typically part of the
picture. It is unwise to try to ignore sexual reactions simply because
they should not be enacted—any more than it would make sense to over-
look murderous countertransference feelings because killing one's patient is therapeutically contraindicated. As Freud and other analysts
have convincingly taught, it is more likely to be what we repress or deny
than what we admit into consciousness that sabotages our good intentions.

CONCLUDING COMMENTS

In this chapter I have discussed some of the more common and taxing
boundary issues that therapists encounter, especially those for which
their formal training may not have prepared them. Both innocent and

intentional challenges to the frame can confront therapists with complex choices. Considering that clinical predicaments involving boundaries are as varied and complicated as the unique individuals who present them, I have covered only a small sample of the innumerable scenarios practitioners face. I have emphasized the value of understanding the unconscious meanings, the interpersonal contexts, and the possible consequences of various enactments at the perimeter of the therapy relationship, and I have challenged the simplistic notion that psychotherapy requires the practitioner's strict observance of self-evident, universal rules. In place of rules, I have talked about how to insist on limits that protect the integrity of the therapist and the treatment with minimal disruption of the therapy process and maximal preservation of the client's dignity. I have also noted instances in which one might decide, for solid therapeutic reasons, to ignore or cross a traditional boundary, and I have tried to show how conventions about the professional frame may differ from person to person and culture to culture on the side of both therapist and client.

NOTES

1. Fortunately, the eventual pathology report disclosed no additional malignancy, and I have been healthy ever since. The two therapist patients who had believed they were always tuned in to my state of mind were chagrined to learn months later through the analytic grapevine that I had gone through this crisis without their knowledge. Because both of them had a frustrating tendency to insist that their ideas about me did not represent transferences but instead were accurate readings of my inner state, I got a certain satisfaction out of the damage to their fantasies of omniscience.

   Some analysts believe that nothing goes on in the therapist that is not registered at some level by the patient. Although I think our clients frequently know a lot about us and often sense our moods, authoritative statements about how much they perceive sound as dubious to me as the older fiction that the therapist can be a blank screen. When I have told this cancer story to other therapists, those who believe that nothing important can be hidden tell me that my patients "must have known" about my diagnosis, or at least my apprehension, and also must have known that I did not want them to bring it up. I would give this belief more credence if I had not had several experiences like the one I just mentioned, in which patients became mortified at what they had missed. Despite the self-betrayal oozing from our pores, two people in intimate relationship are oblivious to a lot about each other at the same time that they know a lot about each other. If one insists that the therapist, given ordinary human blind spots, often misses what is going on in the patient, one cannot simultaneously argue that the patient is always accurately tuned in to the therapist.

2. The ethical situation may be different if one has, for example, done a brief evaluation of a child whose parent one meets in a social context years later. Lazarus and Zur (2002) have argued that in forms of treatment that are not psychoanalytic there may be less reason to be so rigid about sexual contact long after treatment is over. This is a reasonable argument given that nonpsychoanalytic practitioners do not deliberately cultivate a powerful transference.

   In the interest of comprehensiveness and the avoidance of sweeping moralization, I should also note that I know of a small number of former therapist–patient dyads in which sexualization does not seem to have been disastrous, including a few in which a posttherapy marriage has lasted for decades. Very few rules have no exceptions, but I think most contemporary analysts would concur that the problem with admitting an area of gray in the sexual realm is that it opens the door for rationalizations fueled by the power of sexual desires and narcissistic craving.

Chapter 8

Molly

Her full nature . . . spent itself in channels which had no great name on the earth. But the effect of her being on those around her was incalculably diffusive: For the growing good of the world is partly dependent on unhistoric acts; and that things are not so ill with you and me as they might have been, is half owing to the number who lived faithfully a hidden life, and rest in unvisited tombs.

—GEORGE ELIOT, *Middlemarch*

In this chapter and the next, I present two cases in detail. In doing so, I am hoping that the issues I have been raising will be brought to life. When I am in the learning role, I can assimilate only so much in the form of abstract concepts; to understand them, I need to see how they work in a specific case. The woman whose treatment I discuss in this chapter would be considered by most mental health professionals as a good candidate for conventional psychoanalysis or exploratory psychoanalytic therapy: She had impressive ego strength, the capacity to form an alliance, and a strong motivation to change. She also had disabling psychological troubles, most of which were entwined with personality dynamics that had become fixed over the course of her life, but unlike many people with a diagnosable personality disorder, her character structure was in the neurotic range.

In Chapter 9 I present the contrasting case of a client who, on grounds of impulsivity and a borderline–psychotic structure, is typically deemed "inappropriate" for psychoanalytic treatment, yet who eventually thrived on the kind of relationship the analytic literature has been unmatched at describing. Thus, I have tried to show the range of psychoanalytic clinical theory, the differential applicability of different analytic styles, and the use of different parts of the therapist's personality to meet the treatment needs of diverse clients. I hope that both treatments exemplify the values and sensibilities I reviewed in the first two chapters of this book. Both were undertaken when I was just learning how to do therapy and thus are full of the kinds of mistakes beginners often make, but both seem to me to illustrate the clinical lore and empirical evidence that well-intentioned devotion to the patient's welfare transcends specific failings.

One phenomenon that the two therapies portray is the contrasting trajectory of treatment with more neurotic-level versus treatment with more borderline and psychotic-level clients. In most patients who have a capacity to ally with the therapist and whose personality structure can be conceptualized as containing an id, ego, and integrated superego, there is a gradual and contained regression that the client permits once adequate trust is secured. This circumscribed regression benefits treatment by bringing into awareness primal affects and cognitions that have been suppressed by defensive processes and supplanted by maturation into later modes of feeling and thinking. Thus, the therapy of neurotic-level people tends to become most difficult for both therapist and client in the middle phase, when transferences begin to emerge with primitive intensity. In patients with severe disorders of self-cohesion, affect regulation, reality testing, and capacity to trust, therapy is hardest in the beginning phases and gradually gets easier. There is no utility in promoting regression in these clients because archaic affects and cognitions are already overwhelming them. Instead, trying to contain (and helping the client to contain) disorganizing emotions and perceptions gradually promotes growth that both parties find relieving.

On to "Molly." As many analysts have commented, few therapies are devoid of any "parameters" or supportive elements, and my work with Molly is no exception. But in general, I approached her therapy traditionally: I emphasized free association, encouraged use of the couch, recommended multiple sessions per week, and tried to approximate neutrality and abstinence in the best senses. As one of my first healthier patients, Molly taught me about the value of classical work with individuals who are motivated for and capable of the kind of facilitated introspection that demands from the therapist mainly the role of witness. With Molly, I eventually felt (though not in the middle phase) that all I had to do was sit back and watch her make herself well.

ORIGINAL CLINICAL PICTURE

Initiation of Therapy

When I first interviewed her in 1973 as a candidate for psychoanalytic therapy, Molly was twenty-seven years old, had been married three years to a brilliant law student, and was supporting herself and her husband on her earnings as a nurse and teacher of intensive care nursing in a local hospital. She had no children and was estranged from her family of origin, a working-class Irish Catholic family in a small New Jersey city. She had no significant relationships outside her marriage and her professional duties.

Molly was obviously very bright (I later learned that her tested IQ was in the 160s), precise of speech, and controlled. She was quite attractive, though in an artificial sort of way, especially in the let-it-all-hang-out context of the early 1970s. Her bleached hair was neatly coifed, her nails perfectly manicured, her nursing uniform immaculate, her makeup flawless. Her affect was so controlled as to be inaccessible, her body movements were rigid, and her mood was both depressed and anxious. I remember thinking, as she sat primly in front of me smoking one cigarette after another (this was before I routinely asked people not to smoke in my office), that she looked like a china doll, albeit a desperate one.

Molly's stated reason for entering psychotherapy when she did was that she saw that her husband's then ongoing psychoanalytic treatment was producing impressive changes in him. He had been urging her to "get analyzed," and she was willing to see if the process would result in similar progress for her. Possibly more important, though, she implied that Tom was not changing fast enough to have completely stopped abusing her physically and emotionally (he was in therapy for explosivity, among other things, she said). Molly was losing her patience with his mistreatment and was looking for a chance to evaluate her marital situation. She was not forthright about this—she was probably not entirely conscious of this agenda—in our initial meeting; this focus emerged over the first several sessions. She felt entrapped by her husband's apparent psychopathology and was confused about her possible contribution to it. She was also desperate to improve the relationship; it was all she had.

When asked about other areas she might want to work on, Molly mentioned several things. First, she felt sexually inhibited. Although she could masturbate easily to climax, she had never experienced orgasm with penetration or via someone else's sexual ministrations, either with Tom or with previous lovers. In addition, she suspected herself of a tendency to use sex as a weapon or as an expression of other feelings. She had recently and impulsively gone to bed with a virtual stranger when Tom was away, and she was suffering considerable guilt over the infidelity. Second, Molly regarded herself as inhibited in a much more general sense: She was rarely able to identify her feelings, much less find ways of expressing them. She named anger and grief, in particular, as emotional states that were hard for her both to feel and to vent. Third, she mentioned a general tendency to try to please people and to comply with their wishes regardless of her own needs. She said she felt she had never given up the wish to win her mother's love, and that she acted out her efforts to gain that love with virtually everyone. Along these lines she mentioned a tendency to lie, in an effort to inflate her fragile self-esteem as well as to avoid possible rejection by "telling people what they want to hear."

One other factor that Molly mentioned in passing was a history of migraine symptoms that seemed to occur with greater frequency when she was under emotional stress. She hoped to reduce her vulnerability to these attacks. She also hoped to avoid further dependency on medication. As a nurse, she found it easy to obtain tranquilizers and was currently taking low doses of Valium. During a stressful year in college, she had escalated her use of Librium until she was taking 80 milligrams a day, an episode that had scared her deeply. During that year, she had also had her only previous experience with psychotherapy. She had seen a university counselor once a week for several months, having consulted him to alleviate a fairly severe depression at the suggestion of a professor to whom she had turned in a paper detailing her family's ordeal with a devastating inherited illness. She described this counseling experience as lifesaving in that it enabled her to separate from her family and to complete her college education, but she now felt that the therapy had been mostly of a supportive nature ("the glue that held me together"), and regarded it as not intensive enough to have helped her to mitigate what she saw as more fundamental difficulties in her personality.

Later, I learned that she had abandoned this relationship abruptly when her counselor began inviting her to lunch and showing what she suspected was a sexual interest in her. In that era, boundaries were being challenged right and left, and I imagine she was right about this. It was partly to avoid a recurrence of this seduction that she was specifically seeking a female therapist. She also mentioned in this context how her parents, who regarded psychotherapy as fit only for the hopelessly crazy, had virtually exiled her on learning that she had bared her soul—and the family secrets—to "an outsider" (see McGoldrick's, 1996, pertinent essay on Irish families).

Early Clinical Impressions

It was difficult to find specific origins of Molly's presenting difficulties, as most of what she wanted to work on was depicted by her as "always" having been true. Although she evidently appeared to acquaintances to be a model of personal success (she had married an aspiring professional, her own career had progressed rapidly, and she was regarded as a leader by many colleagues), all her achievements coexisted with a chronic undercurrent of depression. She had only one real friend, now several states distant, and no hobbies or diversions. What others saw as an admirable conscientiousness appeared to Molly to be a driven, compulsive need to put the welfare of others before her own. Molly had many obsessive and compulsive qualities (e.g., her isolation of affect and workaholic tendencies), some hysterical features (the combination of sexual inhibition and impulsive sexualization without gratification), significant counterdependent tendencies, and obvious depressive dynamics. Her self-described target symptoms included anxiety, depression, and behavioral and somatic complaints, but overall, I was struck by how well Theodor Reik's (1941) description of the "moral masochist" applied to her. Reik wrote of people who are masochistic in the general rather than the specifically sexual sense; that is, their self-esteem depends on their compulsively sacrificing their own needs to those of others, often at the price of considerable suffering, shame, and abuse.

It became clear to me fairly soon that the specific stress that precipitated her seeking help was the deterioration of her marriage. Although her husband's behavior was becoming intolerable (more so than she admitted for a long time), she could not bear either to leave him or to make credible and enforceable demands that he change. She told herself that he "had problems" and that he thus deserved sympathy and support, not confrontation. It had never seemed unusual to her that she set aside no time for recreation or pleasure, or that in the division of labor with her husband she took responsibility for virtually all chores, from washing dishes to repairing the roof. Her marital situation was only highlighting the inherent problems in a self-defeating personality organization.

Molly seemed to approach the prospect of therapy with a sense of dread only slightly less extensive than her motivation to get her problems straightened out. She nodded solemnly as I articulated some of the goals and procedures of treatment. Her husband had described psychoanalysis as a painful but potentially creative process, and she clearly wanted to be a "good patient," one who was prepared to suffer in the interests of eventual growth. One interesting feature of her style in seeking therapy, which I tried to address in the first session in order to encourage her internal motivation and to forestall a possible flight from treatment, was that in coming to therapy largely under her husband's pressure, she was repeating the very pattern of compliance and neurotic need to please that she was hoping to change.

Molly's mother, who had embraced Catholicism with the special fervor of the convert (from Anglicanism), had proselytized to Molly all her life about the promise of salvation through the Church alone. Molly had responded to this sermonizing with overt deference and covert rebellion (outwardly a good Catholic girl, inwardly a defiant agnostic). Now, her husband held out psychoanalysis as a new orthodoxy, with Saint Sigmund replacing the Pope, and Molly was once more complying with the scenario for salvation and privately suspecting that the whole psychoanalytic ritual was bunk. When I made this connection for her, she denied that it was quite the same now, but she smiled knowingly, as if I was on to something important.

I have already alluded to Molly's use of the defenses of repression and isolation of affect. Reversal, the effort to meet her own needs for care by projecting them onto others and caring for them, was another central defense. Her zeal to care for the sick, the needy, the bereft, was extraordinary. Unable to acknowledge or express the weak, dependent, or suffering aspects of herself, she ministered to these needs vicariously, giving her spouse, her students, and her patients the best care she could. Her defenses were in many ways highly adaptive. Molly could function without emotional upset when surrounded by the dying; she was capable of integrating vast quantities of information instantly and turning them into a coherent treatment plan; she could forego sleep, coffee breaks, and conversation when her work demanded it. But she could not turn these defenses off, and her personal life was suffering from that inability.

Personal History

Molly was the first child born to a young and inexperienced couple (mother was eighteen, father twenty-one) who had met and courted in England, the mother's birthplace, during the war. They were a somewhat unlikely match, in that Molly's mother's background was Scots-Irish and English upper-middle class, and her father's was first-generation Irish American working class. Her mother had completed twelve years of education in contrast to her husband's eight, and she made no bones about having married "beneath my station." Shortly after World War II ended in Europe, Molly's mother followed her soldier to his home state, converted to his faith, married him, and set up housekeeping. She never worked outside the home, but as will become evident, there was so much to deal with at home that this is hardly surprising. Her first child disappointed her by being an active, colicky baby rather than the cuddly, placid one of her fantasies, and Molly remembered frequently being told as much. In fact, most of Molly's earliest memories concern her mother's criticism, sarcasm, reproval, or denigration. Molly learned about three years into our work that her parents had married because her mother was pregnant with her, a fact that we had begun suspecting and that emerged via Molly's careful detective work despite her parents' determined secrecy.

Seven other children followed in fairly close succession. But starting when Molly was still a preschooler, something began to go wrong: One after another sibling began evidencing massive physical and/or mental deterioration. By the time she was a teenager, four had died, all at different ages and with different symptoms, and one was hopelessly retarded. Her parents originally interpreted these losses as some kind of cosmic accident or test of faith; it was not until Molly was in college that her family finally learned that both parents were carriers of an extremely rare congenital disease with meningoencephalitic implications, causing the destruction of whatever brain centers happened to be affected. Although this condition theoretically was caused by a recessive gene and was therefore subject to Mendelian laws (i.e., one out of four children could be statistically expected to suffer from its effects), five out of the eight offspring were afflicted. Thus, throughout her formative years, Molly witnessed the suffering and death of one after another sibling, without even the support of some kind of understanding of their fate. The death of her youngest sister when she was twenty-two and the little girl was five had left her feeling especially bereft. She had privately regarded herself as the "real" mothering figure in this child's life and had hoped that somehow her caretaking would fend off an inevitable death. Her memories of this sister would play an important role in her therapy.

Naturally, the parents' suffering under these circumstances made it hard for them to respond to the particular needs of their eldest. Molly's mother continually put her in the position of caring for the younger children, with a maximum of nagging and a minimum of emotional support. Her father reportedly played virtually no role in her upbringing other than to exhort her to obey her mother. An over-the-road trucker, he was an alcoholic of the melancholy and withdrawn variety, whose drinking seemed to Molly to increase noticeably with the death of each succeeding child. Molly felt closer to him than to her mother, but she saw him as weak and dominated by his wife, and she remembered making a heartfelt resolution never to marry a man who could be so easily pushed around.

Molly's developmental milestones were otherwise unremarkable. A defiant streak appeared early in battles around eating, bedtime, chores, and so on, and never disappeared. Her intellect bloomed early, along with her tendency to use compulsive and intellectual defenses: At age three she had all her Golden Books arranged by category of subject

matter. She always did well in school. Although skinny and slow to mature, she was not unhealthy, except during part of her adolescence,
when she was hospitalized with severe hepatitis, a condition that was
diagnosed quite late because her mother had insisted that she was ma-
lingering. Throughout latency and early adolescence, Molly was mildly
school phobic. Starting on Sunday afternoons she would get increasingly anxious, sick to her stomach, and panicky about leaving home the
next day.

As the hepatitis incident suggests, a predominant motif in Molly's
young life was her mother's criticism and inability to empathize. In an
early session she reported seeing a television show in which a mother
comforted a daughter, to which she had reacted with deep sadness that
she had never had such a relationship. She recalled only two occasions
in which her mother had treated her warmly; both involved her own
failure (once in making a cake and another time in hemming a dress)
and her mother's willingness to set her right without shaming her. The
best guesses she and I could make about the reasons for her mother's
rejection included the degree of stress the woman was constantly
under; her jealousy of an attractive daughter—especially during Molly's
teenage years, given that the war had essentially deprived her mother
of a normal adolescence—and her characterological dependence on the
defense of projection. She would aggressively "interpret" Molly's behavior in ways that did not fit her daughter's experience but looked suspiciously like an externalization of her own feelings and desires.

Evidence for her mother's reliance on projection can be found
in Molly's recollections of her rather unhappy adolescence. A late-
blooming, inhibited, moralistic girl, she was repeatedly accused by her
mother of promiscuous intentions even before she had begun to date.
When boys did start calling on her, her mother would dress seductively,
sit on their laps, and flirt like a schoolgirl. Parenthetically, Molly never
received any information about sex from her parents, beyond vague
warnings and inexplicable giggles, and her experience in parochial
school in the 1950s only aggravated her sense that sexuality was a dangerous mystery.

With this history, it was not hard to see how she had developed a
masochistic personality style. In part, a self-abnegating orientation had
been explicitly taught to her. Her parents had consistently stressed putting others first at all costs. This injunction seemed to include not only
the demand to be her mother's constant and uncomplaining helper but
the demand to *like* being in that role. Molly felt that the Church had reinforced a masochistic message with its admonitions about selflessness,
especially for women. Later, her nursing training had repeated that lesson with an emphasis on how "the Doctor is always right" and "the pa-

tient's needs always have priority." But in addition to these external shapers of her psychology, Molly seemed to have developed the pathogenic belief that if only she could find a way to be "good" enough, she might be able to reclaim what little maternal love and attention she had once had all to herself, before her siblings had arrived.

The unsatisfactory relationship between Molly and her mother would eventually loom large in her therapy. That it would do so was evident in the beginning. In the first session, thinking it would prepare her for possible transference reactions (and acting out my own anxiety and counterphobic wish to get some control over the coming unpleasantness), I remarked to Molly that it is not uncommon in psychoanalysis for the patient to feel toward the therapist strong attitudes that were held toward a parent. "If that's true, then I feel sorry for you!" she replied.

One obstacle to a resolution of her feelings toward her mother (and her family in general) was the sympathy that others—and she, too, to some extent—felt for the woman's plight in losing one child after another. Whenever she felt angry or hurt in relationship to her mother, or even when she disagreed on some minor issue, she would be told by her mother or father that she had no right to criticize a person who had suffered so much. This lack of support for feelings that facilitate separation and individuation, reinforced by a family dynamic in which stark alternatives of conformity and rebellion were the only options anyone understood, left Molly with a Hobson's choice: stay with the family in hopes of being cared for, but at the expense of any autonomy, or cut all ties and sacrifice dependency needs for the sake of individuation. It was a testimony to her ego strength that she had chosen the latter course, but the price she had paid in doing so had been high. Her marital situation was recreating a crisis of individuation: How could she separate herself from a harmful environment without being paralyzed by feelings of loss and guilt?

HISTORY OF TREATMENT

The Beginning Phase:
Strengthening the Working Alliance

The initial contract I made with Molly was for two sessions a week; it was what she said she could afford on her salary. I recommended that she use the couch. (Although there were no clear counterindications, it eventually became evident that my making this recommendation so quickly was expressing not an empathic evaluation of her readiness to work this way so much as an enthusiasm to do what I saw as "real" psychoanalysis.) Molly understood intellectually the nature of dynamic therapy and expected the work to last many months and probably several years. I felt that our major task together would be to increase Molly's access to feelings of need and dependency, to help her to come to accept her longings for closeness as a combination of normal strivings and inevitable by-products of a depriving upbringing rather than as the defects of character she seemed to believe them to be. (This formulation as I view it in retrospect is not wrong, but it also highlights those features of her psychology with which I could readily identify and ignores other areas in which she was significantly different from me.) I hoped that once a process of self-acceptance was under way she would begin to evaluate her life more realistically and find ways to meet her needs for both comfort and freedom. By the end of the first session I felt we had negotiated the beginnings of a good working alliance.

I was hoping that Molly would find a way to increase the frequency of her appointments, an aim that it soon became clear she shared, though not consciously. At the end of our second session she reported a dream that began, "I am checking into some kind of hotel or retreat and although I really want to stay longer, I register for only two days . . . " Except for the couch issue, whenever I was in doubt about what arrangements would be helpful to her, I tried to follow her lead rather than recommending something based on someone else's theory of therapy, as all other things being equal, the overall value of respecting and promoting her sense of agency and her confidence in her own judgment seemed to me to supercede other considerations.

Throughout the three and a half years we worked together, Molly was consistently a conscientious, deeply committed client. She applied her usual hard-working style to her analysis and sustained an impressive rate of growth. Molly spent at least six months getting used to the unfamiliar experience of analytic therapy. Her greatest difficulty was with wondering what to say, worrying about whether she would "dry up" (be unable to associate) in sessions, as in fact she sometimes did. I concentrated at this time on encouraging her to bring up as much as she could, as spontaneously as possible. Molly would lie on the couch with an ashtray balanced on her abdomen and a bottle of soda at her side on the floor, trying to will her thoughts to flow freely. She kept wanting guidelines and rules from me, and almost always when I would ask her just to tell me what she was feeling, she would reply, "Tense." I had to restrain my impulse to exhort her to talk, and I tried to limit my interventions to the exploration of her subjective sense of being "blank" and "empty." Driving to sessions was an ordeal for her because she worried she would have nothing to say once she lay down. But because we usually managed to end up talking about something, she would leave feeling better, a bit cheered that she had survived another appointment and another battle with her resistances to spontaneous expression.

She quickly adopted the habit of writing down any dreams she could remember, because this made her feel "prepared" for a session. (It took, however, about two years before she could associate freely to the elements of a dream and feel satisfied that she had understood something important about its meaning.) She reported recurring dreams of being an alien to the human race, literally a visitor from another planet. We connected these dreams to her sense of not belonging in her family of origin and to the feeling of strangeness she felt in the ritual of psychotherapy. Since childhood, she had also had recurrent dreams of frightening, empty old houses (rather like the ones in horror films or in the movie *Psycho*), and of a giant, terrifying wave that threatened to obliterate her. She would wake up just as it was crashing down on her, sure she was drowning.

Because I had been taught that recurrent dreams are not only particularly important but also particularly difficult to decipher, I did not attempt any interpretation of the house dream or the wave dream. I privately suspected that the house was a self-representation, expressing the sense that her insides were both empty and dangerous, and that the wave symbolized emotion that she believed could overwhelm and destroy her. The reason I did not say even this much was that I thought it would lead to intellectualization rather than integrated emotional understanding. At that point in therapy, Molly was responding to most things I offered with comments like, "That makes sense" or "Sounds logical." When asked whether she might be feeling a specific emotion, she tended to take a doggedly "rational" position; for example, "It doesn't do any good to be jealous; therefore, I'm not."

I basically worked in a very reflective way in this early phase, maintaining a patient, accepting attitude and mirroring her thoughts with an effort to elicit the feeling aspect of them in more detail (Kohut, 1971). Probably what I did *not* do in this stage of the work (i.e., judge, interrupt, explain, advise, criticize, or even interpret—as her husband and earlier her mother had reportedly done) was more facilitative than what I did. The therapeutic relationship seemed to become progressively more secure. Slowly, Molly began to describe emotional reactions to various situations outside the therapy.

The first time she reported being in touch with a feeling as it occurred involved her realizing that she was angry to learn that a colleague had talked behind her back. I suspected there was a transference issue here, in that she must have wondered how much I talked with her husband's therapist, whose office was next to mine, but I did not push this idea because I thought it would only have been intellectualized. Instead, I simply endorsed the progress she was making in noticing how she felt. About four months into treatment, she exclaimed in the most animated way, "Now I know why people call them feelings. You *feel* them. It's, like, *physical!*" A few days after this, she brought in the following poem, which she said she had clipped from a magazine, explaining that it represented her hopes for her therapy (I have no idea how to track down this poem and give the author proper credit):

> If loneliness were just my little rag doll
> and understanding went as far as
> button eyes can see
> then maybe I'd accept my solitude
> and like a little raggedy head
> I'd smile on childishly.
> But thoughts that fill my head are not of cotton.
> Beneath my skin
> I'm as real as I can be.
> I'm thrilled and fascinated. All at once
> The trembling hopes, the long forgotten thoughts
> Are seen through crystal eyes. No more the dunce
> No more the fool, I rise to heights I fought
> To reach and cling there overwhelmed. So pleased
> To see that all the past has meaning now.
> Without great fear and panic I'm at ease
> In my own company. I can allow
> Myself the freedom all the world once asked
> For me to share, without the nagging sounds
> From deep behind my eyes; the heavy task
> Of reasoning, when reason has no bounds.
> All thoughts, all deeds, are simply done with no
> More hesitation. I am free to grow.

Nevertheless, Molly's fear to open up her emotional capacity was often paralyzing. Several times when she came close to crying she would "turn off" suddenly, becoming intellectual and truculent and asking me what good it would do, anyway, to get in touch with unpleasant feelings. She worried, not without cause, that once she began feeling an emotion like grief, it would not conveniently confine itself to the treatment hour but would "spill over" and suffuse her mood outside. To cry had never been cathartic for her; it had always made her feel worse: humiliated and weak on top of the sadness.

The first important break in her emotional dam came at about six months, in connection with her expressing for the first time her grief over her sister Susan's death. She wept as she described it. In the next session, apparently frightened by her sense of loss of control, she asked to sit up, saying it was getting increasingly hard for her to talk without the "feedback" that the sight of my face would provide. I assented to this request without comment except to encourage her to say more about her need to see me. I could have construed her plea to sit up as a resistance; it certainly contained an effort to resist too abrupt a descent into painful territory. Yet I found myself feeling that there was more going on than defensiveness. Despite the fact that she was frustrating my wish to do "real" analysis, I was pleased with her request: For the first time, Molly had not simply complied with "the rules" as she understood them but had asserted her own needs and judgments as more important than accepted psychoanalytic conventions.

Molly and I now began a period of face-to-face meetings that lasted about a year. She had accommodated to the treatment situation more comfortably and was losing her dread of the sessions. She talked more about feelings, with feeling, and began very gingerly to bring up some complaints about her marriage. This effort initially took the form of offering me her husband's ideas, usually those about her, and asking me to confirm or repudiate them. For example, "Tom says I forget my dreams because I'm really hostile toward the analysis. Could that be?" Responding to such questions required a discipline I found hard to maintain. I often felt the temptation, and more than once I succumbed, to address the content of each issue and either agree with or do battle with the absent Tom. Mainly, though, keeping in mind the goal of furthering Molly's sense of agency, I would ask her what she thought and how she felt about what he had reportedly said. Usually her associations to having her behavior "interpreted" led to angry memories of her mother's similar style. I tried to sustain in myself and to encourage in her the conviction that ultimately, she was the only person who could judge how she "really" felt.

As Molly began seeing her marriage as a replay of the painful aspects of her relationship with her mother, she began getting depressed. Although not yet able to stand up for herself, she stopped deferring quite so automatically to Tom's controlling behaviors, and consistent with Lenore Walker's (1980) later observations about the increased danger when a battered woman begins to separate psychologically from a batterer, her increased sense of autonomy reportedly angered him. Twice during this period she came in visibly bruised, and more than once she told me he had threatened to kill her. She learned that his previous wife had left him in fear for her life. I became very anxious, and yet I knew she was not ready to leave the marriage. Resources for abused women had not yet become common, and even if such services had been available, I am not sure she would have pushed past her shame enough to take advantage of them. I had to contain the anxiety for both of us, and I remember having a few sleepless nights.

In the absence of a way she could imagine dealing with her situation, she became more depressed. On her own, she sought out a physician who prescribed the tricyclic antidepressant Elavil, which she took for several months with a concomitant reduction of the worst depressive symptoms. At the same time, signs of growth began appearing. Molly sought out and got a better paying job and decided to use the extra money for a third and eventually a fourth session per week. The issues she worked on included her sense of entrapment, her memories of maternal rejection, and a great deal of material about her Roman Catholic socialization and what she saw as its destructive efforts to turn people, especially women, into "unquestioning, self-sacrificing, antisexual robots."

The transference throughout this first year and a half was benign and idealizing, much as Kohut (1971) described as typical of narcissistic characters, though I did not see Molly as essentially narcissistic. Molly often seemed to test me for similarities to her husband, the Church, and her parents. I generally avoided interpretation lest she experience me as just one more underminer of her capacity to understand herself on her own. Often the sessions were quite chatty. We would talk about her work, her ideas about her ethnic background, her impressions of the world of intensive-care medicine, or anything else that emerged as an interesting topic. She seemed to have been right about needing to see me in order to "take me in" visually.

I remember most vividly a couple of sessions in which we laughed together so hard that we could hardly catch our breath. She was educating me about various quaint practices of the nuns in her childhood parochial school, who had actually told the girls not to wear black patent leather shoes lest boys see in them the reflection of their underpants, and who encouraged their students to sit on half of their desk chair so that their guardian angel could sit on the other half. Molly recalled a time, right after the family had taken Communion during Sunday services, when her younger sister had come down with the flu and vomited in the toilet. Her mother took the doctrine of transubstantiation literally and was so horrified that "Jesus is in the toilet!" that she insisted on bringing a priest to their home to bless the bathroom plumbing.

I was not restricting my activity entirely to empathic mirroring and supportive chatting, however. In addition to gently challenging Molly's habitual defenses, I occasionally "took on" the Church—or at least her internalizations of its teachings, particularly those that equated suffering with goodness—and the previously unquestioned mottoes of her nurse's training. She and I managed to clarify her overriding masochistic pattern, including especially how she would "go on automatic" in any stressful situation, defining it as one in which she should be caring for someone else and shelving her own needs. In this way we slowly made ego alien many behaviors that she had never previously questioned.

After about a year of this face-to-face collaboration, I came to my office one day to find a hastily scrawled note on my desk. In it, Molly explained that Tom's abusiveness had become suddenly intolerable. Consequently, she had taken off abruptly to spend a few days in Ohio with her one close friend. This was the first time she had "abandoned" her husband, and while her reported guilt later was severe, her excitement that she had actually acted on her own behalf outweighed it. Shortly after this incident she asked to use the couch again, saying she now felt ready to "go deeper."

The Middle Phase of Treatment

Back on the couch, Molly quickly began experiencing stronger feelings, and, somewhat to the dismay of both of us, negative ones. The transference took a new direction as she began accusing me of not caring, not helping her, and representing a psychoanalytic orthodoxy that had no relevance to her needs. I could see that the rejecting parent was finally being externalized, but I still found her attacks hard to contain. Her tone at this juncture was often accusing and sarcastic. "Why should I relive my childhood feelings?" she would demand. "They were bad enough the first time!" The amount of observing ego seemed minimal.

I tried to weather this storm without undue defensiveness, but frequently I would find myself encouraging her old habits of intellectualization or trying to redefine her reactions as "really" relating to her mother, father, or husband, because the experience of being berated was so toxic. My own intellectual conviction that this kind of anger in the here-and-now was exactly what she needed to express, along with my belief that all I had to do was to accept it, was only the weakest antidote to my countertransference worries that she would leave treatment and that this would mean I was a failure as a therapist. The siege abated considerably when I made the interpretation to Molly that in attacking psychoanalysis she seemed to be trying to get me to "defend the faith." This comment led her to realize that one of the few weapons she had had against her mother was to attack her orthodoxies and to feel morally and intellectually superior when she evoked her defensiveness. Thus, we concluded, her sarcastic verbal assaults represented a last-ditch effort in the direction of autonomy and the preservation of self-esteem. From that point, much to the relief of both of us, they diminished.

Concurrently, she began to try to talk sincerely about sexual matters. Previously, we had talked *around* them a good deal (what the Church had promulgated, how her mother had acted, etc.), but now she began, haltingly, to put into words her own sexual desires and practices. These included masturbation fantasies, of which she was deeply ashamed, involving various kinds of masochistic subjugation. She was quite relieved when I remarked that such fantasies are common and not necessarily correlated with actual masochistic sexual behavior. Molly was, as in most areas of her life, very *competent* at sexual interactions, very adept at pleasing a partner, but almost totally without responsiveness. She had been afraid to face her own feelings for fear she would learn that she was "really" in some fundamental sense a sexual masochist. An important insight she came to on her own was that her inhibitions about experiencing arousal derived from a fear of losing control, for she suspected that an underlying passivity would emerge. She recalled wryly a joke about a man on trial for necrophilia who protested, "How did I know she was dead? I thought she was just a good Catholic girl!"

Around the middle of this phase, Molly began working on the sexual aspects of her marriage. She and Tom started to tackle the problem of their different needs and preferences as more of a team. They went to erotic movies, bought *The Joy of Sex* (Comfort, 1972), and experimented with new positions. Molly began experiencing excitement, and twice she reached orgasm during intercourse. At the same time, she began asserting herself in all areas of her marriage. She and Tom became better friends, and her life calmed down a good deal. She also gave him an ultimatum: If he physically abused her again, she would leave. This declaration followed considerable discussion in treatment about her sense of entrapment and whether it was as objectively warranted as she had felt.

One of the things Molly started realizing, which also had its inception in her sexual experimentation, was that not everything was her responsibility. Tom's approach to lovemaking was apparently abrupt and lacking in tenderness, and he seemed irritated by her requests for more foreplay or cuddling. She began to reassess her old belief that he was sexually normal, while she was "frigid." She began to wonder whether her sexuality might flourish with a more intuitive, less defensive partner. Mustering up all her strength against her Catholic superego, she decided she would have an affair, and she picked for her partner a colleague in her hospital who had been flirting with her for some time.

In her effort to keep her vow never to take up with a "weak" man,

Molly had always chosen tough, authoritarian mates, her husband being the latest in a series of such choices. Now, having acknowledged her wishes for tenderness and equality, she chose a gentle, reserved man who in actuality appeared to have considerably more inner strength than his compensatorily masculine predecessors. A recently divorced intensive care nurse in her unit, Steve proved to be very much at home in the language of feelings and sharing, and Molly's best-laid plans for a rational experiment encountered an unexpected complication: For the first time in her life, she fell in love.

Interestingly, Molly's decision to look outside her marriage for sexual love and emotional support coincided roughly with her learning that I was pregnant. I privately suspected that she was transferring many of her dependency feelings from me to Steve, in anticipation of a loss like the ones she had suffered when each sibling came along. When I asked her to talk about any responses to my imminent maternity, she insisted she had no reactions, and again, I felt that if I had pushed such an interpretation, it would only have been intellectualized. She did tell me later that on the last session before my six-week break to have the baby, she had suddenly felt like giving me a big hug. This was one of her first direct, open-hearted expressions of positive feelings toward me.

For the first months of a long and very cautious flirtation with Steve, Molly continued to regard the as-yet-unconsummated affair as a temporary relationship that would ultimately dissolve because of expected improvements in her marriage. During this time, however, Tom reportedly made the mistake of becoming verbally abusive, threatening to hit her, and leaving home to punish (and perhaps protect) her for a couple of weeks. Then when he wanted to make up and move back in, Molly refused. She told him he could lie in the bed he had made; she had come to see she was fine without him. She began to pursue a legal separation.

While all this was going on, Molly was also working hard on understanding the connections between her childhood difficulties and her recurring problems. Her complicated feelings about the deaths of her siblings slowly came to the fore and then suddenly intensified around the anniversary of her sister Susan's death. When I told her, in answer to her question, that I had named my new daughter Susan, Molly began an intense phase of grieving, ignited by the abrupt realization that she resented my giving a child that name. She had been "reserving" the name Susan, she realized, because in some strange way she had been refusing to believe that her sister was really dead. Stark dreams of standing over an empty grave accompanied these themes.

Slowly we reconstructed how she had tried to make up for the absence of a loving mother–child attachment in her own history by establishing one with the infant Susan. The fact that she was now in a loving, romantic relationship was making her aware just how much she had missed the feeling of being loved, and how deep were her desires for such a relationship. She began to understand the depth of her connection and now grief over Susan as a derivative of her early privation of good-enough mothering. Then finally a series of memories emerged about Susan, including one about Molly's having dropped her sister, breaking her arm, an accident over which she had always felt unfathomable guilt. It occurred to her for the first time that perhaps she had had some mixed feelings toward this child she thought she had unambivalently cherished; perhaps she had even wanted at some level to hurt her or get rid of her. I tried to help her feel less shame about this normal reaction to sibling displacement. I took her realization as emblematic of her beginning to come to terms with hostile, competitive, and destructive impulses in general, which she had previously handled by repression and whose unconscious existence had darkened her sense of self.

Months later, Molly dated the "pivotal moment" in her therapy, the time at which everything seemed to consolidate and move toward more and more experiences of pleasure in her identity and autonomy, as this moment when she realized she had had negative feelings toward Susan. Having aired and accepted these, along with associated feelings such as shame and envy, she had come to terms with an aspect of herself very different from the constantly helpful *persona* (Jung, 1945) she had adopted, and she decided she was not as evil as she had feared. Unlike her parents and the Church, I regarded the wish to hurt or kill as an inevitable part of being human, and Molly, internalizing my attitudes about such feelings, began to report feeling part of the human race.

The Termination Phase

Once Molly started valuing herself and accepting as part of her personality even her feelings of greed and hatred, her spirits became steadily brighter. The change in mood was evident in both behavioral and intrapsychic changes. In the realm of action, Molly began reporting that she no longer had to please others at any cost but was becoming comfortable simply saying what she felt. She began to develop her own tastes, not worrying about what others considered appropriate or fashionable. She discovered that her difficulty making friends had resulted mostly from her having intimidated potential intimates in her efforts at impressing them and thereby preempting their expected rejection. She let her hair grow in its natural color, started dressing in jeans or comfortable dresses rather than in tweed suits, girdles, and high heels, and stopped compulsively sculpturing and lacquering her nails. There was probably a lot of modeling going on here, in that I rarely wore makeup in those years and dressed casually, but Molly's subjective experience was that she was learning to be herself. Her voice became softer and her manner more relaxed. She developed a sense of humor, and although she never dealt directly in words with issues such as an early oral need, she began making jokes like, "I must be feeling fed. Have you noticed I don't bring a bottle in here anymore?"

In the sexual sphere Molly had become reliably orgasmic with Steve, and, perhaps more important, was enjoying a general sense of pleasure in her sexuality. No more was sex another job to be done. In the somatic realm, she lost her previously chronic sense of fatigue—something she had not mentioned during the intake phase because she had no experience of a vitality with which to compare it and hence could only label her previous condition once it had changed. At the time she began talking about termination, she had not had any migraine symptoms for more than two years. We had not "analyzed" her migraines; they had just disappeared in the process (see Mumford, Schlesinger, Glass, Patrick, & Cuerdon, 1984). After persuading herself that these changes might just be maintainable, Molly cut her therapy sessions down to three and then to two times a week. Again, I could have treated this decision as a resistance, but I felt that developmentally, it made sense for her to decide when she was ready to see less of me, to take more responsibility for maintaining her gains, and to move on.

In the intrapsychic sphere, the changes were reflected in her dreams. The wave nightmare began occurring less frequently after we talked at length about her fears of being overwhelmed with feeling, and it made its final appearance on the night before she mourned Susan's death so dramatically. The dark, empty houses were replaced in successive dreams by brighter, newer structures, and finally became filled with plants. Molly began telling off her parents in her dreams, and concurrent with her nighttime attacks on them was an increasing daytime interest in getting back in touch with her family to see if it might be possible to work out some mutual *modus vivendi*.

Molly began having warm friendships with several of her coworkers. Her relationship with Steve grew and deepened, and her early superstition that "It's too good. Something has to go wrong!" began to be refuted. The two lovers started talking about looking for a better job out of state and applied as a team to a highly respected intensive-care hospital where their skills could be much better used and rewarded. After exhaustive interviewing, they were hired. Molly gave notice to her employer and set a definite termination date with me, three weeks away.

In the last sessions, Molly reviewed her progress and mused about
how she would continue to work on the problems that remained. Her
transference fear that I would try to persuade her to stay in treatment
until it was completed to *my* satisfaction was quickly recognizable as her
expectation that like her mother, I would put her personal judgment
and experience second to my needs. She did ask for a referral to an analyst in the area where she was moving, in case she found herself needing more help, and after pursuing a contact I had in that area, I gave
her two names, both physicians. I thought that as a medical professional herself, she might appreciate a medical analyst and so was unprepared for her dismayed and suspicious expression on receiving the
names. When I asked her what the look meant, she replied, "I don't
want to go to a psychiatrist; they're all Freudians." (My supervisor
found this response highly entertaining, given that her own treatment
had been quite "Freudian.") Thus, Molly's distaste for orthodoxy remained, while her compulsion to comply did not.

A month after our last session I received the following note from
her:

> [Steve and I are] getting on very well. . . . I love him and feel it all
> the time. But I'm taking care of me first.. ..I'm concentrating on
> getting in touch with anger etc. as soon as I feel it at all, or find
> myself acting angrily, etc. I know when I "store" [feelings] it's harder
> to ever deal with them. I'm dreaming like mad, but can't make much
> of them–they're all very long and involved, and I'm not too good at
> analyzing my own free association . . . I bog down and lose the flow.
> Eventually I'll have to work on it, but for now I'm coasting. I feel very
> loved and loving. We sit down and talk about the feelings we're
> having on various things almost daily. Communication is wide open,
> and we both work at it. The fact we've both gone thru bad marriages
> makes us both appreciate acutely what we have now. I've learned to
> accept dependence on Steve as being an integral part of the
> relationship, and because of the type of person Steve is, I'm comfortable
> in the dependency.
>
> We're slowly putting together our feelings about my being a sort of
> stepmother to Steve's daughters. It's sort of ironic I'll be coming in
> contact with a little girl at the age of 5. I know I'll feel very motherly
> to her, and wonder how I'll handle the feeling of picking up with
> Susan after a 7 year interruption. . . .
>
> My parents wrote to me after hearing about Steve etc.–and it was
> a loving letter–I'm planning on keeping them at stamps' length for a
> while, tho. I miss you and hope you're well.

Molly and I agreed when she terminated that all other things being equal, we would have liked to work together somewhat longer. But over the three and a half years in which she was in therapy, she had accomplished significant growth and change, and I felt that Freud's argument in *Analysis Terminable and Interminable* (1937) applied to her. Freud felt that the therapist can often see unresolved issues that might give future trouble to a client, but that it is best to do a piece of work and let the person go, encouraging him or her to come back to work on future issues as they come up and are more emotionally salient. I also felt that Molly needed to achieve a separation that was self-initiated and not all-or-nothing, as she had been unable to do with either her family or her marriage with Tom. Even though it could be argued that she had transferred some unresolved longings from her therapist to Steve, I felt that she was ready to go, and that it was appropriate that she was getting what she needed from a partner in the world outside the consulting room.

POSTTERMINATION OBSERVATIONS

I heard from Molly periodically after she moved away. She would typically send me a Christmas card with a note about her life. She and Steve went through some difficult periods but were able to work together on their problems and to survive some severe stresses, including the loss of their home to fire, with their love intact. Once when they were visiting relatives of his who live near me, they stopped in and had coffee and filled me in on what was going on with them, Steve's daughters, their work, and their many animals. Things seemed to be going very well until about ten years after she terminated, when Molly called me in a state of devastation: She had developed physical problems that had been diagnosed as the symptoms of the family disease. Both of her living siblings were also showing signs of deterioration. Evidently, this scourge did not follow the Mendelian path that had been expected but had sooner or later shown up in every one of her parents' offspring.

I had explored with Molly during the therapy the question of whether she worried that she could come down with this illness. She had said that her physiognomy contained features that were associated with it, but that she was pretty confident she would have shown symptoms by this time if she had been afflicted. I think she and I made an unconscious decision not to investigate the issue any further; it was too upsetting to imagine that after all her struggles to improve her life, she would have to face an early and physically painful demise. Molly had spent some time in her therapy coming to the decision—and grieving over the decision—not to have children. She did not want to pass on the genetic curse. Now she felt terrified and completely defeated. I felt not much better.

For a brief period after that, Molly and I were in frequent telephone contact discussing the implications of her diagnosis. One of the problems she faced was a new version of her old tendency to be more intimidating to people than she realized. We brainstormed together about how she might go about finding a medical specialist who would not be threatened by the fact that this patient might know more than the doctor about an extremely rare condition (Molly had, of course, researched it fully). She finally decided to travel to a prestigious medical-school-affiliated hospital and to interview the specialists there. She found a physician who was willing to be taught by her, to work closely and collaboratively with her, to research the newest information on the disease, and to do everything possible to keep her alive. For several years, they staved off various medical crises. She stayed regularly in touch with me during this time.

A letter from her in 1987 states:

> This is all very hard, but endurable. You know me—I'm tougher as survival requires. . . . No one in my family will begin to face that I'm going to die—not soon, but now I know how. (Of course, I could always be hit by a bus.). . . . Nancy, you know this isn't an unexpected development . . . not to me. I had some early, excellent teachers in living the life you have. I'm going to live longer because of modern pharmacology than many in my family, and I cherish the time here—now how many people do you know who can live life that way?

And she lived several more years that way. I have a pile of her brave, funny, inspiring letters, in which she occasionally reminisced about her therapy, especially about our laughing together over her parochial school experiences. But in the spring of 1991 Molly suffered a respiratory crisis and died. Her psychotherapy had given her more than fifteen years of the pleasures of authenticity, the sense of agency, access to a depth of feeling, participation in a loving and egalitarian relationship, and a sense of self-knowledge and self-mastery. I wish she could have had many more, and I found it hard in her last years to tolerate my impotence to save her life. I still miss her. She would have been pleased, however, that I have told her story here and passed on what she learned in treatment to another generation of therapists.

Chapter 9

Donna[1]

There are many ways and means of practicing
psychotherapy. All that lead to recovery are good.
—SIGMUND FREUD (1905, p. 259)

Although the psychoanalytic literature includes some extended, detailed treatment descriptions of people in the borderline and psychotic ranges (e.g., H. Green, 1964; Sechehaye, 1960; Stoller, 1997), most of the cases currently presented to students in the service of exemplifying psychoanalytic practice tend to involve clients like Molly who can readily engage in a cooperative way with the therapist. Many of the patients that beginning practitioners see are, like the woman described here, much more likely to attach with hostility and devaluation than with an attitude of friendly collaboration.

Because she was one of my earliest clients, the treatment of "Donna" illustrates nicely the way I groped along as a younger therapist and managed to help someone in deep and permanent ways despite my chronic worry that I did not know what I was doing. Her story may also illuminate some of the reasons for my emphasizing certain issues in this book. Our first patients are critical in shaping our individual sense of what factors in psychotherapy matter the most. I think I learned more from Donna than from any other person I have treated. I do not regard her treatment as exemplary in the sense of my having done most things right, but my lapses may make this case all the more useful to present in the context of a book whose main emphasis is that the therapist's tone, expressing the sensibility that informs the interventions, makes more of a difference than any particular technical decision.

An additional reason for my writing about this case is that I have known my former client now for over thirty years and thus have a long-term perspective that follows up both how she was permanently helped and how she remains vulnerable. I also have a not-so-hidden agenda: Despite the scorn currently heaped on what some call the "Woody Allen syndrome"—that is, interminable psychoanalytic therapy—I believe that some patients need a level of devotion that amounts to a commitment to try to remain available for the very long term, if not for life. Most therapists I know have had (often still have) such clients in their practices, including those who do not work psychoanalytically. My eminent cognitive-behavioral colleague Donald Peterson, for example, commented to me years ago, after I had presented the case of Donna to a small group at Rutgers, that he also has had some clients who have checked in with him for repeated periods of treatment over many decades. I regard such devotion as, on balance, socially cost-effective. Especially for more disturbed patients, prolonged access to a caring person on an outpatient basis takes up far fewer resources than the repetitive hospitalizations, psychiatric emergency consultations, crisis interventions, and sometimes jail sentences that are otherwise their destiny.

I have changed the client's name and a few of the demographic details in the following account. But with Donna's permission, I have related what went on in our therapy sessions with as much accuracy and fidelity as she and I could summon.

ORIGINAL CLINICAL PICTURE

Initiation of Therapy

When Donna first came for help to the mental health center where I was working in the autumn of 1972, she was a twenty-three-year-old, second-year student at a local college, majoring in labor relations. She had had several previous contacts with therapists and agencies, including two short hospitalizations and considerable drug treatment (with Navane, Mellaril, Thorazine, and several antianxiety medications in the Valium group), beginning when she was sixteen. At that time, in the context of an intense, fused, sexualized relationship with a girl who was eventually hospitalized for schizophrenia, with whom she had shared an elaborate fantasy about rock stars that bordered on delusion, she was tortured internally with fears of dying and was talking about killing herself. She was significantly overweight, had a handwashing compulsion, was using drugs heavily (marijuana, hashish, methamphetamines, and LSD), and was creating angry scenes at home.

In the seven years between her original adolescent crisis and her intake at the clinic, her problems had for the most part worsened, despite medication, hospitalizations, a stint in a sheltered workshop, and several short psychotherapy experiences that had come to grief in the face of her seemingly impenetrable hostility. She was acting out sexually in gravely self-destructive ways, was repeatedly cutting herself with knives, mostly on her wrists and arms (though once, in a rage at her father, she carved "DAD" into her leg), and was making homicidal threats and physical attacks on people who irritated her. She was also bulimic, but at that time in my career I did not routinely ask about possible eating disorders, and I did not find out that she would regularly binge and purge until five years into our work together, when she casually announced, "By the way, I'm not puking anymore."

As a condition of the state rehabilitation agency's financing her college courses, given her official classification as emotionally disturbed, Donna was required to be in therapy. Hence, she was a reluctant, provocative, despairing patient. Her own description of her presenting problem was, "I am a nervous person. Anxious. Acid trips depress me and I have no motivation to do my work at school." She chain-smoked cigarettes, bit her nails, talked compulsively, craved sweets, and worried that she could easily become an alcoholic or addict of some sort. She was phobic about illness, with a special terror of breast cancer that bordered on a somatic delusion. An admired teacher had referred her, and at his urging Donna was trying to give the clinic a chance to be of help, but she was deeply suspicious of mental health agencies. She also had a profound distrust of both women and Jews; consequently, her female Israeli interviewer elicited a stream of insults and provocations.

Early Clinical Impressions

Despite being heavy, Donna had attractive features and dressed like college students in her general age group. Nothing in her external appearance was off-putting and yet she projected an intense combination of hostility and panicky desperation that made it easy for others to feel intimidated by her. She appeared quite paranoid, gave very concrete responses when asked to give the meaning of proverbs, and talked tangentially and with inappropriate affect. She reacted with an enraged diatribe when asked to complete a fill-in-the-blanks intake questionnaire including items such as "I am the kind of person who _____." For these reasons she had been diagnosed as schizophrenic (chronic undifferentiated) when she first came to me. In retrospect, a diagnosis of paranoid–masochistic character (Nydes, 1963) at a borderline level of personality organization (Kernberg, 1975) seems more warranted, given that Donna has never had fully elaborated hallucinations or delusions. For the first few years of my relationship with her, however, and preceding it, several different examining psychiatrists always chose a severer diagnosis (paranoid, hebephrenic, undifferentiated, ambulatory, or pseudoneurotic schizophrenia), probably because her anxiety in the interview situation disorganized her so dramatically that she sounded flagrantly psychotic. Donna's ego functioning when I first knew her should certainly be considered as at the border of the psychoses rather than at the border of the neuroses (Grinker, Werble, & Drye, 1968).

Personal History

Donna was the oldest of three children born to an upwardly mobile, middle-class Italian couple. Through genealogical research, she has recently learned of instances of severe mental illness in the families of both her parents, including one suicide and one case of adult elective mutism that lasted for decades. Donna's father, who became quite wealthy in the construction business, evidently partly on the basis of connections with organized crime, enjoyed indulging her materially and showing off the family's affluence. She remembers her family's driving around the neighborhood in their Cadillac, enjoying the envy that they assumed they were stimulating. In the context of the prevailing parental myth of the family's great good fortune and superiority, Donna's actual emotional deprivation is particularly poignant.

Her mother, who is still alive, was nineteen when Donna was born and was far from ready to care for a baby. From a couple of conversations I have had with her when she called me because she was worried about her daughter, I have a sense of how deeply she loves Donna. But when Donna was born, she went into a severe, two-year-long postpartum depression. Despite some help from her own mother (whose care Donna still mentions with profound gratitude), she was able to give her infant only the most perfunctory custodial attention. During the span of the depression she never got out of her pajamas. Because she was constantly exhausted, she would leave Donna unattended in a crib for hours, wet and crying. Occasionally Donna's maternal grandmother would rescue her from the worst of this neglect, but she was not always at hand.

Although we did not have then the empirical studies we now have that have convincingly demonstrated the relationship between maternal depression and psychopathology in infants (Cohn, Campbell, Matias, & Hopkins, 1990; Field, Goldstein, & Guthertz, 1990; Tronick, 1989), intuitively I felt it was impossible for Donna to have survived her mother's major depression and consequent emotional neglect without significant emotional damage. Since then, Beatrice Beebe and her colleagues (Beebe, Lachmann, & Jaffe, 1997) have aptly emphasized the impossibility of interactional repair when a baby's mother is severely depressed, noting that a failure of maternal response forces the infant back on its primitive self-regulatory capacities. Their research suggests that maternal depression is therefore a major source of psychopathology in the first year.

Several years into treatment, Donna succeeded in getting her mother to talk without defensiveness about her infancy. She learned that on at least one occasion, her mother had cut her, in a somewhat dissociated state of rage. Donna described her mother as anxious, infantile, and terrified; her depiction suggested a profoundly agoraphobic woman. The year before I met Donna, her mother had separated from her husband, Donna's father, and entered what became a stable, enduring relationship with a female boarder whom Donna originally despised but of whom she became more accepting over time. Since losing her husband, her mother has always been financially strapped. At the time I first saw Donna, she was working in a series of clerical positions where she reportedly supplemented her income by shoplifting and stealing small amounts when circumstances permitted.

Her mother had another girl when Donna was seven and a son when she was twelve. In both instances she again suffered a completely debilitating, lengthy postnatal depression of psychotic proportions. She turned much of the child care over to Donna, who hated the role and vented her resentment on the baby. Both of her siblings have had significant psychological problems. Both, like Donna, have been highly self-destructive and have found it difficult to have a close relationship with another person.

Donna's father, who died of a heart attack in the third year of her therapy with me, had little to do with the domestic life of his family. His work and his extramarital affairs seem to have claimed whatever emotional investment he gave. A big, opinionated, authoritarian man, he frightened his children. Donna feels she was a disappointment to him from the start because she was not a boy. She remembers his insistence on being seen as always right. He seems to have been alternately punitive and seductively intrusive with his daughter. Donna recounted how in her adolescence he would ask her to shower with him, and she described with disgust how he had once kissed her and put his tongue into her mouth. She became terrified and subsequently barricaded herself in her room whenever he approached her. Complaints to her mother about his behavior reportedly elicited the accusation that Donna was "a liar and a pervert."

Donna's childhood was understandably chaotic. Despite precocity in walking and talking, she had recurrent battles over eating, overwhelming fears about being deserted or forgotten, and nightmares about falling off a gypsy wagon. Her description of her upbringing contained no recollections of anyone's respect for, or even naming of, her feelings, with the possible exception of her beloved grandmother. A painful memory from latency concerned the death of her grandfather. She was not allowed to go to the funeral services and was told to "go to bed and think about teddy bears and other nice things." She abused animals throughout her preschool and school years. Separation for kindergarten was traumatic. Once in school, though, notwithstanding a severe problem concentrating, she easily earned B grades because of her superior intelligence. From the preteen years on, she adopted a belligerent identity as a "nonconformist" and hung out with the more alienated students. By age twelve she had developed an intense dependency on her Girl Scout leader, a woman she idealized and looked to for emotional support, who suddenly suicided in a particularly grisly way: She cut her throat with an electric knife. This was a disastrous loss for Donna at a particularly impressionable age, and no one talked with her about it.

Donna's parents, who had had violent arguments for as long as she could remember, finally separated and divorced during her midteens. The breakup of her family seems to have been the immediate precipitant to her entering the symbiotic and sexualized relationship with her girlfriend, in which she first experienced herself as out of control and suicidal. This friendship may have represented an identification with her mother's choosing a woman as a partner, or it may have been a particularly passionate "chum" relationship (Sullivan, 1953), or both. Her bulimia, self-cutting, substance abuse, and violent attacks on others all seem to have originated in this period of family breakup and adolescent transition seven years before I first saw her.

HISTORY OF TREATMENT

I began seeing Donna in April of 1973, in the context of a group for women with schizophrenia that I had been asked to lead in connection with my job at the local mental health center. She was different from the "other" schizophrenic patients in having much more energy—all of it expressed in hostile form, but energy nonetheless. She was then in twice-weekly therapy with the Israeli social worker who had done the intake interview. Several weeks later, when this therapist learned she would have to move, she asked me to take over Donna's individual treatment. I was eager to get experience treating more disturbed clients, and Donna's vitality in the schizophrenic group had been fascinating me for some time. I began working with her at a frequency of two sessions a week, face to face, in addition to seeing her in the group. (Once, several years into her therapy, she wanted to try lying on my couch, but as soon as she did so, she became overwhelmed with a psychotic conviction that she was a murderer, and she gave the idea up fast.)

The Beginning Phase: Developing a Working Alliance

To call the first couple of years of our therapy relationship stormy would be like referring to a tornado as a strong wind. Donna began with me in a rage, based partly on her competition with the other patients in the women's group and partly on her fury about being abandoned by her therapist, with whom she had begun to try to work cooperatively. I noted to myself that it was a good sign that despite her hatred of women and Jews, she had been able to make a positive attachment to this woman. She had also been briefly put on Haldol, to which she had had a severe allergic reaction that her therapist mistakenly suggested might have had a psychological component. This experience had only fortified her antagonism toward the mental health center and mental health professionals in general. She related to me with occasional expressions of dependency and desperation, but mostly with scathing criticisms, attacking my appearance, my clothes, my interpretations, my training, and so on. Because I knew how powerful her personal demons were, this hostility was less difficult to absorb than one might think.

In the first two years Donna asked me a lot of questions about myself, most of which seemed to translate into "How can I expect you to be of any help when everyone else has failed me?" Included with these were specific queries about my politics, my family situation, my professional training, and my theoretical orientation. I answered them frankly and fully, in line with my training to the effect that paranoid clients need a sense of the therapist's willingness to be completely candid. The rationale for this recommendation is that because they project so much, paranoid people may need to be told what aspects of their observations are accurate (so that they learn to feel less crazy) as well as what they may be misinterpreting (so that they can learn that they often get the phenomenon right but the meaning wrong). This style of work also reflects an awareness that paranoid patients experience it as strength when a therapist nondefensively answers a question and as a dangerously weak or sinister evasion when the question is simply explored. Thus, a typical interaction between me and Donna would be, "Why do you always wear your hair the same way? Are you afraid you'd be too attractive if you did something more stylish?" "Actually, I kind of like my hair this way. According to my own sixties-style aesthetic, it *is* attractive. But I gather that you disagree [smiling]." Then I might follow it up with, "Do you have any idea why the consistency of my physical appearance is on your mind today?"

Perhaps the earliest intervention I made that seemed to increase her willingness to try to cooperate with me was my agreement with her assessment that she did not belong in a group of women with schizophrenia. "I know I'm crazy, but I'm not crazy in the same way they are," she protested. Fortunately, I was in analytic training at the time and was learning the difference between a person with schizophrenia and a person whose anxiety under stress reaches psychotic proportions. I presented her to a teacher at my institute, who said, simply, "She's not schizophrenic." I did not take on my professional elders at the mental health center and contest the psychotic diagnosis on which they all agreed, but I was able to persuade my boss that Donna was not a good fit in the schizophrenic group and should be removed for her own sake as well as that of the other members. Donna was surprised and relieved to be supported in her decision to drop it.

Somehow, despite her relentless and sometimes consummately effective attacks, I liked Donna. She was a fighter, and I respected her rage. I could see how she lacked the vacant, confused quality of the patients diagnosed with schizophrenia and how her hostile attacks seemed to be tests of whether anyone could stand her inner life. She spent weeks and months parading what she assumed were the worst aspects of her pathology in front of me, evidently to see whether I would become frightened and helpless (like Mother) or angry and authoritarian (like Father). She was taking illicit drugs indiscriminately, having sexual contact with a large group of male and female acquaintances, and cutting herself frequently. She became pregnant twice and had an abortion in each case. She seemed to be saying, over and over again, "Can you stand who I am at my worst?"

The first time Donna ever responded to an interpretation of mine with anything but skepticism and devaluation occurred about a year into her treatment. I told her she seemed to have a core problem with closeness and distance, and she readily agreed. I was stunned that she had accepted something I had said and for the first time felt I might have something interpretive to offer that would not be spit out. (I had not read Masterson [e.g., 1976] yet, but even without his useful formulations about borderline ego states, I could see that Donna had a central conflict about feeling engulfed and controlled when close, and devastatingly abandoned when given some space.) She then missed the next session. Not showing up was an anomaly for her, for in spite of an initial phase of unreliability, she had become a model patient about coming to appointments. She tended to arrive on time, to talk with agitation and hostility in a very tangential way for about half an hour, to settle down as we zeroed in on a theme, and then to get anxious again and dart out, terminating the forty-five-minute session two or three minutes before its scheduled ending. I was puzzled by her disappearance just when I thought I had finally reached her, but my supervisor suggested that she was needing to withdraw after feeling she let me in too close, and that felt right.

(I never confronted Donna about this pattern of early exiting, because I wanted to support her sense that she had some control over titrating her level of exposure to me and the feelings that emerged between us. After a couple of years, when she was able to stay for the whole session and tolerate my ending it, I commented at that point about how it seemed she was becoming more able to trust that I would keep the boundaries. This tendency to try to understand without interpreting, when I could see the self-preservative and health-seeking aspects of her behavior with me, and then to comment appreciatively when something shifted, was pretty typical of my interpretive style. Fred Pine (1985) has called it "striking when the iron is cold." I thought that if I landed on every nuance of resistance with an interpretation, she would feel minutely critiqued and controlled, and so I reserved much of my interpretive commentary for appreciative retrospective statements.)

The next time Donna showed a capacity to internalize something from me had to do with my setting limits. This incident occurred when I changed jobs and explained that I was willing to continue seeing her privately, if she wished, at the reduced fee she had been paying the mental health center (I did this with the center's blessing; her threats of litigation in connection with the Haldol disaster had made their administrators leery of being responsible for Donna's care). "What if I don't pay?" she immediately challenged. "Then I won't see you," I responded. She then subjected me to a dazzling, ruthless harangue about hair splitting and greed, but in later years she volunteered that her feeling at that time had included a secret pleasure about being treated like a person capable of responsibility. Her family pattern was to pay her no attention until she was in crisis and then to rush in, take over, and treat her like a helpless victim.

At the time, I knew intellectually what stance I had to take, but

mostly I was flying by the seat of my pants emotionally, trusting my supervisor and hoping I was not making any irreversible mistakes. My
main memory of the feeling in the relationship during that early period when the working alliance was still unstable involves Donna's persistent splitting of the world into the good guys, of whom there were
very few, and the bad guys, who were everywhere. Usually her mother
was good, and I, like the rest of the mental health establishment, was
evil, self-seeking, arbitrary, and uncaring. Given the extent to which her
mother had realistically failed her, I was awed by Donna's determination to keep her mother as a good love object. It was Donna more than
any other patient who taught me the truth of the observation that children cling most strongly to traumatizing caregivers (see Main & Hesse,
1990).

A similar limit-setting interaction transpired the next year, when in
a fury I suspected was unconsciously related to my mentioning an up-
coming vacation, Donna took herself, bleeding and threatening suicide, to the emergency service of the mental health center and was hospitalized on the inpatient unit. After a few hours of residency there,
she called and begged me to intervene to get her released before the
mandatory seventy-two-hour period of observation. (Times have radically changed. In that era it was common, when patients signed themselves in for hospital treatment, to insist that they agree in writing to
spend at least three days under observation before being discharged.)
Staff members on the unit had told her they would be willing to let her
go early provided I okayed her discharge. They knew me and would
have been happy to have this angry woman off their hands. I asked to
speak to Donna, and the gist of what I told her was, "You signed yourself in knowing you were committed to being there three days; you can
keep your commitment and get out day after tomorrow. I'll be available
to continue working with you when you do." Again, she was livid at my
failure to rescue her, and gave me heat for it for months, but privately
(she later admitted to me), she felt affirmed as an adult expected to live
with the consequences of her actions.

Late in the second year of our working together, she said she had
something to tell me: She trusted me. From such a paranoid person,
this announcement was deeply moving. But it also ushered in a period
when I became unrelentingly good and all other authorities bad. This
was, from my perspective, only a slight improvement. During her peri-
odic regressions, usually associated with separations, she would appear
at the mental health center demanding immediate emergency treatment and then castigate the hapless staff member on duty for not being more like me (e.g., "You fucking bimbo, MY therapist, Nancy
McWilliams, would NEVER treat me with this asshole insensitivity—

SHE is a PSYCHOANALYST, not a drug-happy, pencil-pushing airhead like you!"). This behavior did not make me many friends. For a while, I lived with my own paranoia—I was certain that she would exasperate all my colleagues into a perpetual state of resentment toward me. For about a year, this fear seemed anything but unreasonable. In fact, several well-meaning colleagues found a way to suggest to me that I was going down the wrong path with this severely ill woman who needed "better management."

Donna was, however, starting to make visible progress at the same time. With some generous medical supervision, she was weaning herself slowly from Thorazine, taking fewer street drugs, and accomplishing some psychological separation from both her mother and her most disturbed friends. She had dropped out of school, but her daily routines were stabilizing. She was cutting herself less often, and her tendency to sexualize in self-destructive ways was becoming less driven and frequent. She had gradually lost some weight. In her appointments with me, she was much less tangential, was occasionally able to laugh at herself, and was less likely to spend the sessions in long tirades. We began to feel a transitional or "play space" (Winnicott, 1971) opening up between us.

The Long Middle Phase of Treatment

As Donna's condition improved, she began to be able to tolerate more time with me and more attention to how she experienced me. She increased to three sessions a week. She now became alternately idealizing and contemptuous toward me, and the sources of her attitudes were sometimes possible to find and discuss. I was becoming excited by her increasing capacity to be interested in our work, instead of treating me as either a satisfier or frustrator of her immediate needs. She seemed to have more capacity to tolerate her feelings without acting them out, to bring them into the consulting room, and to trust me to help her understand them. Her superior intelligence began to feed on the process of figuring out what was going on unconsciously, and she began expressing curiosity about herself. She seemed to be developing some faith in the possibility of change.

Her father died during this period, and she made a sudden marriage within four months of losing him. When she proclaimed her intention to marry a man she had only recently met, I suspected that she was oppositional enough that whatever objections I might raise would only increase her determination to go ahead with the wedding, yet at the same time I felt I would not be doing my job if I said nothing. So I told her my dilemma: "I imagine you know that as your therapist, I'm supposed to raise questions and press you to examine any decision that seems impulsive to me. But I have a feeling that wouldn't feel very help-ful to you." "You're absolutely right," she responded. "Don't say a word." She went on to explain that if I were to register even a whiff of objection, and then the relationship were to fail, it would be too humili-ating to her to admit this to me and get my help at that point. "I'm go-ing to do this no matter what you say," she announced, "So it's better if you save your breath for something I can listen to." I did as I was told, and interestingly, that marriage lasted several years and, although trou-bled, was not altogether unhealthy. She had picked a weak man toward whom she was sometimes both verbally and physically abusive, but he provided a continuity she had never had.

Around the anniversary of her father's death, she went into a pro-found melancholia to which she still shudderingly refers as "the Black Depression." Although virtually unbearable for her, I was hoping it was evidence of a developmental move out of an exclusively paranoid sensi-bility, into what Klein (1935) had called the depressive position and Winnicott (1954) later construed as the "stage of concern." For the first time in her life, Donna seemed to be mourning. She managed to get through this period without medication other than the Valium pre-scribed for her when she had weaned herself from Thorazine, and her determination to tough out a long-deferred, acutely painful grieving process without antidepressant medication was inspiring. If I were treating her now, I probably would suggest that she consider trying one of the newer antidepressants, but at that time, a consult with a psychia-trist friend supported my belief that the available medications could be dangerous. Most of them had the side effect of weight gain, which would have been damaging to Donna's health and self-esteem. In addi-tion, the monoamine oxidase inhibitors required more disciplined avoidance of certain foods than I thought Donna could manage, and the tricyclics were lethal to any impulsive patient who overdosed on them. I can still feel my admiration for how she survived a major de-pression without pharmacological help and without giving up on ther-apy.

This period of grieving for her father coincided with my having a baby, and Donna rebounded from the worst of the depression when I reappeared after a six-week break. She embarked on a legal campaign to contest her father's estate (everything had gone to his new wife) and was able to secure a substantial amount of money for her mother, brother, sister, and herself. It was the first time I had seen her ad-versarial posture put to a legitimate, appropriate, and effective use. (In-terestingly, none of this inheritance ever really reached Donna. A combination of her mother's neediness and her own vast unconscious guilt, which manifested itself in her inability to tolerate and profit from a success, ensured that she ultimately went without—thus recreating her early deprivation.)

Through the first two years of therapy she had been living on disability stipends and occasional maternal handouts. Now, because her income included her husband's modest but regular salary, she volunteered to increase her fee to me. This kind of generosity was one of her most appealing qualities. Occasionally she would bring me a homemade muffin or a bouquet of flowers or a drawing she had done. And despite her periods of desperate regression, she never abused my willingness for her to call me between sessions. I understood her offer to raise my fee as partly a masochistic act and partly a healthy shift away from her predominant identity of helpless mental patient. I accepted the offer (my fee was low enough to suggest that my own masochism was involved), and she seemed to feel an increase in dignity as a result of paying me a more normal rate. I accepted her occasional gifts, as well, without much interpretation in the first years (later we figured out together that she often brought me presents when she was trying to counteract and undo negative feelings toward me). I would have refused any offering that seemed to express a self-destructive level of beneficence, but her generosity never had that character. Unfortunately, Donna was still much too paranoid to work as a paid employee herself. She had held a bank teller job for several weeks, but she had decompensated crazily when given a promotion and had gotten herself fired.

Donna's acting out in our fourth year together took on a more specific and analyzable character. At one point she slit her throat superficially and was able to understand her action as embodying an unconscious identification with her old Girl Scout leader. She began a sadomasochistic affair with a biker whose power impressed her (she had moved, in the transference, from mother to father preoccupations). They engaged in practices like burning her nipples, bondage, penetration with sharp objects, and so on. She did not talk much about this, but she was cutting herself much less. I consoled myself that at least her self-destructiveness was finally object-related. (If I were her therapist now, I would have confronted her more aggressively about her behavior, along the lines that Kernberg and his colleagues [e.g., Clarkin et al., 1999] have recommended. At that point, I was too afraid that nothing I could say would make a difference in her behavior, and I felt that it would be worse if I were to try to stop her and be proven impotent than if I just kept listening and trying to understand. It took me several years to realize how much power I had as a therapist and how valuable it can be to exert it with specific agreements about self-destructive behaviors.)

We had analyzed many aspects of her pattern of self-mutilation (identification with her parents' respective cruelties; repetition of her mother's cutting her in infancy, thus magically keeping her mother with her; identification with self-abusing people in her history; symbolic self-castration; competition with her siblings for the role of the sickest; a cry for help; the firming up of a body ego—"I had to learn about my body by injuring it part by part," she said later; and most centrally, the effort to reassure herself that she was alive, she existed. But in classic psychoanalytic fashion, the symptom did not remit totally until it appeared and was dealt with in the transference. One day she felt misunderstood by me (I no longer remember what I had said or failed to say), and she became furious and incapable of speech. She went into the office bathroom, cut into her wrist, and emerged holding her arm out, dripping blood on my carpet. I lamely suggested that she try to put her feelings into words, but she glared at me silently and left in an obvious rage, only to call me that night in terror that she had finally alienated me for good. I reassured her that I was expecting her as usual at the next session. When we looked together at the incident during that meeting, she was able to see the spiteful aspect of the cutting, evidently the last major unconscious determinant in an overdetermined behavior. The self-cutting never seriously recurred.

Donna did become very involved after that session with having her body tattooed, however, an activity that in the 1970s was rare for middle-class American women. I regarded this behavior as a sublimation more primitive self-mutilatory dynamics. She regarded it as an expression of her artistic, esthetic side, which was beginning to emerge as one of her greatest assets. Both the sadomasochistic affair and the tattooing faded out during the next three years. As Donna slowly got healthier, she became embarrassed about the tattoos all over her arms and would wear long-sleeved shirts. But still later, she decided that they were the concrete evidence of how crazy she had once been, and that she was not ashamed of having been crazy and having recovered. "If they're going to despise me for the visible representation of the fact that I was nuts," she told me, "then I don't want their friendship anyway."

In 1979, Donna began an intensely conflicted but ultimately successful effort to reduce her dependency on drugs of all kinds. She had become seriously addicted to high doses of Valium. She took advantage of the six-week break I took to have my second child by going to a colleague of mine for help in monitoring the slow, systematic elimination of her Valium use. Her only upsurge of violent acting out was during this period: She had become overwhelmed with anxiety after a dosage reduction and again ran to the mental health center demanding some quick medical intervention. When the social worker on emergency duty there said she would have to wait to see a doctor, she swung at her with her spike-studded iron bracelet. It was only the nimble intervention of her biker ex-boyfriend, who had come with her, that saved my colleague from a broken jaw. Donna was taking karate lessons at the time and was a genuine physical threat.

In dealing with this incident in treatment, I told her that the social worker was a good friend of mine. (This was true. I disclosed my attachment in an effort to break down her tendency to split; I was trying to communicate that while this woman may have acted insensitively from Donna's point of view, she was not necessarily a bad person.) Donna felt conscious remorse and shame in the context of being unable to relegate her violent side to the world of the bad guys "out there." Again, it was the experience of a symptom in the transference relationship that made it amenable to change. Around that time her splitting began to be replaced by more ordinary forms of ambivalence; she was able to feel both hatred and love for me within the same hour, and she talked about other people with more depth and nuance.

A synopsis of such a lengthy therapy cannot adequately convey the back-and-forthness of Donna's slow improvement. Even more than most clients, she would go into massive regressions on the heels of any significant gain. I grew to dread the appointment that followed any session in which I felt a strong surge of excitement about her progress. But through all the ups and downs, certain strengths that she had, whatever her ego state, impressed me. For example, like many paranoid people, she was so hypervigilant about my affect that she never missed a thing. Not once did I succeed in getting a stifled yawn by her, in spite of the fact that the perfection of what one of my colleagues calls the "nose yawn" is one of my most cherished professional achievements.

A dramatic example of Donna's extraordinary intuition concerns her feeling for a local eccentric widely known as "Sheet Man," a fairly obvious paranoid schizophrenic who roamed the main street of the community where I worked, wearing a white, sheet-like robe. One day, in a typical tirade about the negligence of mental health authorities, Donna became intensely agitated about Sheet Man's condition. "He used to look at least physically healthy," she insisted. "Now he looks grey and drawn, and his feet are bleeding. He's *changed*. He's in bad trouble and nobody's helping him!" I believed her upset was a displacement of her own feeling that she was not being helped enough. Accordingly, I brought this material into the transference, interpreting it as a displacement of her anger at me for not noticing some aspect of her suffering. I speculated that she was experiencing me as a lot like the depressed mother who did not react to her infantile neediness. Donna grudgingly accepted my analysis of the intensity of her concern. The next day, Sheet Man stabbed his mother to death. Donna began her next session looking uncharacteristically smug, and I had to admit that her astuteness went way beyond displacement.

Some time in 1982 or 1983 I began hearing evidence of Donna's having internalized the self-observing aspects of therapy that I had been carrying alone until then. The first time I noticed this was in her recounting a description of a party at which another guest, to whom she had taken an instant dislike, was bragging about the expense and quality of her jewelry. Whenever another woman competed with her, Donna's automatic reaction was to try to insult and mortify her. This time, though, as she was about to launch her usual sarcastic volleys, she had stopped to wonder *why* the woman was boasting. She asked some questions to draw her out and learned that the woman's father had deserted her family when she was thirteen, and that all she had to remember him by was a bracelet he had given her. "So I understood why she was so hung up on jewelry," Donna declared, proudly. As I was waiting beamingly for the sympathetic statement I expected to follow, she added, "So I realized I didn't have to humiliate her *publicly*. I could just destroy her in my *mind*." Not an insignificant psychological achievement.

Along with these mostly internal developments went a number of positive behavioral changes. Donna became increasingly less dependent on her family of origin, and grew more honest and friendly with all her relatives. Despite our not focusing on it as a target symptom, her bulimia disappeared. Her suicidal and homicidal preoccupations went away. She no longer had crises, emergencies, and malignant regressions. Although her husband divorced her on the basis of the abuse he had suffered at her hands, they have remained close and mutually devoted friends. After the divorce, she lived alone successfully for the first time in her life, an achievement I could not have imagined when I first started working with her.

In 1982 she met a man with whom she developed a much calmer and more loving relationship. After about a year of dating, they were married in the Roman Catholic church as an expression of Donna's rapprochement with a childhood religious tradition that for many years she had virulently rejected. The marriage went well for almost a decade, until her husband suffered a job-related injury and became so habituated to painkillers that he began behaving with the callous undependability and exploitiveness of the severe addict. At that point, long after she had stopped seeing me, she was able with minimal support to take a self-protective and nonenabling stance with him, and when he persisted in not taking her limits seriously, she divorced him. In the good years of their relationship, they had a warm if unexciting sexual connection with none of the former masochistic elements that she had once acted out so flagrantly. In fact, she looks back on that chapter of her life with incredulity.

In the early 1980s, Donna got a dog. Initially she mistreated the animal, but eventually, in the face of its imperturbable affection for her, she became more and more nurturing. For a while after that she went through a grieving process related to her feeling that she should renounce any hope to have a baby. She felt she would not be able to achieve a state of emotional readiness to take care of an infant before her fertility disappeared. In 1986, however, Donna became pregnant, and although we were both nervous that she might have a postpartum depression as severe as her mother's had been, she decided to have the child. After a relatively uncomplicated pregnancy, she gave birth to a girl, whom she was able to mother with remarkable responsiveness. I made a few home visits in the early weeks of her recovery from childbirth and found her attachment to her daughter deeply touching. No sign of serious depression appeared. Both she and her husband were thrilled by parenthood. Eventually, before his accident, they were able to afford a house in a safe neighborhood with other young families.

Donna's daughter is in her late teens now. She was shy and withdrawn as a young child and was diagnosed with some learning difficulties during grade school. Adolescence was hard for her; in response to her difficulties, her mother made sure that she had access to a therapist. Eventually she found her way to a special school for children with cognitive and emotional difficulties, where the staff gave her warm individual attention. In that environment she flourished. She has a boyfriend now and seems to be growing up without any of the florid, self-destructive psychopathology of her mother's young adulthood. It remains to be seen how she and Donna will negotiate her adult separation process, but so far, Donna's combination of anxiety about losing her and irritation at living with a testy adolescent seems within normal limits.

The question of work has been the most problematic of all areas of change for Donna. Throughout our history together, she came up with many ingenious ideas for employment, some grandiose, some quite reasonable. For brief periods she would hold a job, but all her employment experiences eventually foundered on the shoals of her paranoia, especially when she was given any appreciative recognition or promotion by an employer. Her most successful job was as a cook for a local fraternity house in the years before her daughter was born, a part-time position in which she could work mostly alone and as her own boss. In spite of a few weeks of almost crippling anxiety and regression, she managed to keep that job for a long time. The pay was negligible, but the students appreciated her, and the work gratified her not insubstantial creativity. An accomplished cook, she regarded her role as an excellent sublimation of the orality in her nature that had once seemed so frightening.

The Termination Phase

Donna's progress during the early 1980s occurred in the context of a gradually less intensive therapy. In 1981, she and I cut back from three- to two-times-a-week meetings, and in 1983, we changed to once weekly appointments. Both reductions reflected changes in my professional situation (I slowly moved my practice to a town at a considerable distance from her), but they were also synchronous with her readiness. Early in 1984, she indicated that she would like to try meeting once every two weeks, with the provision that if she were to get panicky, she could request that we have a session during the intervening week (a request she never found it necessary to make). About a year later she decided that she would switch to seeing me on an "as needed" basis. She found she rarely needed a session, though sometimes she would call me with a quick question, and sometimes she would call just to hear my voice on my answering machine. She referred unself-consciously to this self-titrated reduction of contact with me as weaning.

I knew for sure that Donna was qualitatively and dependably better by the tenth year of our work. Her gradual cutting down felt like the beginning of a natural and mostly self-initiated separation process. All her presenting problems had either gone away or been significantly ameliorated: the self-cutting, homicidality, suicidality, bulimia, sexual risk taking, addictions, extreme paranoia, and compulsive symptoms. But even more significant from a psychoanalytic standpoint, in that year she came to a session with the following dream:

> "I'm in a mental hospital, but the psychotic patients are on the *other* side of the locked door. I realize I'm not a mental patient; I'm outside. I notice I'm very hungry, so I go to the hospital cafeteria to get something to eat. When I get to the cashier with my food, she tells

me I can't have it. Only the patients are allowed to eat the food. I start to leave, but then I realize that's unfair. I turn back to the cashier and make an eloquent argument that even people who are not sick have a right to eat. She is persuaded, and I get my food and leave the hospital with it."

POSTTERMINATION OBSERVATIONS

As is obvious from the foregoing dream, Donna's therapy helped her to develop a more positive sense of herself as a person who is entitled to nourishment whether or not she is mentally disordered, and as a person who can fight for herself in appropriate, problem-solving ways. Her object constancy and self-constancy improved. Her capacity to regulate her affects increased substantially, with a concomitant reduction of acting out. She was able to see others and herself as whole people with negative and positive qualities; she was able to experience and contain ambivalence. She handled a difficult family situation competently and has been a much better parent to her daughter than anyone was to her. She and I feel that we successfully broke the cycle of recurring trauma that has characterized her family from as far back as she has been able to research.

Probably the nicest personality transformation Donna underwent during her therapy with me was the emergence of her sense of humor. Once the picture of paranoid grimness, mitigated only by occasional biting sarcasm, she now makes brilliantly witty commentaries about her own foibles and enjoys teasing me about mine. Except when she is in a panic, an occasional event that may precipitate a phone call to me, she is one of the funniest people I know. In fact, even when she does panic, her sense of humor does not entirely desert her. She called me a couple of years ago terrified that the father of one of her daughter's friends was going to retaliate in horrific ways for her having harshly criticized his son when he had mistreated her daughter. "What should I do?" she pleaded in her old, helpless way. "Well, you could consider apologizing," I suggested. She brightened up immediately. "I would never have thought of that!" she exclaimed. "That just might work. You see why I still like to keep in touch with you? You're very useful." (This kind of almost flippant advice giving on my part would not have been my style during the therapy, but now that we are many years beyond her termination, Donna and I relate in a more relaxed conversational way.)

In the past decade I have spoken to Donna on an average of four or five times a year, sometimes because something has upset her and sometimes simply because she is thinking of me, wants to know how I

am, wants to catch me up with events in her life, and wants to express
her love and appreciation, about which she is touchingly direct. I find
myself always pleased to hear her voice on the phone. It is hard for either one of us to remember emotionally how difficult our early time together was.

Donna has had a few consultations with other therapists since
slowly separating from me in the late 1980s. The combination of my
geographical distance, her mild driving phobia, and her curiosity
about whether she could work therapeutically with someone else affected her decision. Some of her experiences were disasters, but a couple went very well. The capacity to use others as supportive resources is
clearly one of the major gains of her treatment. As her daughter has
gone through her own adolescent separation and her own reaction to
her parents' divorce, Donna has predictably suffered and has reached
out for help in appropriate directions. She saw a loving, talented former student of mine for many months and on his recommendation participated in a dialectical behavior therapy group (Linehan, 1993),
which she found helpful. She feels good about her accomplishments,
proud of her daughter, and grateful for the changes she has fought so
hard to make.

I believe that Donna made substantial and lasting progress in her
long collaboration with me. She still suffers from many anxieties and
occasional paranoid ideation, and sometimes her cancer phobia recurs.
She is finding her daughter's adolescence a challenge, but this parental
reaction is hardly pathological. Although no one would choose Donna
as a poster child for mental health, neither would a new acquaintance
immediately conclude that there is or had been something seriously
wrong with her. A colleague of mine who ran into her a few months
ago described her as "eccentric and lovable." A few years ago one of
her friends asked if she could come to me for treatment because she admired Donna and had taken her advice to consider therapy as a potential source of help for some of her problems.

The fact that Donna could read this chapter and enthusiastically
agree to its publication in so much specificity seems to me to attest to
her self-acceptance, her pride in her growth, and her mature altruism.
She hopes that her story will inspire the therapists who read it to keep
the faith with their most disturbed and difficult clients and to trust that
a natural striving toward growth will ultimately emerge in the context
of their patient efforts to understand and contain affects that are toxic,
terrifying, and disorganizing. She is also thinking of writing her own
account of her life for publication, something she mentioned to me before I told her I had written up our work.

I have a few other long-long-term clients to whom I remain connected, all of them individuals for whom separation is so profoundly disorganizing that it is better, if possible, not to subject them to that strain. (To me, an obvious application of the primary Hippocratic principle "First, do no harm," is that short-term treatments are contraindicated for those who have profoundly regressive reactions to loss, neglect, and separation.) As I mentioned earlier, most of my colleagues seem also to have a handful of such patients, often individuals they acquired early in their work as clinicians, whom they could never in good conscience rationalize abandoning. Those people who have maintained some connection with me over decades all went through an early few years seeing me at least twice a week and then gradually reduced their frequency of contact to once a week or less. The greatest satisfaction in working with them, beyond the joy of witnessing their individual growth, is the pleasure of preventing the intergenerational transmission of trauma (Main, Kaplan, & Cassidy, 1985).

One of the gratifications of writing about Donna is the opportunity to show off a therapeutic success with a difficult patient. But I want to emphasize that I do not consider my experience unusual. Most psychodynamic therapists have treated their own Donnas, with the same effective combination of patience, fortitude, and the consolations of psychoanalytic theories. For the therapist, such patients offer an entire professional education. Unfortunately, our expertise never gets translated into official mental health statistics, partly because of the private nature of independent practice, partly because a lot of what one essentially does with these very troubled individuals is prevention. One can hardly present solid evidence for the number of suicides one has thwarted, or psychotic breaks that have been avoided, or hospitalizations that became unnecessary, or abused children who never were.

Those of us who have worked any appreciable time in mental health agencies have seen scores of patients like Donna come and go. They arrive in crisis, provoke and exhaust those staff members who try to relate to them and elicit an institutional countertransference involving both controlling and rejecting policies which do them no long-term good and only entrench their despair and hostility toward authorities. They first appear as disturbed adolescents and turn into disturbed adults who have babies to fulfill powerful fantasies about healing through symbiosis. They mistreat their children and deplete the resources of their friends and relatives. They consume the favorite medications of one physician after another. They become "revolving door" patients, whose pathology eats up tens of thousands of dollars (usually the public's) as they undergo emergency treatment and hospitalization when they predictably fall apart at every developmental milestone. Their medical records become as thick as telephone books. Yet once securely engaged in a psychotherapy process, even a psychotically dis-organized person can usually be kept out of the hospital by a devoted clinician. If we are ever to make good on our therapeutic ideals and re-alize our hopes for the prevention of endless cyclic repetitions of psy-chopathology, our mental health policies must make more room for people like Donna.

NOTE

1. This chapter expands on an article about Donna that was published in McWilliams (1986). I am grateful to The Haworth Press for permission to publish the expanded and updated version here.

Chapter 10

Ancillary Lessons
of Psychoanalytic Therapy[1]

It is not the same to know a thing in one's own mind and
to hear it from someone outside. . . . Side by side with the
exigencies of life, love is the great educator; and it is by
the love of those nearest him that the incomplete human
being is induced to respect the decrees of necessity. . . .
                                    —SIGMUND FREUD (1916, p. 312)

Throughout this book I have been emphasizing the centrality of the psychoanalytic ideal of honesty and the deep benefits that
can accrue when patients gradually divulge more and more of their
most private thoughts and feelings to a deeply attached and respectful
other. The experience of speaking from the heart and being taken seriously builds the psychic architecture that supports the capacity to bear
life. In addition to the development of this internal emotional scaffolding, most clients pick up from the therapy experience a number of
helpful pieces of information. I want to talk about some of these in this
chapter.

When we encourage people to listen to their feelings, when we
help them search inside themselves for their own answers, or when we
conceptualize their suffering in a way that allows them to understand it
better and embrace their own humanity, we do so on the assumption
that we all have the potential for attaining a kind of wisdom about life,
about who we are and what we seek, about what is possible and what is
not, about what can be changed and what must be mourned. In psychotherapy, even without any deliberate effort on the part of the therapist
to be a teacher, clients keep learning things that go beyond the details
of their individual histories and conflicts.

Of course, what any individual learns in a psychotherapeutic relationship depends on what kinds of knowledge were unavailable or taboo in that person's family or subculture; thus, for example, one man
acquires the new skill of inhibiting the expression of anger while
another discovers that giving voice to anger can be an effective means
of pursuing a goal. Some of what patients learn in psychotherapy constitutes information and ideas that are completely new to them, as
when one of my clients exclaimed that she had never known that it is
normal to have hostile fantasies toward one's children. And some of it
is information that was "known" at an intellectual level but had never
been emotionally assimilated. Thus, one client of mine remarked, "I
could have told you at the beginning of our work that I was afraid of rejection, but I had no idea the extent to which that affects just about
everything I do. Now I *feel* that fear, and the awareness of the feeling
helps me manage it."

ON PSYCHOANALYTIC KNOWLEDGE

It is widely believed that the "wisdom" of the psychoanalytic tradition is
antiquated, culturally limited, and hopelessly contaminated by Freud's
idiosyncratic and outdated prejudices. Noting that such critiques may
have a grain of truth, Drew Westen (1998) nonetheless observed that
"Freud, like Elvis, has been dead for a number of years but continues to
be cited with some regularity. . . . the majority of clinicians report that
they rely to some degree upon psychodynamic principles" (p. 333). As
psychoanalytic insights have permeated Western cultures, they have
come to be seen as common sense, an osmotic process with both positive and negative effects. On the one hand, analytic ideas have benefited the public at large on issues as diverse as hospital pediatric care,
the child custody policies of courts, and the psychological consequences of prejudice. Terms such as "identity crisis," "defensiveness,"
"denial," "attachment," "introversion," "sublimation," and "Freudian
slip," once the arcane jargon of analysts, are common parlance. On the
other hand, the framing of certain ideas as general knowledge rather
than as the currency of psychoanalysis has contributed to defining as
psychoanalytic in the public mind only those concepts that are problematic or counterintuitive or highly questionable (such as the existence of a death instinct or the universal centrality of penis envy in
women). In this book, I am trying to reclaim their status as part of the
diaspora of psychoanalytic ideas that have come to seem commonsensical in the post-Freudian era.
    Alongside this process of diffusion, the lack of familiarity of most

contemporary psychologists, psychiatrists, and other mental health specialists with primary psychoanalytic sources has created a curious phenomenon: Knowledge that was once the province of psychoanalysis gets periodically rediscovered by people with no analytic background. The early behavioral movement in psychotherapy (e.g., Wolpe, 1964) followed most academic experimentalists in minimizing the role of cognition. As that movement developed, however, many of its practitioners became impressed with the same cognitive phenomena that had fascinated analytic clinicians for decades, especially when they explored problems such as depression (e.g., Beck, 1976), in which painful cognitions are central to suffering.

Given that behavioral, psychoanalytic, humanistic, and systems-oriented students of human nature are all paying close attention and trying to understand the same animal, it is not surprising that careful observers from different traditions come to similar conclusions and propose similar interventions. But this process also smacks of reinventing the wheel. When the behavioral movement in clinical psychology added "cognitive" to its identity, its advocates laid claim to an area in which analytic therapists had legitimately maintained a special competence. Subsequently, professionals with very nonanalytic or antianalytic leanings declared their superior expertise in conscious and unconscious thinking processes. There is currently a virtual cottage industry among academic psychologists in unearthing things that practicing therapists and counselors have known for decades, naming them something else, and announcing that science is now privy to radically new insights. The proverbial man from Mars would find it pretty hard to distinguish Klerman's "interpersonal therapy" (Klerman, Weissman, Rounsaville, & Chevron, 1984), for example, which claims empirically supported effectiveness with moderate depression comparable to that of medication, from short-term dynamic treatments.

In the current climate of enthusiasm for biological psychiatry, a false polarity has been created between "talk therapy" and medication. In fact, psychotherapy and psychopharmacology are inextricably interdependent. On the most concrete, practical level, doctors who want patients to take their pills must rely on basic psychoanalytic principles such as establishing an alliance, expressing empathy, and overcoming resistance. They are also interdependent in the sense that the long-standing assumption of a dichotomy between body and mind, or even between cognition and affect (a dichotomy usually attributed to the dualism of the seventeenth-century philosopher René Descartes), has been exposed by contemporary neuroscience as untenable. Just as we know that brain chemistry affects the way we experience ourselves and our world, we know that certain experiences, including psychotherapy, affect our brain chemistry (Goldstein & Thau, 2003; Schore, 1994; Solms & Turnbull, 2002; Vaughan, 1997).

Whether or not they overtly give information to their patients from a position of informed authority, psychotherapists are always and inevitably involved in a kind of teaching. The most classical interpretation (e.g., "You are afraid your hostile feelings will damage me, as you felt they damaged your mother") carries a covert reeducative message ("Despite what you have concluded, hostile feelings are not so dangerous"). The tone of an ostensibly information-gathering question can send an educative message (e.g., "So you didn't discover masturbation until you were in your twenties?" conveys "Most people masturbate earlier than that; there may be something to look at here"). And in addition to imparting information in these ways, few therapists are such purists about technique that they withhold direct educative influence when they feel a patient is misinformed in areas where the analytic community has knowledge. Comments such as "Unconscious anniversary reactions are very common" or "Children typically blame themselves when something goes wrong in their family" or "No reaction is completely without ambivalence" typify the kinds of messages that may be commonsensical for psychoanalytically inclined therapists but may convey new ideas to the patient.

I talked in Chapter 4 about some ways in which analytic therapists help patients learn to play their part in the complex interpersonal relationship that constitutes psychotherapy. For most clients, perhaps for all but the most therapeutically sophisticated, a certain amount of direct education about the therapy process is critical to its success. Beyond carrying out this orienting function, psychoanalytic therapists tend to avoid being explicitly didactic because their concern is to help patients find their own answers. Some of those answers, however, have a universal quality; that is, they tend to be discovered by anyone who persists in the disciplined effort, facilitated by a therapist, to attain deeper and deeper knowledge of the self and the world. In this chapter I cover areas of knowledge that tend to be assimilated in the normal course of a psychotherapy. I have grouped these insights under the categories of emotion, development, trauma and stress, intimacy and sexuality, and self-esteem. Finally, I have a few comments on the attainment of a sincere disposition to accept and to forgive—that is, the achievement of psychological serenity.

EMOTION

One of the bedrock convictions that informs psychotherapy is that talking helps. If we did not have personal and clinical experience supporting that belief, we could find considerable evidence for it in empirical research (e.g., Pennebaker, 1997; Smith, Glass, & Miller, 1980). Many clients come to us not knowing this; it is one of the things they learn from us whether or not we ever lecture them on the value of self-expression. "How is talking going to help?" is one of the most frequently asked questions of the analytic therapist (see Luepnitz's [2002] beautifully written case-study answers to this question). Most practitioners work out some response to this query, even if it is only to say, "Perhaps you are afraid that talking will only make you feel worse," an empathic effort that also conveys the possibility that in the long run, talking can make one feel better. And our clients indeed learn over time that it helps to talk, especially about things to which they have never given voice before.

A related lesson that many of our clients learn in therapy is that diffuse and disturbing emotional states can be named and integrated smoothly into awareness. Sometimes when therapists see themselves as "uncovering" feelings that have been buried by a defense, they are in fact labeling an emotion for the first time in the client's memory. What the clinician may think of as mirroring may be taken in by the patient as new knowledge. That is, the therapist may assume that he or she is simply restating, with some accent on the feeling tone, what the client has just expressed, but the client's sense may be that a previously unformulated perception has now been given shape and color (see D. B. Stern, 1997). The person's experience is not so much one of being "reflected" as of being *organized* by the power of words to give form to chaos. What Bollas (1987) called the "unthought known" becomes realized, stated, and emotionally integrated. The "alexithymic" (lacking words for feelings), psychosomatically troubled patient (see Krystal, 1988; McDougall, 1989; Sifneos, 1973), who seems to take forever to make the slightest progress, is still learning in that painful slowness that feelings have names that can be spoken aloud and shared with another person. Judith Kantrowitz and her colleagues (Kantrowitz et al., 1986), in a follow-up to a comprehensive, longitudinal study of outcome in psychoanalytic treatment, noted significant and lasting changes in affect availability, tolerance, complexity, and modulation.

In a project of obvious interest to analysts, Shedler, Mayman, and Manis (1993) studied a group of people who all looked very healthy on self-report questionnaires and then asked experienced clinicians to differentiate those who seemed genuinely healthy from those who seemed to present a facade or illusion of adjustment based on defensive denial of underlying vulnerability. They found significant health risks associated with the group they viewed as having "illusory mental health." The highly defended, therapy-resistant individuals identified blindly in this study by skilled clinicians comprise a clinically familiar group of patients whom McDougall (1985) has referred to as "normopaths" and "anti-analysands" and Bollas (1987) has characterized as suffering from "normotic illness." They lack imagination, think concretely and pragmatically, and seem deficient in most functions that we now understand as within the purview of the right brain. In therapy, such patients take a famously long time to learn to express feelings, yet they arguably gain more from the experience than those clients who begin their treatment knowing something about what they feel.

I have often been struck by the phenomenon of the gradual disappearance of chronic physical complaints during an extended psychotherapy or analysis, without their having been "analyzed" at all, their departure being presumably a result of the systemic relief that comes with finding what Cardinal (1983) eloquently called "the words to say it." The body no longer needs to express what the mind can encompass. Other therapists have echoed this observation, and there is also considerable empirical research supporting it. In 1965, Duehrssen and Jorswick reported that individuals who had experienced psychoanalytic therapy had fewer hospitalizations over a five-year period than those in a control group, a robust finding confirmed two decades later by a review of fifty-eight empirical studies on the relationship between psychotherapy and health care utilization and cost (Mumford et al., 1984). In a recent study conducted in Germany (Leuzinger-Bohleber, Stuhr, Ruger, & Beutel, 2003), investigators found a dramatic decrease in health care utilization and costs after psychoanalytic treatment, and noted that such costs continued to decrease even after treatment ended.

I described in Chapter 8 how the patient I called Molly discovered that feelings are "like, *physical!*" in her first year working with me and how she noticed suddenly, after three and a half years of therapy, that her headaches had disappeared. At the other end of the continuum of expressiveness are clients who have trouble tolerating strong feelings without acting on them or dissociating or withdrawing into a deeply schizoid state. By the end of treatment, such individuals develop a sense of comfort with their emotional world and learn that they can bear and handle emotions that they previously experienced as taking them over in frightening, alien ways. Long before the development of cognitive-behavioral protocols for anger management, there was a psychoanalytic literature on the processes by which people learn to bear their feelings and contain them (Krystal, 1978; Russell, 1998; Spezzano, 1993; Zetzel, 1970).

Clients with affective lability, including those who have histrionic and hypomanic tendencies and more florid versions of borderline personality organization, learn to modulate their emotions and to see the connections between one state of mind and another. Thus, the patient I called Donna in the previous chapter was greatly helped when she could tolerate feeling her emotions instead of acting them out in ways like self-cutting, addictive behaviors, bulimia, and sexual risk taking, and when she could reflect on such states of mind reliably enough to talk about them at her next therapy appointment. Her discovery that she could hold an affectively powerful idea in her head and not act on it was pivotal to her slow but impressive recovery.

She is not alone in having learned at a deep level that feelings and behavior are two different things. Many much more self-controlled people come to therapy not appreciating this difference. They arrive in our offices having convicted themselves of heinous thought crimes and regarding their negative emotions as evidence of their depravity. It is a rare person with whom one must be so heavy-handed as to lecture about the difference between a sexual or hostile fantasy and a seductive or aggressive behavior, but virtually everything about the therapist's demeanor exemplifies the distinction between feelings and actions. In the spirit of Silverman's (1984) argument that therapists help their clients more when they go *beyond* interpretations of affects or impulses and help the person learn to find pleasure in a previously disavowed state, I have been known to say to patients things like, "It's progress that you can now *admit* to hating me, but I'm hoping you'll come to *enjoy* that feeling." Most therapists probably make similar comments now and then in the hope of reducing their clients' misery about emotions that are universal and, unless enacted destructively, not only harmless but also connected with a deep sense of aliveness and even joy. Having something welcomed as a vital, expectable part of subjectivity can reduce the shame that ordinarily goes with exposure and conveys that private experience is not dangerous. It can also increase the sense of aliveness and authenticity that makes even painful affects worth feeling.

People also tend to learn in therapy that different and even opposing emotional states may coexist. "I'm trying to figure out whether I'm feeling gratitude or resentment toward you," one of my clients recently remarked, as she explored her complex reaction to a useful but wounding comment I had made. "But then, maybe they're not mutually exclusive." Through their work with us, our patients learn that it is impossible to avoid negative feelings, that ambivalence is ubiquitous, that the limitations of any individual are intimately connected with his or her strengths. These are not always welcome lessons; the attractions of simplicity, of owning one side of an affective tension while externalizing the other, or of persevering in the search for the perfection in self or other, for example, are profound. But they are valuable lessons. As we

have seen all too dramatically in recent years, people can be so determined to invest their own position with all goodness, and that of the
enemy with all badness, that they may willingly, even ecstatically, anni-
hilate themselves and others in the service of retaining that illusion
(see Eigen, 2001, 2002).

What Goleman (1995) has called emotional intelligence parallels
what analysts have traditionally termed emotional (as opposed to intellectual) insight (Hatcher, 1973). The fact that this concept has struck so
many in Western cultures with the force of an epiphany suggests that
certain kinds of wisdom that the psychoanalytic community takes for
granted are not common knowledge elsewhere. Numerous reflections
about affect management and emotional maturity get transmitted to
our clients. They learn to differentiate normal grief from pathological
mourning and sadness from depression. They learn that separation
anxiety is unavoidable. They learn what their individual consciences
can tolerate and what they cannot. They come to understand that feeling things deeply is not equivalent to "showing weakness" or "feeling
sorry for oneself." They learn that all feelings and motives are selfish in
the purely descriptive sense, and that there is no shame in acknowledging the personal motivations for even the most ostensibly "selfless"
acts. They learn to take their feelings seriously.

DEVELOPMENT

Ever since Freud speculated about children's progress through an or-
derly sequence of psychosexual stages, psychoanalysis has embraced a
developmental theory. From the earliest years of the psychoanalytic
movement, psychodynamic therapists have been in the habit of viewing
personality styles and psychopathologies as expressing "fixations"; that
is, we envision patients as stuck for some reason in a normal developmental predicament long past the time when it would ordinarily
have been resolved or transcended. For example, Freud saw the famous triad of traits observed in individuals with obsessive–compulsive
personalities—orderliness, obstinacy, and parsimony—as holdovers from
the childhood drama of toilet training, a maturational crisis in which
those responses and their opposites are naturally elicited.

The developmental models of theorists such as Erik Erikson, Peter
Blos, Harry Stack Sullivan, Margaret Mahler, Jean Piaget, Melanie
Klein, Donald Winnicott, Thomas Ogden and others have framed psychodynamic thinking for decades. Given their bias toward construing
problems developmentally, psychoanalytic thinkers have been enthusiastic consumers of research on attachment, infant psychology, and

early parent–child relationship. The assimilation of these theoretical and empirical bodies of work by practitioners, directly or indirectly, has contributed to a sensibility that informs day-to-day interactions with clients. Not surprisingly, by talking about their problems again and again with someone who views them through a developmental lens, clients learn to see themselves as grappling with maturational challenges rather than as stymied with unrelenting, static realities.

Therapists joke among themselves about "doorknob communications" or "exit lines" (Gabbard, 1982)—that is, significant disclosures made by clients at the end of an hour (often an hour in which nothing seemed to happen), when the patient is going out the door and there is no time to process what has been said. There is a therapist analogue to this behavior that I have noticed in myself and that other practitioners have told me they recognize. We make casual "asides," often at the end of sessions, that are intended to convey something important without requiring the patient to respond. These remarks are frequently comments on normal developmental phenomena, intended to allow clients to see a problem in a more normative, less pathologizing light. For example, most clinicians find themselves making occasional comments such as "Idealization is a normal part of the courtship phase in a relationship," or "In pregnancy, one can feel much more adult and competent *and* much more childlike and needy," or "Retirement does present challenges to one's sense of identity," or "It's natural at your age to be working on issues of intimacy," or "That kind of moral rigidity is common in adolescence," or "Kids who are mistreated tend to hang on to the idea that they're bad; they'd rather believe they could improve their situation by becoming 'good' than recognize the terrifying reality that their caretakers are negligent or abusive."

I come from a family of teachers, and my own temperament inclines toward the pedagogical; I would not be surprised to learn that I do more of this than many therapists. Like most practitioners, I make a lot of educative "asides" with patients who are struggling to keep their sanity, because people with psychotic or symbiotic psychologies are often very confused about ordinary developmental conflicts and tend to mix up their normal strivings with their sense of being crazy. But I also find myself making such comments occasionally with higher-functioning people, especially when they confront some new maturational challenge about which my profession—or simply my age—has given me some understanding. For example, I sometimes say to people who are exhausting themselves caring for a dying parent,

> "It's my experience that no matter how devoted you are, no matter how much time you spend at the bedside, you'll probably find your-

self feeling after the death that you should have done more. I
doubt that heroic care-taking now will protect you from later self-
criticism. That just seems to be an integral part of early grief. I've
known people who were models of dedication, who were holding
their loved one's hand at the moment of death, who still castigate
themselves that they didn't say 'I love you' one more time."

Patients have often expressed gratitude later for these kinds of remarks. Development through the life cycle is hard enough, even *with* an
understanding of the issues that go with each new adaptation; consequently, most clinicians occasionally give their patients a kind of
"heads-up" on what they are about to face.

The therapists frequently comment, often in the context of individualized interpretations, on familiar, developmentally informed psychoanalytic observations such as the back-and-forthness of recovery from
one's symptoms, the normal human need for attachment, and the relative stability of one's basic temperament and attachment style. We hope
that these observations will be internalized, and that after the treatment is over, they will operate in the service of a client's capacity to
maintain gains and handle future challenges with grace. The woman
who learns at twenty-seven to understand a depressive reaction as expressing a reactivated identification with her deceased mother, who
was twenty-seven when she was born, will not be surprised when she
has a depressive reaction on reaching the age her mother was when she
died. Ideally, her knowledge about the power of unconscious anniversary reactions will permit her to grieve more effectively when she has
another, and to comfort herself in ways that would not be possible without that knowledge.

Whether or not the clinician is as explicit as I sometimes am about
the maturational contexts of clients' problems, the analytic therapist's
developmental frame of reference tends to be transmitted to patients
and to be assimilated by them. A common sign of this assimilation is a
patient's sudden appreciation of the immaturity of his or her childhood self. When we reflect on events from early in our lives, we may
feel a sense of continuity between who we were as children and who we
are now. Yet talking about childhood experiences in therapy often trig-
gers in patients the startling emotional realization of *discontinuity*, of
the changed adult perspective from which they can now view their
developmental unreadiness to have coped with the stresses of their
younger years. As they revisit their childhood feelings, they begin to
differentiate their adult self from the self of childhood and can take
some distance from attitudes that originated in their early lives. A
revelation frequently heard by therapists involves a client's encounter

with a child of the age at which a person experienced some significant stress or trauma. "Seven-year-olds are really *young*!" one of my clients exclaimed after visiting a beloved niece, recalling the desperate precocity she had summoned up to deal with her molestation at that age. Compassion for the child in ourselves and others requires some appreciation of how very different the emotional world of childhood is and of how many transformations have attended our passage from then until now. Such compassion is another nonspecific lesson of psychotherapy, about which I say more shortly.

TRAUMA AND STRESS

The psychoanalytic tradition has always embraced an epigenetic epistemology in which development interacts with stress and trauma. We have learned a great deal about traumatic experiences, psychological stress, and human vulnerability over the years (see, e.g., van der Kolk, McFarlane, & Weisaeth, 1997). We know, for example, that the assumption that all children are resilient and will bounce back, without help, after a loss or dislocation or divorce is wishful thinking. We appreciate the intense nature of attachments and the pain that attends the loss of loved ones. We know that people do not thrive in corporate cultures in which they feel unappreciated, overworked, relentlessly criticized, and vulnerable to being fired at a moment's notice. We know that trauma can damage the brain (Fonagy & Target, 1997; Thomson, 2003) and lead to retraumatization by flashbacks and reenactments. Many people in Western culture do not share our views; some are passionately convinced, for example, that combat experience strengthens character instead of damaging it, sometimes irreversibly.

Our patients assimilate these painful realities as they confront their own vulnerability in our offices. A man I treated who had always defensively minimized the implications of his life-threatening allergy to shellfish began wearing a medic-alert bracelet as he became able to take seriously the fact that he could go into anaphylactic shock and die if he were ever misinformed about the contents of a casserole. A client of one of my colleagues, a woman with a similar kind of bravado, began getting medical screenings such as Pap smears and mammograms once it penetrated her consciousness that she could not necessarily ward off cancer by force of will and healthy living. Psychotherapists do not get much credit for the amount of prevention we do (largely because we cannot prove what would have happened in the absence of treatment), but the responses of these two individuals to therapy support our conviction that by helping our clients to become more

honest about their fragility and limitation, we prevent many serious afflictions.

In this context it is interesting to consider the possible implications
of the recent finding (Jeffrey, 2001) that the mortality rate for psychoanalysts, at least male ones, is lower than that of virtually everybody
else, including other male professionals, physicians, and psychiatrists.
Most of us in the field infer from this research that having undergone
psychoanalysis conduces to physical well-being. But it is also possible
that, in addition to the health benefits we have derived from putting
feelings into words and reducing our defensive response to our fragility, analysts have learned vicariously to avoid the stresses that we see
dominating the worlds of our clients. In the United States, the widespread social sanctions for living one's life in ways that are not humanly
supportable amount to the endorsement of a cultural psychopathology.
In recent years, I find myself increasingly challenging my patients' beliefs about how far they can stretch themselves. I wonder out loud
whether they will regret not having spent more time with their young
kids; I question their taking a job that requires them to be on call night
and day; I ask how they expect to enjoy a life that includes working
sixty hours a week and caring for two preschool children, a teenage
stepdaughter, a dog, a home, a boat, and a pair of elderly parents.

The assumptions that psychoanalytic therapists make, on the basis
of their own intensely scrutinized experience and their observations of
the intimate lives of others, about what is a manageable life seem to be
increasingly at odds with what is expected in the more materially ambitious subcultures of contemporary technological societies. And it is
small comfort that recent political, economic, and social psychology
scholarship is confirming psychoanalytic assumptions that the pursuit
of happiness via material accumulation is doomed (see Lane, 2000).
When Erich Fromm (1947) made his famous observations about the
"marketing" orientation attendant on the twentieth-century phenomenon of national and international commerce (he described the emergence of a kind of person who experiences self and others as commodi-
ties and seeks self-esteem by "packaging himself" or "selling himself" as
someone of superior attractiveness, fame, and resources), I doubt that
he could have imagined the lengths to which that kind of driven psychology could be extended. The increasingly common medical exhor-
tation to "reduce stress" is a pale antidote to all the economic, technological, and social forces that heap stress after stress on contemporary
families. Whatever progress an individual makes in psychotherapy
toward examining what feels personally true and right, above and beyond what is culturally normative, creates some healthy resistance to
unreasonable but pervasive environmental demands.

With respect to trauma—that is, to overwhelming experiences that go beyond the realm of stress—the main lessons that most patients with traumatic backgrounds seem to derive from psychotherapy include that they can protect themselves from many things they once had no control over and that not every situation amounts to an occasion to be retraumatized. Because the transferences of clients with histories of traumatic abuse tend initially to be intense and relatively undiluted by observing capacities, it is hard for such individuals to take in the possibility that a therapist sincerely has their best interests at heart. Trauma survivors mix us up more dramatically with the people who have hurt them than most patients do. The slow process of differentiating the present from the past has always been the heart of the therapy experience for such clients. In addition to the volumes of clinical writing on the process from anecdotal and theoretical points of view, we now know from physiological research that psychotherapy strengthens the activity of the prefrontal cortex so that it will not be so easily invaded by traumatic memories (LeDoux, 1992).

Survivors of trauma also tend to learn in psychotherapy how to avoid situations in which their agonizing memories will be unduly stimulated. Even though psychoanalytic therapists tend to try to avoid giving instruction, it is common for us to advise explicitly in this area. On September 11, 2001, many of my friends and colleagues were telling their clients, "Don't let your kids sit at the television watching the trade towers fall again and again." I have asked more than one dissociative patient, "Are you sure it's a good idea to watch 'Sybil'?" Our clients internalize our own conviction that they can protect themselves from retraumatization, that they are not doomed to repeat the past, and that they do not deserve to suffer any more damage beyond the insults of mortality and vulnerability that are inevitably a part of life.

INTIMACY AND SEXUALITY

In psychoanalytic therapy, we learn from first-hand experience that a relationship that is confined strictly to talking can be intimate to a degree that surprises, comforts, nourishes, and moves us. The increased facility we develop in articulating very personal thoughts and feelings transfers elsewhere, whether or not we entered treatment to improve our ties with other people. It is a rare individual who goes through intensive therapy and fails to learn something about how to enrich his or her friendships and love relations. An expanded capacity for emotional intimacy is thus a frequent by-product of analytic therapy; sometimes, an increased aptitude for sexual intimacy emerges as well.

Research conducted in the past couple of decades reveals that many people, at least in the United States, complain of waning desire for the person with whom they wish to have a sexually fulfilling partnership. Whether straight, gay, bisexual or transgendered, individuals who have gone to sex therapists in recent years have been expressing vague feelings of deprivation and sexual apathy more often than they have been asking for help with concrete sexual malfunctions (Leiblum & Rosen, 2000). Even though the capacity to integrate sexual excitement with emotional commitment is not always an explicit goal of those who come to psychotherapists for help, the knowledge that it is possible to combine familiarity with passion often emerges from a therapeutic experience.

Therapists hear more stories about people's sexual and intimate lives than just about anyone else—even bartenders, hairdressers, and taxi drivers. We become impressed by how sexually diverse people are. While many cultures observe the myth that "all cats are the same in the dark"—that is, that most people follow a standard pattern of sexual arousal and that the essence of being a good lover is knowing various ingenious ways to activate a universal pattern—therapists become fascinated with how markedly individuals differ in areas such as level of drive, pattern of arousal, content of sexual fantasies, types of identification called on in sex, location of erogenous zones, influence of sexual fears and wishes, history of sexual trauma, preferred degree of intensity or languor and activity or passivity, and ways of integrating sex with strivings like aggression, dependency, and wishes to see and be seen, to possess and be possessed, to use and be used, and so forth. We notice how people differ in their defensive uses of sex: to vent hostility, to enact unconscious guilt, to master trauma, to repair interpersonal ruptures, to solicit comfort, to restore self-esteem, to compensate for distance, and to ease boredom, among others.

It seems to be easy for us as individuals to feel that we are either "normal" or "abnormal"; that is, to presume that most other people are like us or to presume that our personal inclinations are aberrant and impervious to another person's understanding. The truth about most things is probably somewhere in the middle; that is, we all resemble each other in certain basic ways, and we are all unique in others. Psychotherapy helps us to articulate what is unusual or special about ourselves without feeling shame that we are beyond the pale of human experience. The tendency for individuals to assume either ordinariness or waywardness may be especially true in the domain of sexuality: We are all sexual beings and we are all at least a bit idiosyncratic in our sexual tendencies. Many individuals learn in psychotherapy that they cannot make glib assumptions about either their own sexuality or that of others. Therapists probably communicate in subtle ways something about the uniqueness of individual erotic organization, if only by asking patients for concrete details when they talk about sex. The appreciation of sexual diversity and the capacity to own one's unique sexuality without apology are frequent "nonspecific" outcomes of analytic therapy, outcomes that open the door to improvement in the negotiation of sexual relationships.

People learn to talk graphically and matter-of-factly about sexual issues in psychotherapy. Sex may be the only area of life in which each of us has to find a way, without the help of our elders, to communicate what we need. Our parents may have been good sex educators when we began asking questions in the preschool years, but when puberty throws us into a transformed awareness of the demands of our bodies and makes our concerns much more personal and pressing, the developmental exigency of separation militates against our going to even the most enlightened parents to get practice in talking about what we are feeling and desiring. Few people have had the opportunity to talk nondefensively about sex to a person in authority before they come to a therapist, and they consequently listen for the clinician's perspective on it with a particularly sensitive ear.

Individuals trying to enrich their sexual lives may find ways to express their idiosyncratic sexual nature to their partners and to learn from their partners what is specific to their own pleasure. They become less inhibited about asking for what turns them on, because they are less inhibited generally about verbalizing, and they burden their mates with fewer expectations that they should "just *know*" what is wanted, without words. They learn that sexual and emotional intimacy usually require struggle and negotiation. Cultural images of couples falling wordlessly into wonderful sex or living happily ever after once they have found their true soul mates are not good sources of education about sex and intimacy.

Several popular books by psychoanalysts have addressed this issue in recent years, presumably because therapists see a general need in their clientele to find and explore their conflicts over closeness and because they have witnessed the ongoing value to patients of attaining more understanding in this realm. Harriet Lerner (1989), in a book aimed at women, described the back-and-forth patterns of committed couples as a "dance of intimacy." Stephen Mitchell, in the posthumous book *Can Love Last?* (2002), argued that intimacy can be more terrifying to us than isolation. Deborah Luepnitz's (2002) writing on the topic draws inspiration from a parable cited by the philosopher Schopenhauer, who implicitly compared human beings to porcupines on a cold night: We need to get close in order to be warm, but then we prick each other and move apart so as not to get hurt. Then we start to freeze and move closer again, and the cycle repeats.

The realization that emotional and sexual intimacy is both wished for and feared is a frequent outcome of psychotherapy, as is the sense that one has some power to improve relationships by giving voice to one's desires and encouraging one's partners to do with same. In a related vein, people learn in treatment that the solutions to their difficulties will not lie in the transformation of their partners but in coming to terms with the partners as they are. They often comment about having come to understand deeply that an individual's bad qualities are inextricably connected with his or her good ones ("I learned that people come in packages," one of my friends reflected), and they develop an appreciation of the people who live with them for tolerating their own less winsome attributes.

SELF-ESTEEM

The development of a reliable and realistically based sense of self-esteem is another common therapy result that evidences an in-depth learning process. With treatment, people can come to understand and accept themselves as they are, to maintain reasonable standards by which to evaluate themselves, and to tolerate criticism and failure (or success, for that matter, the tolerance of which can also be difficult) without anxiety or loss of a sense of self-regard (cf. Strenger, 1998). What is learned in psychotherapy that contributes to stable and resilient self-esteem differs from one person to another, depending on individual psychodynamics.

Some people (most notably depressive, masochistic, and classically obsessional individuals) come to therapy with savage inner voices that constantly remind them of their defects, failings, errors, sins, and illusions. For them, what must be learned in treatment is that they are not as bad as they feel, that there is nothing particularly special or unusual in their version of limitation or sinfulness, and that their relentless contrasts between their own psychology and that of a fantasied ideal person are unreasonable. As their harsh superegos are softened by the repeated process of exposing their hated qualities to a nonshaming therapist, such patients learn to console themselves instead of attacking themselves. They lose the conceit that they are uniquely bad, and they become comfortable with being good *enough*.

Others (notably people with significant narcissism or psychopathy) come to therapy with an inner feeling of emptiness or an unrealistic sense of entitlement that leaves them chronically envious of others whom they see as having what they lack. The more successful people in this clinical group may brandish the insignia of worldly achievement (money, fame, power) and yet confide that all their attainments still do not feel like "enough." The less successful individuals in this category come to treatment because they are mired in a resentful, depressive funk. They want to figure out what it is they are not "getting" about how to live their lives. They value appearance more than substance and seem unfamiliar with the pleasures that come from drawing on inner resources. Kernberg (1984) notes that they are more at risk than people in other clinical categories for alcohol and drug abuse.

What the subjectively "empty" client tends to learn in therapy is that self-esteem is not fed by the accumulation of trophies or conquests or chemical highs but by the development of a sense of internal motivation. He or she learns to look inside for what feels true rather than outside for what feels transiently diverting, and to accept what *is* rather than striving for a perfectionistic ideal. This shift does not result from moral instruction. Rather, something about the process of extracting meaning from the smallest clinical incidents contributes to the capacity to be in the moment and to enjoy the here and now without continually comparing it to some fantasied better time. In Chapter 3 I commented on how much is learned, especially by clients suffering from a sense of emptiness or fraudulence, from the therapist's willingness to acknowledge mistakes and limitations without seeming devastated. The fact that the therapist maintains a robust sense of self-esteem in the absence of perfectionism can make a strong impression on this kind of patient.

When I work with a person who seems morbidly empty or defensively false in some elemental way, my criterion for a good session is whether it contains a grain of emotional authenticity. Patients in this group have a bad reputation among mental health professionals because of their apparent self-absorption and their indifference to the therapist's humanity, and yet the moments when an "empty" client finds a compelling and genuine way to speak can be profoundly moving to both client and clinician. Compared with other patients, the progress of these individuals seems slower, and their acknowledgment of progress slower still, but over time they do take in the therapist's sincere interest, emotional honesty, and relative incorruptibility, and what has been a very chilly inner world begins to be warmed by that internalization. "I've learned that I feel better about myself when I'm working, even at a stupid, low-class job, than when I'm manipulating the system to get disability," one of my former clients commented, with some surprise.

When patients who suffer from subjective emptiness spontaneously describe what they have learned in therapy, many of their comments suggest that they have learned more by example than by conversation or self-scrutiny. They may come to identify with admired aspects of the therapist and thereby increase their sense of self-worth. More than one of my patients has told me that my habit of ending sessions on time or my insistence on being paid promptly has given them inspiration about the possibility of behaving with self-respect. Others have told me that they have learned from me how to listen. And one man told me at the end of treatment, much to my surprise, that the most enlightening aspect of his therapy had been my matter-of-fact refusal to behave fraudulently with his insurance company.

FORGIVENESS AND COMPASSION

It is common to enter psychotherapy with a powerful hope, sometimes conscious and sometimes not, that we can resolve our own problems by somehow changing our parents, our partners, our bosses, our family members. It is painful to acknowledge at the emotional level that the only person we can reliably change is the one who came to therapy. It constitutes a major renunciation of childhood wishes, and typically involves a long grieving process, to give up on the project of transforming others, making them finally hear us, getting them to be responsive, having our own subjective reality vindicated. We learn the difference between "fixing" someone or something and finding a way to deal with our situation. We learn that accepting limits is more liberating than endlessly protesting them, a lesson that is worth all the grief involved in resigning ourselves to disappointing realities.

Many people with no personal experience of psychoanalytic therapy suspect that it is an exercise in whining, an ritualized invitation to blame one's childhood caregivers for one's own mistakes and failures of will. Parents worry that a child who sees a psychotherapist will expose all their worst failings and will be encouraged to see them as fools or monsters. It is true that early in treatment, many patients get in touch with complaints about family members and become keenly aware of all the ways in which the authorities of their youth fell short of a parental ideal. But over time, as disappointments are mourned and accepted, the converse attitude begins to emerge. Parents and other authorities come to be viewed as people who did their best in the context of the hand they were dealt. As clients feel more like adults themselves, they come to understand that grown-ups are only human. The infantile demand that the universe be fair comes to be replaced by the consoling appreciation that although life is not fair, it contains opportunities for creativity, pleasure, and satisfaction.

Crimes have to be acknowledged before they can be forgiven. Usually we know intellectually when we begin therapy that our parents had parents, that they once were children who were damaged by the shortcomings of others and by the accidents of their histories. But in order to *feel* forgiving toward those who have failed us, it helps to admit and explore the emotional consequences of the failures. And we have to have found comparable failures, or the potential for them, in ourselves. Psychoanalytic therapy encourages us to speak our grievances, to express in the transference our anger at the felt perpetrators of the wrongs we have suffered, to feel our grief about what has happened, and, finally, to come to terms with the reality that although our past cannot be changed, our future can be shaped by our growing sense of agency.

In psychoanalytic therapy we learn to regard our own problems and limitations with less self-criticism. Instead of attacking ourselves, we work to change what can be changed and we develop the capacity to comfort rather than to attack ourselves for what cannot be changed. As we develop more acceptance of ourselves and our shortcomings, we also find ourselves able to be more compassionate toward others. In fact, Young-Eisendrath (2001) writes about increasing compassion for self and others as a treatment goal of equivalent value to the alleviation of suffering. Neville Symington (1986, p. 170) explicitly connects self-esteem with the capacity to love. Although it is true that in short-term treatment and in work with more damaged patients it is unrealistic for the therapist to expect a client with a life full of misery to transform into a paragon of magnanimity, it fits my clinical experience that a conspicuous outcome of open-ended psychoanalytic therapy is the capacity to forgive both oneself and others.

NOTE

1. Much of this chapter appeared previously in McWilliams (2003). I am grateful to the APA Press for permission to adapt it here.

Chapter 11

Occupational Hazards
and Gratifications

I have been a fool for lesser things.
—BILLY JOEL, "The Longest Time"

There is nothing I would rather do for a living than be a psychotherapist in independent practice. I feel nourished by ongoing opportunities for in-depth learning, I have control over my time commitments and my conditions of labor, I am confident about the value of what I do, and I feel consistently moved at being in a position of sacred trust. Every patient or supervisee is different, and the work is rarely boring. Still, these privileges come with a price tag. For those readers who have been aware since childhood of a compelling wish to be of use to others, it may be valuable to learn about the disadvantages and limitations of the role of professional helper—the editing of one's more grandiose rescue scripts cannot start too early. For those who feel less of a sense of calling and who are unsure if they are temperamentally suited to be a psychoanalytic therapist, this chapter may be useful in evaluating whether they are headed in the right direction professionally. I first cover some discomforts and disappointments of the role, and then I indicate its substantial gratifications.

OCCUPATIONAL HAZARDS

Practical Professional Liabilities

It used to be common in my department at Rutgers for faculty members without clinical practices to comment, with disapproval and possibly envy, on the cushy life of the psychoanalytic practitioner. In their

260

fantasies, we sit around all day treating the "worried well," saying "Hmm" at regular intervals and collecting hefty checks at the end of each hour. We do not extend ourselves to read the empirical literature (about this they are right—most therapists read what other therapists write rather than what academic researchers report), we see wealthy patients indefinitely whether they need it or not, and we do not have to account for ourselves to anybody. If this rendition was ever accurate, it has certainly not been so in the thirty years I have been practicing. In reaction to comments such as these, it has been hard for me not to retort, "Yeah, it must be really hard to have tenure, a secure job, a free office, a secretary, graduate student assistants, photocopy facilities, a dependable salary, paid sabbaticals, benefits, no loss of income if you're sick, and nobody calling you at midnight threatening suicide." For the perks of academia, I might even read more of the empirical literature.

There are significant practical disadvantages to being in the psychotherapy business, as there are to being in any profession—many of them intimately related to its advantages. With every patient we confront the unknown. We cannot recycle our last performance; we have to start from scratch with each new individual, figuring out how to enter into meaningful conversation with this person, how to be of help. We have daunting responsibility and sometimes less than adequate power to carry it out. We may be faced with frightening and even dangerous expressions of psychopathology. If we misspeak, our words may become engraved in our patients' minds and come back to haunt us again and again. We are repeatedly confronted with our limitations and failings, we suffer a chronic internal pressure to be as genuine and honest with ourselves as humanly possible, and we have to put a lot of time in before we see the kinds of in-depth change that originally made this work so attractive to us—which sometimes does not crystallize in a manifestly visible way until after we have finished seeing a particular client.

If we practice in an agency setting, we may have all the problems of working in a dysfunctional institution: destructive office politics, unsympathetic administrators, a crazy boss, arbitrary policies, changing rules, and bureaucratic impingements of sometimes dizzying proportions. Attention to keeping the files litigation-resistant may be much more scrupulous than attention to patient care. In the United States, therapists in agencies have to adapt to insurance-driven requirements to fill out one form after another that has almost nothing to do with how people are really helped (converting analytic therapy to the language of "target symptoms" and "level of functioning" is a skill that many have mastered but few can enjoy). And the workload can be crushing. Even in well-run organizations, current pressures for rapid patient turnover demand that therapists attach to, and separate from, many more clients than a caring professional can possibly invest in emotionally. A colleague of mine recently commented that employees who stay for many years in agency settings these days tend to be either saints, hacks, or those who have never completed the process of getting licensed for independent practice. And given the limitations of short-term work, such pressures deprive agency therapists of the confidence-building experience of seeing significant personality change or the mature assimilation of new capacities in the people they treat.

Those of us in private practice have the advantage of setting our own fees and work schedules, but our income is rarely stable. Patients come and go, and even those who stay a long time may change their frequency of appointments. When we are ill or have an emergency or get called for jury duty or take a vacation, we receive no compensation. Whatever our official or "regular" fee, the softhearted among us, who are legion, tend to lower it when a client makes the case for financial need. Unless we can get coverage through a family member, those of us in the United States spend a sizable portion of our income on health insurance. We must rent an office, furnish it, pay for malpractice insurance, publicize our availability, cultivate referral sources, keep up with professional developments, manage our billing and record keeping, and make provisions for our patients' welfare when we go away. Given that the most reliable source of referrals is a satisfied customer, if we are not good at our work, we are not likely to get many clients. These are not overwhelming problems, but they do require us to be reasonably astute businesspeople, an aspect of professional life that is often at odds with our personal inclinations and tends to be neglected in our training programs.

Finally, the sedentary nature of our work gives us insufficient exercise. Therapists not only sit all day, they tend to sit *still* all day. Those who treat children are advantaged in being able to sprawl on the floor and draw or to play in sand trays. Those who treat mostly adults have no such physical outlet (though between sessions I go up and downstairs one time whether I need to or not). And the strain on the body of sitting still so long is hard to relieve by careful attention to posture; I have not yet found a sitting position that is good for my back that signals to the patient that he or she can relax with me and let it all hang out. When I sit up straight with both feet on the floor, my posture says "military officer" or "parochial school teacher," not "relaxed confidante." I was not surprised to learn recently that therapists are second only to truck drivers in their incidence of back and neck problems.

Affective Exhaustion and Indirect Traumatization

Absorbing all the emotionally infused messages that come one's way in the course of a day as a therapist is tiring in a way that goes far beyond ordinary weariness. I am always struck by how much energy I have at the end of a vacation day or even after a full day of teaching, compared with how spent and inert I feel after working all day with patients. Emotional exhaustion is an insidious kind of tiredness; in the here-and-now of the clinical hour I am completely unaware that it is creeping up on me. My conscious experience while working is that I am alert, interested, and connected as I process the material of each session, sifting with interest through my associations, images, and emotional responses to my clients' communications. Except for people in the borderline range who assail me with storms of affect, patients do not exhaust me in the moment. Just as some athletes report that they are not aware of feeling tired until a game is over, I am not conscious of being emotionally used up until I leave the office.

My daughter Helen, once she got old enough to tell the difference between an adult who is listening actively and one who is merely adopting an interested expression, used to accuse me of having a "listening disability" (which she was happy to abbreviate, DSM-style, as "LD") after a day with patients. She was right. Having treated the children and spouses of a number of therapists, I have noted that a common complaint from this group is that the parent or partner so revered by colleagues and patients for an attitude of boundless interest and compassion is, at home, a paragon of inattentiveness and irritability. Considering how affective exhaustion plagues even those of us with limited and self-regulated caseloads, I can only imagine what happens to therapists in agencies who are expected to treat huge numbers of individuals and families. They must either learn not to care or burn out fast, or both. One of my consultation groups includes three therapists who work at college counseling centers. At high-stress times of the academic year, they all talk wistfully about how nice it would be to run a little flower shop.

Part of this depletion is doubtless the result of simple hard work and ceaseless discipline; being so constantly tuned in uses up the emotional energies critical to maintaining empathic contact. But part of it may be connected with the fact that therapists have few opportunities to talk about all that they absorb, to excrete emotionally a portion of the affect that they soak up all day. Like mothers who become starved for adult conversation after spending the day alone with infants and toddlers, therapists can feel used up and desperate for a different kind of relating. Even in institutions, the role of therapist is isolating; all the projective and introjective identifications that invade one's consciousness cannot easily be exorcized. Moreover, confidentiality obligations decree that when we do get opportunities to share our experiences with colleagues, we cannot simply spill. By staying constantly mindful of our clients' rights to anonymity, by using pseudonyms and changing small details that might be identifying, we work even when we are off duty, carefully protecting the privacy of the people whose secrets we keep. In analytic writing, there is frequent mention of the danger of burnout (e.g., A. Cooper, 1986).

Another consequence of having other people's emotions put into us so unremittingly is that we find ourselves feeling strong reactions we would rather not have. Even loving takes energy, but it is especially unpleasant to experience boredom or irritability or hatred toward a client. With those for whom we feel a consistent sympathetic concern, we are not relieved of painful affect states; we may have strong negative reactions to the people our patients describe to us. It is easy to hate faceless individuals who are represented as making a beloved person's life difficult. Therapists of adolescents have to battle regularly with their temptation to identify with their clients and thus construe their clients' parents as idiots or monsters. In treating people in a relationship, when I work with one member of the couple and have permission to talk with a colleague treating the other, it is rare that we can speak with genuine harmony about the dynamics between the two parties. Instead, despite our good intentions, we find ourselves siding with our respective patients and criticizing the partner under the other's care.

Sometimes one works with individuals who are much more interested in persuading a therapist that their child or spouse is beyond hope than in seeing how to ameliorate some of their difficulties. This need to insist on the pathology of the other is particularly distressing to witness when a parent is determined to see a child as bad no matter how that child behaves, especially when the parent seems too psychologically fragile to be confronted directly about his or her projections. Treating a child often involves having to witness the pain of that child in less than ideal families who may be doing their best but are nevertheless damaging. So often we want to transform a whole family system or to give a client or a client's relative a mind transplant, yet we must be content with small adjustments. Perhaps adapting to limitations is inherently tiring, as it involves a piece of mourning in the renunciation of more ambitious but unrealistic goals.

Like many therapists, I am an unregenerate voyeur: I love to witness what is private, hidden, concealed from public view. I read *People* magazine. I gossip. I savor the juicy anecdote. I thought, when I began training as a therapist, that this lamentable yet robust part of my personality would be deeply nourished in the work. I regret to report that feasts for one's voyeurism lose most of their spice when one cannot share them with others. The more spectacular and distinctive is the material divulged by a patient, the more potentially identifiable the person, and thus the stricter the prohibition against talking about that person's disclosures. And since "You did *what*?!" is rarely a therapeutic intervention, one is constrained from sharing voyeuristic excitement even with the individual for whom there is no confidentiality barrier. So much for hopes of a rewarding sublimation of voyeuristic urges.

In a more serious vein, when one is managing a lot of worry about clients—those tempted by suicide or enmeshed in abusive relationships or addicted to danger or beset with a frightening illness, for example—there is not much comfort to be had. The same sensibility that inclines toward helping is aggrieved by helplessness. It is impossible to promote growth in people psychoanalytically without caring about them, and caring has its associated torments (see Gaylin, 1976). People outside our field, who may imagine that we develop a thick-skinned imperturbability to suffering, are usually unaware of the affective density of our daily lives. Those of us who work with victims of trauma can be particularly undone by that commitment, so much so that there is now a growing professional literature about secondary or vicarious traumatization (Greenson, 1967; Herman, 1992; Kogan, 1995; Pearlman & Saakvitne, 1995).

Guilt, Rational and Irrational

Clinicians can rarely help people as fast and as much as they wish, and sometimes they have to tolerate not helping them at all. Not everyone can be reached by psychotherapy, not every person who wants help finds psychoanalytic approaches congenial, and not every therapist–patient dyad works out well. The "fit" between patient and therapist is a delicate and critical matter over which one has little control (see Kantrowitz, 1995). The downside of hanging one's self-esteem on making a difference—and that is how most therapists' superegos seem to be constructed—is that failing to have a positive effect evokes in the therapist a depressive aftermath. It feels wretched to fail with a client, especially after a long time and a significant emotional investment.

A certain amount of omnipotence is probably an asset in a practitioner. My early determination to believe that I could help anyone I tried hard enough to understand and treat probably facilitated the recoveries made by some of my most difficult patients. Authoritative confidence generates hope, and hope is itself powerfully therapeutic (Frank & Frank, 1991). But there is a line between normal omnipotent strivings and grandiose denial of unpleasant realities, and stepping over that line is an occupational hazard specific to the psychologies of many therapists. Those of us with particularly strong wishes to rescue come to be familiar with a painful kind of self-criticism.

Statistics on the lethality of major mental illnesses suggest that anyone, no matter how skilled, who works long enough with seriously disturbed people is going to treat someone who suicides. The anguish of the therapist whose patient has died this way is monumental. Clinicians who go through this traumatic event would be well advised to get some help with it—if possible, from a professional with experience talking with practitioners whose patients have killed themselves. It is common to get somewhat paranoid after the suicide of a client, to worry that everyone in the mental health community is now talking about the bad therapist who could not keep a patient alive. The dynamics of this reaction involve turning against the self all the rage and criticism that a suicide induces (feelings that have the client as their natural object) and then projecting those attitudes on to one's colleagues.

Probably the only professional experience worse than failing to prevent suicide is treating a person who commits murder. A colleague of mine, asked by a loving and concerned woman to examine her increasingly paranoid husband, saw the man once, tried to develop an alliance, and urged him to consider being hospitalized and getting started on a course of antipsychotic medication. The patient's managed care company, responding to the man's articulate and persuasive protests that he was fine, refused to support hospitalization. In the week before his next appointment, he killed his wife in a gruesome and highly publicized way. No one could fault the therapist for how he had approached this problem, but of course the therapist blamed himself.

At least this practitioner had the consolation of having tried to do the right thing. Imagine how he would have felt if he had underestimated his interviewee's homicidality—an easy thing to do when a person is trying to hide his destructiveness—and had recommended weekly outpatient therapy. As I noted in Chapter 3, all of us make mistakes, and usually they are rectifiable and can even be growth-promoting. But sometimes they are just plain disasters. Given the centrality of guilt dynamics in most clinicians, especially the unconscious origins of many aspirations to be a therapist in wishes to undo fantasied crimes of childhood, it can be hard for practitioners to forgive themselves for their limitations. A friend of mine, an attorney whose practice includes defending therapists who have been the object of a complaint, reports being regularly astounded by how readily most of his clients feel guilty when they have not done anything wrong and by how masochistically they are ready to submit to harsh disciplinary measures when they have.

Problematic Relations with Others

One small annoyance for most psychoanalytic therapists is the defensiveness with which people outside the field may initially relate to them. "You're not analyzing me, are you?" they say, with a nervous laugh. I sometimes feel like Miss Manners (Judith Martin), who complains that whenever she goes to a dinner party, the people seated near her become self-conscious about whether they are using the right fork. Usually I find that individuals who make these anxious, half-serious witticisms can be put at ease by a joke along the lines of "I never work when I'm not being paid" or by the more serious response, "You have no idea how much more you'd have to tell me before I could even start to do that." A colleague of mine handles these situations by teasing: "Yes, you are totally transparent to me, and I can see everything wrong with you—but I'm still willing to have dinner with you!"

More difficult is the self-consciousness of individuals who are connected in some way with a patient. They may suffer distressing fantasies about what the clinician is hearing about them (often when the therapist has no idea that they are the "Jane" or "John" of whom the client speaks) or they may feel critical of the therapist who does not seem to be helping their friend fast enough. Sometimes therapists find themselves the target of unexpected, incomprehensible behaviors and attitudes that can only be understood as stemming from others' connections with their clients. It is oddly lonely to spook people or to irritate them without knowing why, or—if one does suspect why—without being free to bring up the issue that may be causing the awkwardness.

Much more problematic is the painful sense of being misunderstood by people closer to us, including our friends and colleagues. It is a little discussed but significant occupational hazard that we regularly hear from our patients what others have supposedly said about us. Individuals in psychoanalytic treatment are likely to have a keen ear for anything they learn about their therapist and to listen intently to other people's representations of him or her. Sometimes they seem to report what others say fairly accurately, and sometimes their account of what was said appears full of transferential feelings that distort the tone or content of a remark. Patients are not always goodwill ambassadors for their therapists. Even relatively honorable clients have been known to dissimulate under the press of strong emotion. One patient of mine confessed that she had *made up* a professional-sounding, pejorative "diagnosis," dumped it on her husband, and attributed it to me.

I mentioned in Chapter 8 how my client Donna used to go to the emergency service of the local mental health center with some regularity, especially when I was on vacation, and then attack her interviewer

savagely for not being more like me. I once heard through the grapevine that the head of that agency had made disparaging comments
about my competence on the basis of her provocative and threatening
behavior. I could hardly blame him, but it pained me, and there was
nothing I could do about it (until now, when I can vent about it and
transform the experience into something useful to others—see Lepore
& Smyth, 2002). At the time, the only consolations I had were my vivid
and detailed fantasies about suing him for slander.

When one gets reports of derogatory statements allegedly made
by a friend or colleague, it is hard to tell, without the context, what has
really been said or meant. Because of our commitment to confidentiality, we are not free to do what we encourage our patients to do—namely,
to ask the quoted person, "Did you really say I'm a nut case? If so, that
hurts my feelings." Thus, we cannot process our responses and detoxify
them. It is an irony of being a therapist that for all that we cherish both
genuineness and straightforward emotional expression, our occupation
sometimes prohibits our behaving with either one.

For those therapists who live and work in a small community, ordinary daily activities can take on aspects of living in a fish bowl. If one
practices in a university setting, a school, a corporation, a religious
community, a rural village, or a small town, one feels a chronic pressure to be like Caesar's wife, always above reproach. Even in big cities,
psychotherapists are sometimes seen in nonprofessional roles by curious clients or their informants. Individuals who want to become therapists usually understand ahead of time that they must behave with discipline inside the consulting room, but they rarely anticipate the extent
to which they must do so outside it. Therapists differ as to whether
they behave in uninhibited ways outside the office and just let the chips
fall (i.e., they figure that anything a client witnesses or learns about
their nonprofessional self is just grist for the therapeutic mill), or
whether they try to maintain reasonable decorum whenever they are in
public. Probably most of us do some combination. Whatever our adaptations, we must manage a degree of resentment about the extent to
which we are under scrutiny. Self-consciousness is an occupational hazard of anyone in an important or high-profile role—clergy, business
leaders, celebrities, politicians, teachers, and so on—but most would-be
therapists fail to anticipate the extent to which their modest, workaday
life excites gossip, envy, hostility, and the other side effects of power.

One social problem specific to therapists is the invitation to an
event involving—or potentially involving—one or more clients. It can be
stultifying to attend a party at which one is constantly aware of being
studied and sized up. Some therapists ask to see the guest list when invited to a social get-together so that they can decline to go if a patient

will be there. Some talk the issue over with the person in question and reach an agreement about how they will behave toward each other at the occasion. Some decide which to do based on the patient's preference alone. Most of us probably make very client-specific assessments, such as "Does this woman have enough trust to come back and talk about anything that bothers her about my behavior?" or "Have this man and I been working together long enough that he can tolerate some dents in his idealization of me?" or "Will this teenager's history of sexual abuse mean that seeing me out of role feels like a retraumatizing violation of taboo?" Therapists sometimes find themselves envying people who can rely on their uncomplicated personal dispositions when deciding whether or not to accept an invitation.

At the once preeminent and now tragically defunct Menninger community in Kansas, therapists and patients had no choice but to run into each other virtually everywhere. Topeka is a small city, and the Menninger Clinic was one of its main employers. Most of the psychiatrists, psychologists, social workers, and nurses there were in therapy or analysis in the service of their training; of necessity, they were in treatment with colleagues in the same tiny community. Other patients came to Topeka for its high-quality, long-term hospital treatment. Everyone at the medical center, patients and practitioners, ate at the same cafeteria. It was common to see someone walk up to a table with a tray of food, notice a patient there, and do a graceful swivel over to another group of diners. Parties must have been a real challenge.

Theoretically, therapists are as entitled as anyone else to "have a life"—that is, to relax and enjoy their own activities outside their professional zone. Yet many therapists I know have had to constrict their extra-office involvements in some way because of trying to protect a therapeutic relationship. A friend of mine gave up a satisfying political involvement because a client, a woman with a borderline psychology and a history of obsessional stalking, joined his group of activists and began coming to meetings and volunteering for various activities. The people who assigned the work, having no inkling that the therapist and patient had another connection, would put them on the same committees and talk about one of them to the other, something the patient obviously enjoyed and the therapist could barely stand. In her sessions, she would try to get him into political conversations, and she was too defensive to see how her determination to join his organization was the first sign of another obsessional attachment, this time in the transference. The therapist, who was feeling "stalked" by the client and was wearying of making excuses to others about why this or that committee was suddenly unattractive to him, finally opted out of the organization. He could have insisted, as a condition of her continuing treatment with him, that his patient not participate in a group in which he was active, but he felt that this woman would have a paranoid and traumatized reaction to being asked to leave. These kinds of dilemmas are more common than most of the literature on therapy and professional development suggest.

Working Overtime

Many people who become therapists note that from childhood on, they seem to have fallen easily into the role of someone to whom others came for understanding, consolation, and advice. Often, it was their enjoyment of the stance of confidante that sparked their interest in becoming a therapist. And many clinicians like to help people above and beyond their professional commitment to do so; they are attracted to roles as volunteers, contributors to their communities, mentors to disadvantaged children, and so on. Yet once employed as a therapist, most of us find it tedious to be sought out by individuals who want an out-of-office consult on their personal problems. I get at least one instant message a week on my computer from someone I don't know, with a question about psychological symptoms or interpersonal relationships. I used to try to address each writer respectfully, to find out where he or she lived, and to make a referral to a therapist in the area. But this took a lot of time and rarely eventuated in the person's seeing the colleague. Now I simply do not respond to unfamiliar instant messages.

Working overtime with close friends is not usually a problem in the sense of creating resentment at being overextended. The therapist knows them well, cares deeply about them, and enjoys being of help. But with people one knows only casually, being the object of uninvited confidences and requests for help can become quite burdensome. The amount one has to know about the context of any difficulty and the personalities of the people contributing to it is so vast that outside the office, in the absence of having taken a good history and done a clinical interview, therapists are not much better at giving advice than anyone else. The sense of foreboding upon hearing the words "Oh! There's something I've been meaning to ask a psychologist [psychiatrist, counselor, social worker]" is familiar to most of us. We fear becoming stuck between, on the one hand, seeming rude if we try to deflect an unsolicited solicitation and, on the other, getting trapped interminably with a person who takes our politeness as an invitation to go on and on.

And then there are the people who want to complain about their therapist, or their spouse's or child's or friend's therapist, who ask loaded questions designed to support them in their conviction that the treatment is doing no good or the practitioner is incompetent. "What do you think of a professional who tells a patient X?" is a particularly unwelcome overture. We all develop more or less graceful ways of side-stepping requests to give free treatment to the anxious acquaintance or ammunition to the critical one. But therapists find it painful to frustrate others and acutely dislike these Hobson's choices between over-working and avoidance.

One variable that contributes to therapists' working outside the office is the fact that we get better at being empathic over time, and as we mature professionally, any natural concern we have for other people becomes expressed with progressively more effectiveness. We pick up on facial expressions and body language and often invite more disclosure from others than we really want to deal with in our off hours. For example, I once arrived with some colleagues for a conference in a distant city after a long and tiring plane ride. I was first in line at the hotel reception desk, when I noticed that the woman assigning rooms to newcomers was looking pretty worn around the edges. "Hard day?" I asked, while she consulted her computer about the availability of no-smoking rooms. She immediately launched into the details of her impossible afternoon, warming up to my sympathetic interest with voluble enthusiasm. A colleague who was waiting behind me tapped me on the shoulder and whispered, "When the session is over, I'd kind of like to get to my room."

It is easy to get used to being in the role of therapist and to go on automatic pilot in nonprofessional relationships—at the price of the intimacy that would be genuinely nourishing after the depletions of the work. This may be especially the case for therapists with significant institutional responsibility, who find themselves the object of regular transferences reactions, especially idealization and devaluation, not just from their clients but also from their supervisees and employees. Because opportunities for real mutuality become slimmer for those in authority (people who cultivate relationships with powerful others usually have an agenda more complex than friendship—it really is lonely at the top!), it is a particular loss when an experienced therapist cannot suspend the habits of the self-controlled listener in relationships of potential equality and reciprocity. A colleague of mine who directs a training institute writes:

> I have found with colleagues that it is very easy, once habituated by years of practice, to relinquish one's own desire in a personal relationship, even in a friendship, and privilege the desire of the other—as one does in a professional relationship. I have had to practically re-train myself to be an ordinary person who can take up space, have needs, say

what *I* want or how I feel about something between us after having become so accustomed to suspending these very ordinary aspects of reciprocal relationship in the service of the patient's therapy. (personal
communication, August 4, 2003)

Addiction to Authenticity

A seldom-discussed occupational hazard, but one my colleagues tell me
they recognize when I mention it, is the phenomenon of being ruined
by the practice of psychotherapy for chitchat, small talk, and cocktail
parties. The effort to stay in touch with what is authentic, emotionally
important, and nondefensive can become so habitual that ordinary
banter becomes an ordeal. I noticed a few years ago that when a friend
says something teasing, ironic, or dryly humorous to me, it may take
me a while to "get it." I don't think I have gotten dimmer over the years
or have lost my sense of humor; it is just that my default position is to
take seriously anything that is said to me.

When I am with patients, all kinds of things come at me that it
would be professionally disastrous to laugh at (the "suicide attempt" of
a friend of one of my clients, who tried to cut her wrists with a plastic
butter knife, comes to mind here). Keeping a straight face, or at least
maintaining a relatively bland expression when listening, becomes so
automatic that it is difficult not to extend this attitude into social relationships. Perhaps this phenomenon explains why so many therapists
are regarded by others as humorless, dull, or preoccupied. And some
people are put off balance by the obdurate sincerity of many of us in
this profession. When they want to be glib or light or unchallenged in a
particular defense, our automatic disposition to take them seriously
can make them uncomfortable and turn us into caricatures of the
caring–sharing-type professional.

Hostile or Insensitive Professionals

With the current vogue for both pharmacological and cognitive-
behavioral interventions and the popularity of accusations that psychodynamic treatments are not "empirically supported" or "evidence
based," analytic therapists are frequently treated by other professionals, even those in mental health disciplines, as ideologues, dinosaurs,
or idiots. Once, during a social event at an American Psychological
Association convention, I was getting to know a psychologist from a
distant state with whom I was enjoying dancing. I asked what he did
and was interested to hear about his work with people who had suffered severe brain injury. Then he asked me what I did, and I answered

that I was an analyst. At this point he physically let me go, as if I might be contagious, exclaiming, "Well, it's a dirty job, but I guess *somebody* has to do it!"

It has always been true that nonclinical psychologists and researchers tend to look askance on anything remotely Freudian, but at least they used to leave practitioners more or less alone. In the past couple of decades, even professors who teach abnormal psychology have tended to have very little clinical experience themselves—pressures to pursue grants and to publish research have become so intense that no one can afford the luxury of treating a few patients. As a result, it is rare that issues of psychopathology and psychotherapy are presented to undergraduates in a manner sympathetic to the nature of clinical practice. Most contemporary therapists find themselves quite distressed over the misrepresentations currently purveyed to students, and gravely worried about the extent to which public policy has been and continues to be influenced by individuals with no sense of what the work is like.

In a parallel development, in recent years I have heard an increasing number of stories about how the patient of a devoted analytic therapist was told by some putative expert—a medicating psychiatrist, a family member, a teacher, an acquaintance—that the kind of treatment he or she is undergoing is ineffective or even "unethical"—a waste of time and money. It is painful to encounter so much contempt, especially when it threatens a patient's hard-won trust. Fortunately, most individuals in psychoanalytic therapy see the evidence that they are being helped and therefore shrug off other people's undermining opinions. But therapists typically do not like being on the defensive; they would rather just go about trying to help people than trying to justify their existence. Being misunderstood by other professionals is aggravating and potentially destructive.

There used to be a kind of professional courtesy—perhaps honored more in the breach than in fact, but the ethic certainly exerted some influence—to the effect that one respects and supports the work of other practitioners. If one's patient went into crisis and needed to be hospitalized, the personnel at the medical center would listen respectfully to the therapist's evaluation of what was going on and would work with the patient with the objective of returning him or her to outpatient treatment with the primary therapist. In well-run institutions, these considerate practices are still the norm. But in many, probably as a result of the strain put on medical center employees to see more and more people and to handle them faster and faster, such thoughtfulness seems extinct. Many of my colleagues have found that when their clients encounter hospital bureaucracies, their own work is treated as a "failure," and the patient is urged to seek a different kind of treatment or to abandon therapy altogether. Or the person may be put on medication without a phone call to the referring therapist to find out what drugs he or she has taken previously, and with what effects. To tolerate the mistreatment of one's patient by overworked or hostile professionals is difficult.

There is also a troubling phenomenon, much discussed by therapists but rarely addressed in the psychoanalytic literature, that I should note here, namely, the competitive and even scornful ways in which psychoanalytic professionals can treat each other. More than once I have seen a practitioner given a kind of dismissive "public supervision" on presenting a case at a conference. The worst sin of psychoanalysts, aptly dubbed by Clara Thompson (M. Green, 1964) their "pernicious habit," is the substitution of *ad hominem* interpretations for criticisms of substance (e.g., "He's just acting out his narcissistic entitlement," or "She's obviously got a hostile father transference going"). How individuals who, in the consulting room, are the soul of patience, the model of empathy, turn into such boors in public forums is an interesting question. Possibly their mistreatment of one another has something to do with the buildup of hostility based on the kinds of experiences discussed previously, in which one learns of negative evaluations by others through confidential channels and cannot address them directly. I would urge readers not to make things worse by treating colleagues, psychoanalytic or otherwise, with contempt. Bad-mouthing other therapists rarely does anyone any good; for one thing, one never knows who within range of hearing may be in treatment with a person being criticized.

Similarly, although therapists must act in accordance with their professional ethical codes and state laws when they have evidence of unethical practice, I would recommend thinking very hard and getting consultation before encouraging clients to sue or to make formal complaints against prior therapists. I have seen little good and much harm come from efforts at retribution, including the retraumatization of patients being cross-examined by attorneys for the therapists they have tried to bring to justice. There are many countertransferential attitudes that may tilt a therapist toward exerting subtle or overt pressure on a client to seek justice, including wishes to see oneself as being more virtuous than others, wishes to simplify something complex, and an unconsciously contemptuous disposition to see patients as helpless children who lack any responsibility for the situations in which they find themselves. Moreover, once a therapist adopts an advocacy role, the patient is no longer free to look at a decision from all possible angles without anxiety about disappointing the (presumably morally superior) therapist.

I have also heard many stories about conscientious practitioners who have spent months or years undergoing a burdensome investigation simply because an angry client decided to punish them. Those of us in the helping professions tend to side instantly with underdogs, and when we are told about a clinician's alleged failings, it is natural to want to seek reparations on behalf of the person who describes suffering at the hands of such a therapist. I have yielded to this temptation myself, and I regret it. Except where one is bound by legal or ethical codes, it is better for many reasons to give other practitioners the benefit of the doubt. If one is sincerely concerned that a colleague may be doing harm, the ethical statements of most disciplines advise therapists to raise the concerns with the colleague directly before involving a third party.

Narcissistic Aggrandizement

Now that psychoanalysis has fallen off the pedestal on which it sat during much of the previous century, the dangers of therapists becoming too full of themselves are less severe. Still, as I noted in Chapter 8, this profession is one in which we may go through our workday dealing with clients who have made us the center of their emotional world or who are looking for someone to idealize. I have told the following story in a previous article (McWilliams, 1987), but it remains emblematic for me of the "aha!" experience of realizing how my own sense of myself was becoming corrupted by the narcissistic gratifications of my therapeutic role. I had recently been elected to a board of education. I had been quiet for a while, learning the ropes. Then an issue arose on which I felt I had legitimate expertise. I waited patiently for an opening and then inserted what I felt was an astute, tactful, well-timed statement, the kind to which my supervisees often react with appreciation. Instead of being a show-stopper, my comment was received politely and then ignored. My internal reaction was, "Wait a minute! *I spoke!*" This was a genuine wake-up call.

From that time on, I have been championing the idea that therapists, for their own sakes as well as for the well-being of their clients, ought to make sure they have regular and frequent opportunities to be among people who do not know or care what they do for a living. Being an involved parent of young children is a good counteractive to therapeutic omnipotence, as is having friends who will tell you off and keep you honest. The frequency with which their grandiosity is inevitably reinforced in the practice of their art may also be another part of the explanation for the presumptuous, arrogant, and disdainful attitudes with which analysts, at their worst, have been known to treat each other and other professionals.

Loss

In psychoanalytic therapy, we make strong attachments to our patients. We think about them between sessions, develop vivid images of the people in their lives, and hold our breath and root for them when they take risks to act in ways that would not have been tolerated in their family of origin. When they leave treatment, even in a jointly planned termination after a rewarding collaboration, we mourn—not in a desolate way but with the bitter-sweet sentiment of recognizing that the benefit of the work requires of us to let the client go. Some therapists have compared this response to that of a loving parent who sheds a tear on a child's first day of school, graduation, or wedding (see Furman, 1982). This kind of mourning is private and a bit lonely, but at least it may co-exist with positive feelings and pride in a job well done.

When a patient or ex-patient dies, the therapist's mourning has none of the foregoing consolations. It is especially lonely, and it can be complicated by the idiosyncracies of the profession. Unlike the grief accompanying the death of someone in our family or friendship network, the pain of losing a confidential relationship is not recognized and eased by common rituals and shared norms of consolation. I remember with particular sorrow the bereavement services for Molly, the client I described in Chapter 8, which were, serendipitously, held in my own community, despite the fact that she had moved out of New Jersey and had been living in Virginia for many years. She and her husband had been visiting his relatives in a nearby town when she died of an acute flare-up. On a previous visit to her in-laws, she and her husband had visited me in the building where I live and work. Her husband appeared on my doorstep one morning years later, saying that while he had not recalled my name, he remembered the house. He stated, rightly, that he knew I would want to know about Molly's death. He asked if I would go to the wake with him, as he expected it to be attended mostly by relatives of hers whom he disliked. He explained that he wanted to have with him someone who had loved his wife for who she was, unlike her parents, who had insistently pushed her to fulfill their own thwarted ambitions. Molly had never told her relentlessly critical family members about her analysis.

There he and I were, as her friends and family came to pay their respects, obviously depending on each other for emotional support, incidentally broadcasting the fact that I was someone of importance in the life of the deceased. Every time another mourner asked me how I had known Molly, I said something vague ("We were both professionals in the same area some years ago." "Oh, are you a nurse, too?" "No, but I'm in a related field . . . ") and then I would look around desperately for a distraction. Because it was a full-time job trying to maintain her confidentiality while supporting her husband's self-discipline (he was afraid he would attack her bereaved parents), my own grief went mostly unexpressed. The next morning, I deliberately arrived at the funeral service a few minutes late so that I would not have to socialize and could stand quietly in the back and weep at the premature loss of a woman I had admired deeply throughout her long therapeutic struggle with the legacy of a difficult childhood.

On the topic of mortality, Michael Eigen is the only analyst I know of who has seriously discussed with his supervisees the stress imposed on therapists by the obligation to stay alive. At least in long-term work, a contract for therapy implies our ongoing availability. The fact that the therapist survives (Khan, 1970; Pine, 1985; Winnicott, 1955) is a major ingredient in the healing process, especially for people with deep convictions about their toxicity. When we receive a suffering person into a therapeutic collaboration with us, we enter into an implicit covenant to do our best to be there for the duration. The encouragement to patients to let us become important enough to counteract some bad effects of their histories imposes on us the responsibility to stay as healthy as possible. When therapists do become sick, especially terminally so, their resources for handling illness are taxed by myriad professional decisions related to their patients' welfare. As I noted in Chapter 6, the flipside of being powerful enough to modify longstanding psychological processes is having to manage the burdens of that power.

GRATIFICATIONS

Most of the gratifications of being a psychoanalytic practitioner, especially the most important ones, are not immediate. There is some prestige at the start of one's career in simply having the role of therapist (I remember finding ways, when I was starting out, to drop the phrase "my patients" periodically; after a long and somewhat infantilizing career as a student, it made me feel unambiguously adult). And it is a pleasure to earn some money and to start to recoup the debt accumulated during training. It is gratifying simply to make a living by doing something so meaningful and positive, something about which I felt a special sense of wonder when I was first practicing. Beginning therapists have frequently told me that it feels "unreal" to be paid for something they would do for free if they could afford it.

In the early months and years of practice, aside from the gratifications just noted, the main reward is the steep learning curve about human psychology and the skills of helping. Although ongoing education about people and how to help them provides pleasure throughout one's professional life, it is especially important at the beginning because the deeper and more intrinsic satisfactions of the work have not yet emerged. Most people going through training in psychotherapy do not work with people long enough to see their clients grow in significant, life-changing ways; they must take it on faith that this happens.

The short-term therapies they do in the training years may be deeply helpful (cf. Marmor's, 1979, argument that psychotherapy does not have to be long in order to be deep), but credible evidence of their lasting effect may be scant. Even the rare person who later seeks out the counselor once seen at an agency, expressing gratitude for the long-term effects of their conversations (this does happen), does not show up for years. Training programs tend to be tilted toward breadth rather than depth, exposing students to the widest possible range of clients rather than supporting them in intensive work with just a few. This may be the better choice, but it slows the process of students' solidifying a sense of competence to make a real difference. This satisfaction and some others of substance are discussed in the sections that follow.

Ongoing and Personally Relevant Learning

There is a continuing fascination for the practicing therapist, at the emotional as well as the intellectual level, in learning about the uniqueness of each person's internal, subjective world. This gratification begins right away. Psychoanalysis is not boring. Even when it feels boring, the therapist gets fascinated with why a sense of boredom is invading the therapeutic space right now. Every patient is different. Every patient opens up a new window on how a life can be lived. Every patient teaches us something about ourselves and our families, if only by providing a contrast with what we have always considered (consciously or not) "natural" or "normal." Thus, we learn more about ourselves as we learn more about each client. The fringe benefit to practitioners of an increasingly elaborated self-understanding may be singular to psychotherapy as a discipline, although I have heard actors speak of a similar benefit from their profession.

In the absence of information to the contrary, we all tend to project our own dynamics on to other people. We look at their behavior and understand it in terms of what it would express if we were to engage in it. Sometimes we are right, and sometimes we are glaringly wrong. Given that human beings have a great deal in common, most individuals can get through life reasonably well generalizing from their own psychology and acting on the assumption that they can comprehend the motives of others by reference to their own. Therapists, however, cannot afford significant misunderstandings. Our professional development depends on our learning to discriminate our own dynamics from those of other individuals and on questioning our automatic assumptions that our personal ways of experiencing are the norm. Thus, we are impelled toward a lifelong effort to develop an increasingly comprehensive understanding of ourselves. This impetus toward self-knowledge includes some pain and shame, but it ultimately benefits us in ways that go well beyond our clinical roles.

Parenthetically, the process of differentiating self from other and correcting beliefs based on projection goes on at the macroscopic, organizational level as well as for each person. As psychotherapy matures as a field, we keep finding that sweeping generalizations, assumptions that X "always" means Y, are suspect. However attractive a one-size-fits-all theory may be, it rarely accounts for all the data without strain. Theories tend to be syntonic with the psychologies of their developers (Atwood & Stolorow, 1993) and most enthusiastic adherents. Over the past decades, psychoanalysis as a field has increasingly embraced theoretical diversity (Gill, 1994; Jacobson, 1994; Michels, 1988; Wallerstein, 1988, 1992) and has slowly corrected its early tendency to overgeneralize. Freud was quite dogmatic about some of his ideas, probably because his individual dynamics made them seem "natural" or "normal" to him. One famous[1] attempt to correct misapplied Freudian theory is Heinz Kohut's (1979) seminal article, "The Two Analyses of Mr. Z." In this paper, Kohut accounts for an analysand's dynamics according to a paradigm (self psychology) significantly at variance with the oedipal explanations in which he had been trained, and demonstrates how much more accurate and ultimately therapeutic was this alternative way of viewing his patient.

A more delimited example of getting it wrong collectively, based on projection, may be the fourth edition of the *Diagnostic and Statistical Manual of Mental Disorders* (DSM-IV; American Psychiatric Association, 1994) criterion of "impulsivity or failure to plan ahead" for the diagnosis of antisocial personality disorder. Although some psychopathic people are impulsive, many are chillingly predatory or "reptilian" (Meloy, 1988), planning their crimes with attention to every detail. The idea that, as a class, antisocial individuals are impulsive probably represents a projection by the comparatively nonpsychopathic professionals who constructed the DSM-IV. In other words, it is natural for people without many antisocial tendencies to say, "If I were to commit a heinous act, it would have to be in a state of high impulsivity." Finding their way into the frighteningly sadistic, alien inner world of the criminal psychopath would be a more disturbing experience than generalizing from their own psychologies. Evidence of a similar blind spot in many people without personal experience of trauma is their readiness to believe that individuals with traumatic histories are dissimulating when they dissociate. A nontraumatized person may implicitly reason, "If I were to engage in such dramatic behavior, it would be an act."

The professional experiences of therapists keep filling in these kinds of blind spots, counteracting our tendencies to project. Psychotherapy is an ongoing education in humility. We do not understand, we cannot understand, we need to learn from the patient (Casement, 1985) and from experience (Bion, 1962; Charles, in press). We have to tolerate the modest position of not knowing. Intimate exposure to so many different personal stories, so many different kinds of suffering, so many different assumptions about what life is about is inevitably broadening for therapists. Beyond putting a brake on our projective inclinations, it satisfies our voyeurism in ways that are ultimately good for us. Ella Freeman Sharpe (1947) spoke for most analytic therapists in noting:

> I personally find the enrichment of my ego through the experiences of other people not the least of my satisfactions. From the limited confines of an individual life . . . I experience a rich variety of living through my work . . . all imaginable circumstances, human tragedy and human comedy, humour and dourness, the pathos of the defeated, and the incredible endurances and victories that some souls achieve over human fate. Perhaps what makes me most glad that I chose to be a psycho-analyst is the rich variety of every type of human experience that has become part of me, which never would have been mine either to experience or to understand in a single mortal life, but for my work. (p. 122)

As therapists, we are confronted with aspects of ourselves that we would rather not see but that prove critical to our maturation. We have "aha" moments when we suddenly grasp something unique about a client, something that illuminates how much we did not know before this revelation. And we are affected in far-reaching ways by our emotional immersion in each patient's subjectivity. Recent research in neuroscience (e.g., Cozolino, 2002; Damasio, 2000; LeDoux, 1998, 2003; Schore, 2003a, 2003b; Solms & Turnbull, 2002) reveals that when two people are regularly in sincere emotional connection, their respective brains are slowly changed. As they work out their unique synchronized pattern of relationship, new neural networks are laid down in each party, especially in the areas of imagery, affect, and deep structure specific to the "right mind," the brain hemisphere that psychoanalytically savvy researchers such as Solms and Schore have equated with the Freudian unconscious. Our brains literally "grow" from intimate exposure to the minds of others. As devoted therapists of every era have observed (Aron, 1996; Ferenczi, 1932; Mitchell, 1997; Searles, 1975; Sharpe, 1947; Stone, 1961; Szasz, 1956), our patients heal us as we heal them. In fact, as one of my colleagues commented recently, it may be that the therapy has to change something in the therapist *in order* for the client to be healed. Maroda (2003) writes:

> People change through deep, intimate relationships, where their defenses slip away, their most primitive feelings emerge, and they have the opportunity to know themselves, and also to feel differently. Most people have limited access to this experience. It occurs when they fall in love or when they have a child, or when they wholly give over to the analytic process. We, on the other hand, have an ongoing opportunity to participate in this type of transformative intimacy. (p. 21)

Aging Well and Living Longer

One of the advantages of psychotherapy as a profession is that the longer one practices, the more wisdom one accrues, and the more comfortable one becomes with the craft. Although beginning therapists can often be as effective as seasoned ones, they may attain their successes at the price of more emotional wear and tear than will someday be the case. Fortunately, the fact that therapists ripen nicely over time is appreciated in the culture generally, not just by practitioners themselves. In an era of increasingly accelerating change, when many in the workplace fear they will be replaced by machines or newly fledged experts, it is a blessing to have a career in which it is assumed that years of experience correlate with proficiency and maturity of judgment. Unlike athletes, dancers, and heavy laborers, therapists do not age out of their profession, and barring Alzheimer's disease and other senile dementias, there is no mandate to retire. Some therapists continue seeing patients, publishing original ideas, and contributing to conferences well into their nineties.

I mentioned in the previous chapter the interesting finding that psychoanalysts live longer than members of any other profession (Jeffrey, 2001). Being a psychodynamic therapist involves a commitment to undergoing a significant amount of personal treatment. We know that the emotional expression characteristic of psychoanalytic therapy conduces to good physical health (Penneybaker, 1997) and decreased vulnerability of the immune system (Penneybaker, Kiecolt-Glaser, & Glaser, 1988). It is fortunate for those of us with this vocation that in bestowing the benefits of therapy, nature makes no apparent distinctions between those who enter treatment for training purposes and those who come to relieve their suffering. In addition, the fact that our work is meaningful, stimulating, and valuable must surely be good for both our longevity and our productivity at older ages.

The Gratifications of Helping

To my mind, the ultimate satisfaction in being a therapist is the opportunity to earn a living by being honest, curious, and committed to trying to do right by others. I see scant evidence that "selfless" altruism exists, but human beings do seem to have a built-in need to cooperate and help one another out (Slavin & Kriegman, 1992). While many professions involve service to others, the vocation of psychotherapy allows for a particularly intimate, organic, integrated kind of helping that makes one's work meaningful and fulfilling, no matter how tiring. I am grateful that such a role exists in my era and culture, a role that allows me to earn a living by doing what I enjoy doing and find consonant with my temperament.

Many economically comfortable people I know view their work as a burden, partly (I assume) because it does not so clearly meet their need to feel that they matter. Especially in the recent financial climate, they may be pressured, overworked, and anxious about job security. Their wishes to add value to life, often expressed as a feeling of wanting to "give back" to the community, are often not met via their professions. So they join service organizations; donate to charities; sit on boards of nonprofit agencies; volunteer for causes; and involve themselves in churches, political activities, and the arts. Their lives pull in many different directions, and the danger of their becoming overextended is great.

As a practical matter, most people I know have considerably less control over their work hours and conditions of labor than I have. They may make a lot more money than I do, but they do so at the cost of adequate free time and a sense of autonomy. They often feel they have to dress in a particular way, drive an impressive car, present themselves with a certain polish. I would find such pressures oppressive. But more important than the practical advantages of being a therapist, I feel a kind of fluidity and inclusiveness in my work that I think is rare, at least in the modern and postmodern eras. Via the role of psychotherapist, my work life, my charitable impulses, my limitless curiosity, and my longing for authenticity are all connected. The more I can be fully myself, the better I do with my patients. I think there are many of us who value this feature of our jobs as therapists, and I sometimes wonder if some of the negative stereotypes of psychoanalytic clinicians are related to unconscious envy of these more ineffable satisfactions.

Frieda Fromm-Reichmann, a gifted analyst appreciated by older clinicians for the influential text on psychotherapy I mentioned in Chapter 3, is known to most people as the psychiatrist who successfully treated the psychotic illness of the young Joanne Greenberg, author (originally under the pseudonym Hannah Green) of the autobiographical *I Never Promised You a Rose Garden* (H. Green, 1964). Fromm-Reichmann, who was reared as an orthodox Jew, was inspired in childhood by the writing of the great sixteenth-century rabbi Isaac Luria on *tikkun*, the collective task of rescuing the sparks of the divine that were shattered at creation (see Hornstein, 2000). Luria taught that to help another human being is inherently redemptive. According to the principle of *tikkun*, "To redeem one person is to redeem the world." This kind of faith and the satisfactions of acting in accordance with it are fundamental to the commitment of most analytic therapists.

I mentioned in Chapter 8 that when I saw my client Donna with her new daughter, I was astounded at how emotionally attuned and competent she seemed to be with the baby. She nursed her effortlessly, held her in an obviously soothing position, and in every way behaved like a devoted and sensitive parent, unlike either her psychotically depressed mother or her abusive and negligent father. I asked her how, given what she and I had come to understand about her own traumatic early years, she made sense of her capacity to be such a responsive mother. This very troubled woman, who had never heard of Winnicott or his notion of psychoanalytic holding, thought a minute and then responded, "Two things. One, I'm a primate. Two, I'm only holding her the way you've held me all these years."

Although we fail with some clients, most of our patients get better. They become more honest with themselves, lose disabling symptoms, learn more effective ways to cope with problems, improve their relationships, become more playful, develop a wider range of emotions and feel them more deeply, regulate affect better, comfort themselves more effectively, and feel more grounded, resilient, and alive. Over the long haul, they usually reward us with their gratitude (see Gabbard, 2000), but we are often grateful to them, as well. Watching a client grow psychologically is the closest analogue we have in professional life to the experience of watching a beloved child change into a self-assured adult. There is nothing like it.

NOTE

1. Infamous, to some. In this seminal essay, Kohut described a man he had allegedly treated from a more "classical," oedipally informed point of view. He then described how "Mr. Z," who found the results of that analysis disappointing, had returned several years later for more treatment. In their second therapeutic collaboration, Kohut conducted the analysis according to the precepts of his emerging self psychology, and the man reportedly did much better. After his father's death, Kohut's son revealed to the psychoanalytic community that Kohut himself was Mr. Z. He had presented his own dynamics and his own failed response to a classical analysis as if he had been the therapist of a patient like himself. Whether this was a forgivable disguise in the service of making an important point or an ethical travesty has been hotly debated ever since (see Strozier, 2001).

Chapter 12

Self-Care

A certain kind of therapist may almost disappear as a
definable individual, in rather the way that some self-
sacrificing Christian ladies become nonentities; people
who are simply there for others, rather than existing in
their own right. When psychotherapy is practised every
day and all day, there is a danger of the therapist
becoming a non-person; a prostitute parent whose
children are not only all illegitimate, but more imaginary
than real. . . . It is essential for the therapist to find some
area in which he lives for himself alone, in which self-
expression, rather than self-abnegation, is demanded.
—ANTHONY STORR (1990, p. 186)

I have included this chapter on the care of the therapist in
response to statements I have heard from beginning therapists to the
effect that they wish someone had told them these things before they
had to find them out the hard way. Many of the points I make, especially in the earlier part of the chapter, involve commonsensical, things-
your-mother-told-you observations such as the importance of getting
enough sleep, but I have gone beyond mother in trying to spell out the
ways in which specific deficits in care of the self can have problematic
implications for one's work. I also take seriously the fact that therapists
suffer indirect traumatization when working with clients who have traumatic backgrounds. We have learned to emphasize self-care issues with
our traumatized patients, but we have tended to be considerably less
conscientious about care of ourselves.

Psychotherapists are highly motivated to take care of other people.
They are notoriously less keenly devoted to taking care of themselves. If
our personal inclinations to care for others at our own expense—that is,
our masochistic tendencies—were already not enough of a problem,
many of us have undergone training in which we got relentless mes-

sages that the client's needs are preeminent and the practitioner's secondary. This song is sung loudest in professions that idealize self-sacrifice, such as medicine (especially nursing), social work, and religious vocation—all disciplines in which psychotherapists may get their initial training. I have suggested in the chapters on boundaries that the construal of the needs of clients as inherently in conflict or competition with those of therapists, such that caring for one means depleting the other in a zero-sum game of rivalry for limited resources, is specious. Therapists tend to work more effectively when they attend to their legitimate personal needs.

Contrary to the assumptions with which many of us were indoctrinated, altruistic behavior is not incompatible with self-concerned behavior. I have come to believe, consistent with psychoanalytic ideas about motivation and recent empirical studies about life satisfaction, that genuine and effective altruistic actions depend on a high degree of self-regard. Even that universal image of selfless generosity, the nursing mother who happily feeds the baby without regard for her own needs, does not exemplify a one-way transaction. Nursing mothers benefit from the breastfeeding relationship in a symbiotic and reciprocal way: As the baby takes the milk, the uncomfortable pressure in the mother's breast decreases. She feels better. Not to mention her sensual pleasure at holding and exchanging gazes with her baby. Thus, this most asymmetrical of human relationships nevertheless provides mutual benefit to the participants.

In the paragraphs that follow, I summarize some of the practical wisdom about self-care for therapists that I have amassed in a long career not only doing therapy but also training others to do it. Because newer practitioners have frequently told me that some remark of mine about how to take care of oneself is a new idea to them, the advice that follows is relatively concrete. Notwithstanding some of my confident generalizations, let me acknowledge at the outset that everyone is different, and that some of my counsel will thus not suit some of my readers. Although some functions will overlap, I have somewhat playfully grouped my recommendations under the topics of care of the id, ego, and superego, respectively.

CARE OF THE ID

This section addresses care of one's body, emotional capacity, and basic human needs. Many therapists overwork, minimizing their need for adequate sleep, rest, recreation, and "downtime." I have mentioned some of the symptoms of overextending the self in previous chapters, but let me summarize here a number of areas in which therapists are wise to acknowledge the reality of their physical and psychical limits and to restrain their masochistic tendencies.

Sleep and Rest

First, therapists need to get enough sleep. Probably the single worst state of mind to be in when trying to listen to a client is the feeling of a desperate, consuming drowsiness. Watching the minutes creep by at a snail's pace while willing the eyes to remain open is agony. Some patients, most famously those with narcissistic psychologies or dissociative defenses, induce a narcoleptic response in therapists, and coping with this is hard enough without being physically exhausted on top of the tiredness created by projective identification and affective contagion. One's thought processes can be compromised by sleep deprivation, leading to a painful awareness of not having done one's best work, and patients are, understandably enough, usually injured when they notice they are putting their therapists to sleep.

It is important not to work too many hours, and to have some sacrosanct periods of unscheduled time. People who prize their freedom on weekends and in the evenings should not let those periods be eroded by accommodations made for the convenience of clients; they will find themselves more resentful than is healthy for either themselves or the patients they are trying to oblige. Adequate vacation time, when one can exit for days or weeks the strain of constant affective attunement, is also critical to therapists' well-being. In the era of the wireless telephone, it can be tempting to "cover" for oneself when on vacation, but for most people a vacation is not restful unless it is genuinely a break from the work.

When I was first practicing, I had several clients who had disastrous reactions to separations, and to spare them pain, I tried to be constantly available. I soon learned that the long-term cure for profound separation anxiety is not avoiding separations but leaving and returning reliably enough that abandonment begins to be associated with an eventual reunion. Separation, exemplified by breaks, needs to be fully explored, talked through, and felt rather than avoided. And as I argued in the chapters on boundaries, it is often better for patients to become angry at their therapists' limitations than to feel guilt about overworking them.

Clinicians who work in agencies that make excessive demands on their physical and emotional resources—and with the health care crisis of the United States, this situation has become more and more common—must cope as well as they can and forgive themselves when they find it impossible to care fully about everyone on their caseload (see Altman's article, 1993, or book, 1995, covering the psychological stresses on therapists of working in highly strapped agencies with impoverished clients). Ideally, they should also find ways to be honest with the organization that employs them, giving voice somehow to their belief that the level of demand is inhumanly high, and they should resist whatever shaming comes their way by administrators who need to believe that the stresses they inflict are reasonable. This can be a false economy. It is hard not to identify with the aggressor and internalize the agency's idea of a manageable work schedule. Especially in the early years of practice, when one's career is advanced by pleasing authorities who want to believe they are not asking the impossible, overwork may be the best adaptation. But it is important not to lose one's sense of proportion and to come to define that degree of sacrifice as legitimate. Sometimes it helps to gripe to colleagues in comparable positions, and it cannot hurt to apologize to the patients who are getting less attention than they need because of institutional pressures on the therapist.

Health

Therapists must take care of their health in the long as well as the short term. I mention this because I have known psychoanalytically oriented clinicians who make the assumption that if they are in decent emotional shape, they will be fine physically, an article of faith that is not without merit. But some people who believe that good mental health equates with good physical health slip over into a kind of omnipotent denial, in which their realistic human fragility is ignored. In particular, it is dangerous to rationalize skipping regular physicals and routine preventive screenings. Analytic types are famous for interpreting the symptoms of their cancer as somatization or conversion until it is too late.

It is also important to cope with illness sensibly. Working in a closed room with people who bring their minor ailments to their appointments entails occasionally contracting their respiratory infections. One can usually keep working with a cold or a mild infection; attending to others distracts from physical discomfort and does not retard recovery. More serious maladies require time off. Because practitioners recovering from illness or surgery tend to feel guilty about abandoning their clients, they may be tempted to return to work prematurely. The fact that those of us in private practice lose money for every hour we miss contributes to a tendency to go to work when we are not well enough to function on all cylinders. It is better to forgo the income and recuperate, and not only for one's own sake. Patients need models of adults who take proper care of themselves, and therapists need to stay the journey with them (see Schwartz & Silver, 1990, for a collection of articles about illness in psychotherapists).

The sedentary nature of psychotherapy requires its practitioners to make time to exercise. People like me who are allergic to treadmills and formal exercise routines can still take up walking, running, biking, swimming, and dancing. Those who do not trust themselves to maintain a regime can fortify their resolve by planning regular physical activities with a friend or colleague. Some consulting dyads find walking consultation and supervision sessions as helpful as the sitting variety. Exercise can also be combined with play (see below). For years I went to weekly tap dance lessons with four other over-fifty Astaire and Rogers wannabes. We were truly terrible, but we had a great time.

As noted in the previous chapter, back and neck problems are ubiquitous among therapists, and once one's spinal structure is compromised, everything after that is damage control. Because prevention makes more sense than visits to the orthopedist or chiropractor after the fact, it is wise for therapists to walk around between sessions and to sit in a chair with good back support. Some of my colleagues swear by orthopedic chairs, but readers who decide to go this route should note that although a professionally constructed orthopedic device is worth the expense, it should not be ordered sight unseen. Some well-designed chairs are not a good fit with some posteriors, and when they are "off" in some way, they can feel like machines of torture. My response to the challenge of protecting my back is to sit in a recliner with good lumbar support and to lie back when my patients use the couch until I am virtually supine, too.

Finances

Therapists working privately must make enough money to cover the occasional illness, absence, and unpaid cancellation. It is thus important for them to set a fee sufficiently high that unexpected losses from these sources and others can be absorbed. Although practitioners' fees are usually stated in terms of an hourly rate, or per-session charge, that income also covers time for reflection on the clinical process, obtaining consultations, reading literature and attending conferences that increase one's competence, record keeping, telephone calls, and other duties outside the patient–therapist contact hour. And it must provide the clinician with sufficient resources to allow for adequate sleep, exercise, medical care, and relaxation.

Many beginning practitioners have a hard time simply stating an adequate fee to their clients, but usually they learn fairly quickly that if what they ask for is in a standard professional range, most of their customers do not blink. For patients who need or want to negotiate, it is better to state one's "regular" or highest fee and compromise from there than to have started the conversation with a generously reduced amount. Therapists can often guess on intake who will need a break on the price of treatment, but when one offers a reduced fee before the patient has spoken, the bargaining process that may ensue anyway can move toward a charge that will not even make a dent in the office rent.

In Western cultures where the standing of a profession and the money it commands are associated, especially in an era of insurance-company pressure to reduce payments to "providers," it is important to assert the value of psychotherapy even when offering low-cost services. One way to do this is by naming the fee from which the charge has been reduced. In fact, in the interests of retaining respect for psychotherapy as a profession and educating the public about the realistic cost of professional time, many American therapists working with clients on managed care plans mention their regular fee even when accepting the typically negligible rate offered for mental health treatment by the relevant corporation. No one becomes significantly wealthy on a clinician's hourly wage, even those who fill all their hours with patients paying their regular fee (and I know very few in this situation). Yet a therapist's income does allow us to make a comfortable living, to afford a nice home, to go out to eat now and then, to take interesting vacations, and to pay the costs of higher education for a couple of children.

I have known some colleagues who have overestimated their expected income from therapy and have found themselves overworking to get out of debt. Especially for people going into private practice, it can seem reasonable to set an hourly fee and to calculate a yearly total based on that fee without factoring in emergencies, interruptions, holidays, periods when referrals are scant, and the occasional lowered charge for clients who come upon hard times. Because it is tempting to estimate one's income more generously, especially in the years when training debts must be paid off, I should mention the importance of taking care not to become overextended financially. The sense of pressure to extract the maximum monetary benefit from every clinical hour can interfere with therapeutic decisions, such as whether a client needs an increase in session frequency and whether one treats a person's request to terminate as a resistance or as a developmentally appropriate achievement.

Sublimations

Given the discipline with which therapists must operate in the consulting room, sometimes in the face of affective pressures of almost unbearable intensity, they need extratherapeutic outlets for those aspects
of themselves that they diligently suppress in the clinical hour. The nature of the impulses and feelings that must be vented elsewhere varies
somewhat depending on the patients currently in one's caseload and
varies greatly from one practitioner to another. Freud's term for direct-
ing one's problematic drives into areas where they are either harmless
or socially useful is "sublimation," a concept he took from physics,
where it refers to a change in the form of matter (e.g., the transformation of ice into steam) without going through an intermediate state. I
have always found it a felicitous metaphor for the positive use of psychological energies that might be destructive if emitted in the direction
of clients.

A fair proportion of psychoanalytic therapists, including me, have
exhibitionistic strivings that we take care to contain during our clinical
work. For us, teaching is a great relief from the discipline of psychotherapy. We can say what we think without worrying about all the complex effects that our ideas might have on a client, we can enjoy the
performance aspects of a role markedly different from the quiet and
absorbent therapeutic stance, and we do not have to mute our expressiveness for fear we will overwhelm someone's stimulus barrier. As for
voyeurism, I commented in the previous chapter on how disappointing
psychotherapy can be as a gratification of that tendency, given that one
cannot talk about what one has seen. But other outlets for voyeurism,
such as reading biographies and novels, seeing plays and films, and
gossiping with friends about nonconfidential topics, lack this limitation. Such activities play a critical role in the mental economies of
many therapists.

Some of our mature and reasonable narcissistic needs are met by
clinical practice, in the form of both appreciative patients and the satisfactions of a job well done. As I noted in Chapters 8 and 10, however,
reinforcement of our infantile grandiosity is an occupational hazard
and may be avoided by putting ourselves in environments in which our
neurotic omnipotence is undermined. But in addition to arrangements
designed to prevent or reduce pathological narcissism, we may need
opportunities for ordinary narcissistic gratification that are not met by
our work. Especially when struggling with clients who relentlessly devalue, therapists would be well advised to tell the people who care
about them that they need occasional affirmations that they are appreciated.

In looking for what other writers had said about the need for emotional support from their friends and family members, I ran across this quote from Ralph Greenson:

> The psychoanalyst must have the opportunity to stop being a psychoanalyst when he comes home. He should feel free to react as a spontaneous, wholehearted, whole person when he leaves the office. . . . He needs a place where he can expose his frailties and not only not be punished for it, but even have them looked upon as endearing qualities. It is easy to love and admire a bright man, but only a truly loving wife can love one who is a fool at home. And the psychoanalyst needs this. His work takes so much out of him emotionally that if he really is wholehearted in his work, he becomes depleted. The analyst needs some emotional sustenance when he comes home. (1966, pp. 286–287)

Subtracting the patriarchal assumptions from Greenson's statement, his point is still valid. When both partners in a relationship work, especially if they both work as psychoanalytic therapists, they need to negotiate ways of supporting and refueling each other.

The other area in which sublimation is often called for involves aggressive feelings, fantasies, and impulses. There is a place for some of our aggression in the ordinary course of therapy, but not for much of it. Every confrontation we make has to be tactful enough not to wound unduly the person we are trying to influence. The seriousness of their work and the chronic need to be tactful with clients can create in therapists a hunger for outlets for their aggression. Enjoyment of the fantasy scene in the movie *Analyze This,* in which the therapist character played by Billy Crystal shouts in exasperation, "Get a life!" at his whiney patient is a good example of such an outlet. So is pleasure in the movie *What about Bob?*, whose consolations are clearly in the "it could always be worse" category. Clinical stresses can stimulate among therapists a mordant wit comparable to the famous black humor of surgeons, coroners, pathologists, and morticians. Practitioners condole with each other about "patients from hell" and trade stories about common clinical miseries. These mutual consolation and letting-off-steam functions are fringe benefits of being in an ongoing supervision or consultation group or in a work situation with other colleagues.

Therapists whose needs to confront and compete are frustrated by the demands of their occupation may find considerable relief in sports, political involvements, detective novels, competition in the professional arena, and other pursuits where aggressive themes figure in with less subtlety. A colleague of mine who is a potter enjoys the satisfactions to her aggressive side of throwing clay onto the wheel. I have known therapists who are rabid sports fans, others who enjoy gardening because they love plunging the spade into the dirt, and others who maintain a huge collection of true crime literature. There are many ways to sublimate aggression, and many reasons for therapists to do so. If challenging patients are not stimulating enough to one's hostile side, American insurance companies can do the job quite reliably.

Play

Therapists, especially those in small communities, may find it hard to get completely away from their work and give themselves over to recreation. Of course, this is what vacations are for, but there is also a certain amount of ongoing, day-to-day playfulness without which life can feel like an interminable series of obligations. Sex provides the handiest play space for many adults; therapists who keep the erotic part of their lives awake and vital can withstand considerable stress with good cheer. Although it is a misunderstanding of Freudian theory to believe that people must have a sexual outlet or else risk neurosis (Freud emphasized accepting erotic feelings more than engaging in sexual behavior), a satisfying sex life, especially in the context of emotional intimacy, can certainly put life's stresses and disappointments into perspective.

Other preferences for play are more individual. Some therapists have musical enthusiasms, some are sports fans, some develop hobbies, some are film buffs, some spend a lot of time with their grandchildren. Some practitioners I know go to casinos several times a year to play blackjack, where they enjoy the bantering that can go on at a table of motley, unconnected strangers—nothing feels further from the delicacy of the clinical interaction. Activities such as this that offset the isolation of practice can be particularly valuable. Whatever one's mode of play, it is important not to let work swallow it up. When one's children are small, time for oneself is scarce; nevertheless, for people working as therapists and simultaneously rearing infants and toddlers, it can be critical to mental health to set aside a few hours a week to be doing neither.

CARE OF THE EGO

In this section I cover aspects of self-care that support one's sanity, competence, and professional growth. Readers will hear in it my background assumption that nourishment of the ego is as important to well-being as taking care of the more basic id needs.

Ongoing Psychological Education

In Chapter 4 I presented a comprehensive argument about the importance of analysis or therapy for therapists as a source of learning. Let me add here that it is an invaluable pressure release to have a confidential setting where one can talk about the stresses of clinical practice and figure out what personal buttons those stresses are pushing. Arranging for regular supervision or consultation with a trusted senior colleague, long after licensing requirements for supervision have been met, is worth the investment. Even scheduling a weekly lunch with a friend in the field with whom one can talk about cases can make a significant difference in one's competence and comfort with the work.

Not surprisingly, given the isolation of clinical work and the sociable nature of many therapists, groups in which participants present cases to each other are popular vehicles for ongoing learning. I know people who have stayed in the same group for more than thirty years and still enjoy and profit from the experience. Both leaderless peer groups and those led by a senior practitioner are good sources of ongoing education. They keep their members honest and assuage the loneliness of practice. The special virtue of such gatherings is that they multiply the amount of expertise in the room by the number of individuals present. Even when describing a highly unusual case, presenters generally find that someone in the group has been challenged by similar clinical phenomena.

I remember, for example, one meeting of my Wednesday group in which the patient being presented had come for treatment because of an overwhelming reaction of disgust toward anyone chewing gum. Although a "pathological disgust disorder" exists nowhere in the DSM, another member of the group had had a similar client, a woman who would become helplessly nauseated whenever she noticed a human hair on a piece of furniture. Some problems for which an individual seeks therapy are idiosyncratic enough to have escaped formal diagnostic classification. To help the people who suffer from them, we need to pool the knowledge of a number of practitioners.

There is no such thing as becoming so experienced that there is nothing important left to learn. Especially for people with general practices, there will always be patients who require a new area of understanding, whether it involves their psychological symptoms, the implications of their physical condition, the subtleties of their gender and sexual orientation, their race or ethnic background or nationality, their religious attitudes, the subculture in which they currently live, the stresses of their work life, or their unique historical experiences. Ongoing familiarity with other people's work also keeps practitioners stimulated, exposes them to different styles of doing therapy, and involves them in a network of individuals who can refer to one another, discuss political issues pertinent to the profession, and trade information about therapeutic resources.

Conventions, conferences, and workshops provide other valuable sources of professional nourishment. Postgraduate institutes and training programs can be especially rewarding. For those of us in the human-services sector who are continually extending to others our interest, our empathy, and our sustained emotional investment, the experience of taking in what others have to offer feels like replenishment, an antidote to the emotional depletion that is the cost of caregiving. Even in states that do not require continuing education credits for clinicians, meetings that offer practitioners new skills or ways to understand clients are well attended. Presenting one's own work at professional conclaves is also a useful experience; among other benefits, it offers good training in organizing data and seeing what pieces are missing.

As one develops as a therapist, the learning curve begins to flatten out. At first, this is a relief; finally, we have lost the driven feeling of racing to learn the basics. Then it becomes troubling to lose the energizing effect of intensive, rapid-fire assimilation of knowledge. Experienced therapists report periods of noticing they are starting to go through the motions rather than feeling inventive in their work (A. Cooper, 1986). As Emmanuel Ghent (1989) noted, "When interpretations begin to sound like clichés . . . we are well on the way to the analytic "burnout syndrome" (p. 170). A sense of flatness in their professional life should alert therapists to the need for exposure to some new ways of thinking and working.

Privacy

I talked in the preceding chapter about the fish-bowl-like aspects of professional life, especially for therapists in smaller communities. This is one of those occupational hazards that is often ignored or minimized by people starting out. But because it can exert a suffocating effect on one's sense of comfort and spontaneity, it deserves attention. To whatever extent possible, therapists would be wise to preserve an arena in which they can be themselves without worrying that they will then have to deal with their clients' reactions.

When I moved to the small community where I now live and practice, my prior experiences with feeling too visible prompted a decision not to treat anyone from my new town or the suburb that surrounds it. That policy has stood me in good stead in many ways, including some I had not anticipated. I could run for the board of education without putting my patients in the awkward position of having to decide whether or not to vote for me. I did not have to face the complications of treating friends of my children. I could join the local Rotary club and not worry that if I laughed at a risqué joke, some client would be scandalized. I could run downtown without makeup and in jeans without a big risk of meeting someone who would be jarred by my nonprofessional appearance. (Of course, this will happen anyway, but less frequently.)

This decision to protect my privacy turned out to be particularly valuable when I was diagnosed with breast cancer. I was able to let my neighbors know about this, to draw on the knowledge of community members about good doctors and facilities, to receive emotional support that was critically sustaining, and to express my apprehensions without worrying that the information would go automatically to my patients. As it turned out, none of them learned that I was dealing with cancer until after I had been treated, at which point I knew how good my prognosis was. (Parenthetically, this fact speaks well for the discretion of the therapeutic community. Some of my patients at that time were therapists, and many of my colleagues—who were also theirs— knew about my diagnosis.) It would have been difficult for me to address my patients' anxieties at a point when my own were so high, and at that time I was especially grateful for a private sphere.

I realize that not everyone is in a position to make this kind of decision. Some therapists live in isolated communities where they either treat their neighbors or go hungry. And even for those who have the option, it is hard to say no to referrals when one is starting out and trying to pay the bills, or when a particularly appealing patient comes along. I offer my personal solution to the problem of exposure as an example of a general principle that individual therapists can find their own ways to implement. For many, the best they can do for themselves is to have some retreat where they can go, outside their place of practice, and feel either anonymous or known only to their intimates.

A sense of humor is a must when privacy is compromised. One of my colleagues told me the story of a patient he had originally treated as a four-year-old who came back to him when she was about fifteen. She lived four houses away in a small suburban neighborhood. One day in session she seemed to be having difficulty getting started, and with the practiced intuition of the seasoned therapist, he asked her if there was anything she was having trouble telling him. After some embarrassed silence, she asked if he could do her a favor. "Sure," he responded. At this point she blurted out, "Please don't go out to get your newspaper in the morning in your boxers."

Self-Expression

Therapists are carefully trained to subordinate their own expressiveness to that of their patients. Perhaps one of the reasons analysts generate so many disparate and colorful theories, models, and metaphors is that after hour upon hour of deferring to their clients' self-expression, they need an outlet for their own. Preserving an area in which one's own expressiveness may flourish seems to me a critical aspect of self-care. Individual differences in how to make room for one's creativity are vast, but the process serves a similar function whether the avenue of expression is stand-up comedy or playing in a string quartet.

It is not uncommon for psychotherapy professionals to have talent in the arts. Many of us play an instrument or sing or paint or write poetry. Some therapists (Irving Yalom, Alan Wheelis, and Christopher Bollas come to mind) write fiction, often stories about therapy that allow the author to express feelings and fantasies that are pervasive but unexpressed in the clinical hour. Other clinicians seek training in more explicitly spiritual arts, such as meditation. Some become involved in social and political movements that feed their desire for generative activity. Although there are outlets for one's creativity in the clinical hour, doing therapy is a responsive, derivative process rather different from the opportunity to initiate a creative act.

Professional writing may also meet the need for creative expression (see Slochower, 1998, and the compilation of empirical studies on the therapeutic value of writing edited by Lepore & Smyth, 2002). Michael Eigen, one of the most self-revelatory psychoanalytic authors of recent decades, has stated that he writes out of a profound personal need:

> The voice that comes out in writing speaks from the depths of one's aloneness to the aloneness of others. Psychoanalysis is a writing cure, not only a talking cure. Writing helps organize experience of sessions, but it also helps discover and create this experience. (1993, p. 262).

In writing, we can speak in a voice that we mute when we are with patients. When I am immersed in crafting an article or book chapter, I go into a unique zone, a state of consciousness that is both unfocused and preoccupied, where some deep part of me that seeks expression feels at home. Stephen Mitchell was described at a memorial service as having been happiest on Wednesday mornings, his carefully protected time for working on books and papers. I find that most therapists just starting their careers think of professional writing as a very distant activity for more senior people, but they also have important things to say and can usually find professional outlets for doing so. Once the process of writing an article, submitting it, responding to critiques, and rewriting it is demystified, it can become rather addictive.

CARE OF THE SUPEREGO

In this last section, I discuss ways that therapists can preserve their sense of integrity and pride in their work and protect themselves from situations in which they may feel either morally compromised or at risk of having their integrity challenged. There is a lot more to doing this than simply observing the ethical codes of one's discipline.

Doing Right by Family

In an earlier part of this chapter I talked about the dangers of overwork and overextending oneself financially. The time when it is most critical not to work excessively is the period when one has young children. Unlike Ralph Greenson, few of us (of either gender) have wives who will eagerly fill in the gap created by our absorption in work. Numerous psychoanalytic writers have commented on how typical it is for therapists to cheat family members of time and emotional availability. Storr, (1990, p. 187) for example, notes that the domestic lives of therapists suffer both because "professional discretion means that the therapist is virtually unable to discuss his work with his family," and because psychotherapy is so emotionally consuming that if the workday is too long, nothing emotional is left over. For people with a compelling interest in helping others, doing well by one's children is imperative not only on its own merits but also on the grounds that their self-respect is intimately connected with doing right by those they love.

Awareness that one is short-changing one's family can turn into a long-term, painful guilt about not having lived up to one's values where it counted most. I have treated a number of people in their fifties or sixties who felt this kind of remorse, and their anguish about what cannot be recovered or undone is excruciating. Unfortunately, the years when children are most in need of their caregivers' emotional resources tend to coincide with the period in professional development when training debts are still unpaid and money is scarce. Younger therapists are also more likely to be working in settings in which they have minimal control over their time, and they may also be preoccupied with the various rites of passage involved in becoming adequately credentialed. Nonetheless, to whatever extent it is possible, therapists starting a family

should consider trying to work fewer hours, to avoid taking on unusually difficult clients, and to tolerate the absence of some material comforts in favor of the benefits of more participation in their domestic
life.

Exposing One's Work

For an analytic therapist there is a constant refrain in the back of the
head: "Am I being defensive here? Am I rationalizing my own needs
and calling them my patient's? Do I have to do more work on myself in
this area?" Especially now that the perfectionistic ideal of the "fully analyzed person" has been exposed as a myth, the profession requires an
unceasing introspective process with both burdensome and liberating
effects. Many of the recommendations in the previous section, especially about making space for ongoing learning, apply also to maintaining one's sense of integrity. A good yardstick for whether one is being
true to one's values is to imagine describing specific actions to an admired colleague. If it is hard to imagine telling him or her what happened in the consulting room, there is probably something questionable in one's behavior.

In addition to asking the private question of whether they would
be comfortable revealing their clinical interactions to a trusted colleague, therapists should put themselves regularly in situations where
they do share the details of their work. Talking about one's cases to
others in a safe environment is the best check on movement toward the
famous "slippery slope" (Guthiel & Gabbard, 1993, 1998) of exploitation. I have heard many presentations by therapists troubled by feeling
sexual arousal toward a client or imagining taking advantage in some
other way (e.g., being tempted to pump a stockbroker patient for investment tips). It is natural to struggle with these issues. Supervisors, consultants, and colleagues can help the therapist tolerate and even enjoy
these inevitable feelings and temptations, while throwing their support
behind therapeutic discipline.

Risk Management

The following comments, as well as those about risk management in
the chapters on boundaries, are more applicable to American practitioners than to those in places where the zeal to sue or seek reparation
is less culturally supported. One essential defense against having one's
integrity impugned involves careful, enlightened record keeping. To
protect their patients' confidentiality, most therapists keep in their files

the bare minimum of information allowable by their employer and the civil laws governing practice. Many psychoanalytic therapists used to work without keeping notes at all (e.g., Reik, 1948). Not only was note taking considered an intrusion on Freud's "evenly hovering attention," but the burglary of Daniel Ellsberg's psychiatric file during the presidency of Richard Nixon had also broadcast loud and clear to therapists the message that the less the material on hand, the more protected the client. Laws have changed, however, and it is my understanding that there is now legal precedent in the United States for considering a lack of patient records as *prima facie* evidence of malpractice.

It continues to be important, in the interest of patient protection, to keep notes minimal. But for the therapist's protection, it is critical to record anything about which a question could be raised if the therapist were to have the bad luck to be the object of a complaint, and to make clear what the clinical rationale was behind the therapist's stance. With depressed patients, it is vital for therapists to record that they assessed for suicidality and addressed that issue proactively if the patient seems at risk. Similarly, with clients who are angry and whose backgrounds involve violence, clinicians need to assess for homicidality.

When in doubt about any clinical decision, or when handling any issue in a way that could raise questions from a critical outsider, therapists should consult with a colleague and record the fact of the consultation in the patient's file. Most ethics bodies consider an appeal for consultation as an exculpating or mitigating feature of the clinical record. Countertransference feelings and fantasies should not be put into the patient's file. Ethics boards have not kept up with developments in psychoanalytic practice and often hold therapists to rules of professional conduct that were promulgated in the "blank slate" and "analyze away your countertransference" eras of clinical history.

It is also a good idea to have a friendly relationship with an attorney—not just a competent generalist but someone knowledgeable about mental health law, a comparatively rare specialization. Many state associations of psychologists, psychiatrists, and social workers have a legal authority available to answer questions from therapists confronted with tricky decisions (what kind of letter to write to the insurance company, whether to see the spouse of a patient who is considering divorce, how to respond to the client who wants to see files that the therapist is sure will upset him or her, and so on). Especially before responding to anything in writing, it is well worth the money to run one's options by a qualified lawyer. Finally, and most crucial, in the instance of any complaint or query from a professional board, or letter from a client or past client where one suspects a complaint could follow, therapists should call an attorney before making any response.

In these litigious times, attendance at risk-management workshops every few years is also advisable. Some insurance companies offer a reduction on the cost of malpractice coverage for therapists who present evidence of continuing education in that area. Let me repeat here my opinion about the usefulness of Lawrence Hedges's (2000) book on this topic, which is written specifically for American psychoanalytic practitioners. With the recent changes in laws about patient privacy, it is wise for practitioners to stay abreast of more current writing and teaching on risk management, as well.

Doing Right by Colleagues

Psychotherapy is hard work, and we owe some sympathy and consideration to others who make their living this way, even if their practices and guiding assumptions are markedly different from our own. Behaving well with other people in the field makes sense on its own merits but will also reward the therapist who has behaved with civility. Other practitioners tend to be grateful for being given the benefit of any doubt that they are proceeding with integrity. As I noted in Chapter 1, analysts are now paying a heavy price for the high-handed way in which some of them have treated the rest of the mental health community.

As I mentioned in the previous chapter, word travels fast on the clinical grapevine, and an attack on a colleague, even one in a distant state, may very well reach his or her ears. A field in which we depend on each other for referrals, medication consults, placement in therapeutic settings, and other professional assistance is not a field in which it is wise to make enemies gratuitously. We should be especially careful about assumptions we develop about colleagues that are based on patients' accounts. What we hear in the consulting room should be understood as the client's truth, but this is not the same thing as an "objective fact." Patients, like all of us, have complex unconscious reasons for framing or constructing things as they do, including the wish to simplify the world by the defense mechanism of splitting. When they are trying to feel goodness in the therapist, they are very likely to experience and report badness from others.

I want to take this opportunity also to discourage snobbery toward members of therapeutic disciplines other than one's own. It is one of my pet peeves that psychologists, who know how injured and outraged they become when subject to condescension from psychiatrists, can frequently be heard expressing their sense of superiority over social workers. Every discipline from which therapists are drawn has its strengths and weaknesses, and we therapists have more pressing matters to worry about than our relative status vis-à-vis one another. For example, we need to work together to educate the public about the nature of psychotherapy and to challenge the myth that "evidence-based" therapy consists only of short-term interventions. From this perspective, it has been politically disastrous for the American Psychological Association to put so many of its resources into trying to get prescription privileges for psychologists, a stance that was guaranteed to alienate psychiatrists at a time when we all need to be working together to defend the talking cure from its detractors.

The supposition that others are competent and well intentioned until they prove otherwise is good preparation for most professional encounters. Even in contexts in which one feels naturally on the defensive, such as during an evaluation procedure in a training program, things tend to go better when a therapist assumes that the motives of others are honorable. In evaluation scenarios, it is common to project one's hostility about being examined, leading to persecutory images of one's examiners. More than one candidate I have coached has reported doing better in a formal case presentation via the exercise of deliberately imagining a friendly audience to counteract such images.

Many years ago, when I went through the oral part of the New Jersey psychology licensing process, the case I had written up was a woman I had treated in four-times-a-week analysis, on the couch. I was examined by a prominent behaviorist and a well-known client-centered therapist. This committee made me nervous. They were cordial, but at one point, I almost lost my sense of being a competent grown-up. The behaviorally oriented examiner asked me whether I would ever refer a client for behavioral treatment. "Oh, yes!" I said, ingratiatingly, wanting to demonstrate my respect for her orientation. "For what?" she asked. At that point, my mind went blank. I could not think of any circumstances in which I would refer someone to a behaviorist except for the rare instance when the patient's chief complaint was an uncomplicated phobia, and I knew that a behaviorally oriented practitioner would bridle at the idea that all she was good for is the extinction of simple phobic reactions. So I gulped, decided to assume good intentions and an appreciation of honesty in my audience, and said, "I guess I answered you too quickly, in my effort to show my open-mindedness. As I think about it, I have to admit that a more truthful answer is that I'd try a psychoanalytic approach with just about anyone who came to me, and I'd refer only if it didn't seem to be helping." Both my examiners hastened to assure me that it was okay for me to feel strongly about my own theoretical framework. Thus, they got a chance to express *their* open-mindedness, and I felt better having been candid.

Honesty

This brings me full circle to the theme of honesty with which I started this book. When I was very young, my mother, who had a lot of wisdom about things psychological, counseled me that I could get away with saying just about anything to anybody if I could figure out how to say it. It was a valuable message for someone who eventually decided to spend her life mastering ways of talking straightforwardly to individuals who may be both defensive and difficult to understand. To me, part of the appeal of psychoanalysis as a field, and psychodynamic therapy as a career, has always been the ongoing effort in both the science and the art of analytic practice to tell it like it is. I appreciated Freud for insisting, in a time and place when sexuality was mentioned mostly in whispers, that sex is a drive in women as well as in men, and for finding ways to say so that got him taken seriously. Later, I was delighted that Bowlby called our attention to the centrality of dependency needs in human motivation. Still later, I admired Kohut for making us look realistically at our ongoing narcissistic requirements. Currently, I am grateful to the relational theorists for bringing out of the analytic closet the fact of the therapist's participation in the transference–countertransference atmosphere of any treatment.

Winnicott (1960) wrote about the universal need of the young human being to maintain the sense of a true self in the face of whatever adaptations and compromises his or her environment required. He was talking more about preserving or recovering one's basic sense of vitality than about honesty as a moral position, but the two are intimately related. People tend to feel better when they can be true to themselves, especially if they can be understood by others on that basis. For the patient, one of the greatest satisfactions that emerges in a psychoanalytic therapy is the sense that he or she has been accepted, psychological warts and all. But the virtue of nurturing the true self applies to ourselves as well as to our clients, and it is inseparably bound up with our ability to do our job. Creating the right conditions for truths to emerge and become explicit is the essence of the psychoanalytic project.

Appendix

Annotated Bibliography

The following list is not comprehensive or exhaustive. The selection below, which contains my own favorites for introducing newcomers to the psychotherapy profession, probably overrepresents books in my own discipline (psychology) and underrepresents those from the literatures of psychiatry, pastoral counseling, and social work. I have included a few classics that are conceptually more difficult or less accessibly written because of their importance in the field, and I have exercised a bias in favor of books with verbatim excerpts or extensive case material that illustrate the author's argument and provide readers with specifics about interventions.

BOOKS IN THE CLASSICAL PSYCHOANALYTIC TRADITION

Appelbaum, S. A. (2000). *Evocativeness: Moving and persuasive interventions in psychotherapy*. Northvale, NJ: Jason Aronson.—Lots of verbatim transactions with clients; Appelbaum's emphasis is on reaching the affect.

Greenson, R. R. (1967). *The technique and practice of psychoanalysis*. New York: International Universities Press.—Still a classic textbook on traditional psychoanalysis. Gives the reader a sense of the process from which psychoanalytic therapies were adapted.

Hammer, E. (1990). *Reaching the affect: Style in the psychodynamic therapies*. New York: Jason Aronson.—Like Appelbaum, emphasis on tone and affective communication, though here relative to different personality types.

Levy, S. T. (2002). *Principles of interpretation: Mastering clear and concise interventions in psychotherapy*. Northvale, NJ: Jason Aronson.—Very compact, accessible distillation of classical interpretive technique. Available in paper.

Schafer, R. (1983). *The analytic attitude*. New York: Basic Books.—Excellent, well-written treatment of psychoanalytic tone and context.

Schafer, R. (2003). *Interpretation and insight: The essential tools of psychoanalysis*. New York: Other Press.—This book came out just as I was about to send mine off to the publisher. I have not yet read it, but Schafer's clinical writing is always accessible, intelligent, and empathic, so I am recommending it on faith.

Weiner, I. B. (1998). *Principles of psychotherapy* (2nd ed). New York: Wiley.—A thoughtful, eloquent, and readable classic.

BOOKS IN THE OBJECT RELATIONS TRADITION

Casement, P. J. (1985). *Learning from the patient*. New York: Guilford Press.—A humane, humble, thoughtful exploration of what doing psychotherapy involves.

Charles, M. (in press). *Learning from experience: A clinician's guide*. Hillsdale, NJ: Analytic Press.—Not many people can make Bion user-friendly, but Charles's small volume is superb at explicating him, Klein, Winnicott, and other object relations luminaries and connecting their theories with the daily challenges of practice.

Luepnitz, D. A. (2002). *Schopenhauer's porcupines: Intimacy and its dilemmas: Five stories of psychotherapy*. New York: Basic Books.—So readable that it has crossed over into the popular market, this description of five very different cases treated by the author is a highly realistic representation of current psychoanalytic practice. In the process of telling her stories, Luepnitz illustrates the applicability of object relations theories such as those of Winnicott, Lacan, and Klein to everyday clinical decisions.

Scharff, D. E. (1995). *Object relations theory and practice: An introduction*. Northvale, NJ: Jason Aronson.—Readable text, strong on theory with practice implications.

BOOKS WITH A SELF PSYCHOLOGICAL OR INTERSUBJECTIVE ORIENTATION

Basch, M. F. (1990). *Doing psychotherapy*. New York: Basic Books.—Very good basic text with detailed clinical excerpts.

Buirski, P., & Haglund, P. (2001). *Making sense together: The intersubjective approach to psychotherapy*. Northvale, NJ: Jason Aronson.—Well illustrated explication of the approach pioneered by Stolorow, Atwood, Orange, Brandchaft, and others.

Shane, E., Shane, M., & Gales, M. (1997). *Intimate attachments: Toward a new self psychology*. New York: Guilford Press.—Puts self psychological technique in an elaborated developmental context. Explicates different dimensions of intimacy and relational configurations between client and therapist and their implications for treatment.

Stolorow, R. D., Atwood, G. E., & Brandchaft, B. (1987). *Psychoanalytic treatment: An intersubjective approach.* Hillsdale, NJ: Analytic Press.—A slim, passionately written primer on the intersubjective model of therapy.

Wolf, E. S. (1998). *Treating the self: Elements of clinical self psychology.* New York: Guilford Press.—A readable primer deriving mostly from Kohut's work.

INTERPERSONAL AND CONTEMPORARY RELATIONAL TEXTS

Fromm-Reichmann, F. (1950). *Principles of intensive psychotherapy.* Chicago: University of Chicago Press.—Old-fashioned in its language ("the psychiatrist," "the doctor," use of the masculine pronoun) but still very valuable, especially for people treating patients in the psychotic range.

Hoffman, I. Z. (1998). *Ritual and spontaneity in the psychoanalytic process: A dialectical constructivist view.* Hillsdale, NJ: Analytic Press.—Not an easy book for the beginner, but an important one in understanding contemporary approaches to therapy.

Teyber, E. M. (1999). *Interpersonal process in psychotherapy: A relational approach.* Belmont, CA: Wadsworth.—Good, accessible text, expensive but available in paper.

Karen Maroda is currently working on a book on technique from a relational point of view. Her writing is always energetic, intelligent, and readable.

INTEGRATIVE TEXTS

Bender, S., & Messner, E. (2003). *Becoming a therapist: What do I say, and why?* New York: Guilford Press.—Very specific, easy-to-digest, detailed book that answers the question in its title. The result of a collaboration between a relative newcomer to the field and an experienced therapist/teacher of therapy. One of the most practical books out there.

Bocknek, G. (1993). *Ego and self in weekly psychotherapy.* New York: International Universities Press.—Well written primer on doing once-a-week therapy, integrating ego psychology, self psychology, relational theory, and developmental theory.

Gibney, P. (2003). *The pragmatics of therapeutic practice* . Melbourne, Australia: Psychoz Publications.—A beautifully written and accessible paperback, blending ideas from individual, group, and family therapy seen from psychoanalytic and systems perspectives. An incisive statement of the esthetics and dynamics of psychotherapy itself.

Hedges, L. E. (1983, rev. ed. 1995). *Listening perspectives in psychotherapy.* Northvale, NJ: Jason Aronson.—Important book about adapting one's listening to the kinds of issues that are central to different kinds of clients, respectively. Integrative also of philosophical traditions and psychoanalytic therapy.

Josephs, L. (1995). *Balancing empathy and interpretation: Relational character analysis*. Northvale, NJ: Jason Aronson.—Brings therapeutic attempts to influence pathological personality structures into the relational era. Integrates classical and current ideas.

Roth, S. (1987). *Psychotherapy: The art of wooing nature*. Northvale, NJ: Jason Aronson.—Well written, empathically expressed ideas replete with case examples.

Rubinovits-Seitz, P. F. D. (2002). *A primer of clinical interpretation*. Northvale, NJ: Jason Aronson.—Reviews classical and "postclassical" approaches to interpretation, including the approaches of Kohut, Hoffman, Schafer, Spence, the intersubjective theorists, the "radical relational" school, and pluralistic approaches. Readable question-and-answer format useful for the beginner.

Schlesinger, H. J. (2003). *The texture of treatment: On the matter of psychoanalytic technique*. Hillsdale, NJ: Analytic Press.—An erudite but relatively jargon-free exploration of the psychoanalytic therapy process from a systems point of view. Rich illustrative material.

Stark, M. (1994). *Working with resistance*. Northvale, NJ: Jason Aronson.—Usefully frames psychotherapy as a grief process. Lots of explicit examples of Stark's interpretive style. Especially valuable in discussing how to work with clients with issues of entitlement.

Storr, A. (1990). *The art of psychotherapy* (2nd ed.). Woburn, MA: Butterworth–Heinemann.—Unintimidating, gracefully written primer that covers basic issues and discusses adapting one's style to the personality structure of patients. Covers hysterical, depressive, obsessional, and schizoid personalities. Storr was very influenced by Jung.

Wachtel, P. L. (1993). *Therapeutic communication: Knowing what to say when*. New York: Guilford Press.—Eloquent, thoughtful integration of psychoanalytic and cognitive-behavioral approaches, with many specific examples.

CONTROL–MASTERY TEXT

Weiss, J. (1993). *How psychotherapy works: Process and technique*. New York: Guilford Press.—Straight-talking explication of psychoanalytic therapy from the point of view of the clinicians and researchers in the San Francisco Psychotherapy Research Group.

SUPPORTIVE PSYCHOANALYTICALLY ORIENTED PSYCHOTHERAPY

Karon, B., & VandenBos, G. R. (1981). *Psychotherapy of schizophrenia: The treatment of choice*. New York: Jason Aronson.—I understand that this book has become hard to get. But those who can find it will appreciate its passionate commitment to understand psychotic patients and its practical strategies for helping them.

Pinsker, H. (1997). *A primer of supportive psychotherapy.* Hillsdale, NJ: Analytic Press.—Very clearly written, specific advice for therapists working with patients who respond to supportive techniques. Numerous explicit quotes illustrating the aims of supportive treatment.

Rockland, L. H. (1992). *Supportive therapy: A psychodynamic approach.* New York: Basic Books.—The first major text on therapy with those people for whom more exploratory work contributes to too much regression or anxiety.

Ann Appelbaum is currently writing a book on supportive therapy that promises to be excellent.

PSYCHOTHERAPY WITH BORDERLINE PATIENTS

Kernberg, O. F. (1975). *Borderline conditions and pathological narcissism.* New York: Jason Aronson.—A difficult read for the beginner, this seminal description of borderline personality organization was the basic text in borderline-ness for a generation of therapists. Emphasis on alternating ego states and lack of identity integration.

Kernberg, O. F. (1984). *Severe personality disorders: Psychotherapeutic strategies.* New Haven, CT: Yale University Press.—Less hard to read than the above; especially valuable for its description of the structural interview.

Masterson, J. (1976). *Psychotherapy and the borderline adult: A developmental approach.* New York: Brunner/Mazel.—Comes at understanding borderline dynamics from more of a developmental model inspired by Mahler's work. Valuable for its communication of the differences between neurotic depression and depression in borderline clients, and also for its depiction of the engulfment/abandonment conflict.

Yeomans, F. E., Clarkin, J. F., & Kernberg, O. F. (2002). *A primer of transference-focused therapy for the borderline patient.* Northvale, NJ: Jason Aronson.—A manualized psychoanalytic approach to working with borderline patients that is comparatively easy to read and implement.

BRIEF AND MANUALIZED PSYCHOANALYTIC THERAPIES

Book, H. E. (1997). *How to practice brief psychodynamic psychotherapy: The core conflictual relationship theme method.* Washington, DC: American Psychological Association.—An empirically derived, easy-to-learn version of psychoanalytic brief therapy.

Luborsky, L., & Crits-Christoph, P. (1990). *Understanding transference: The CCRT method.* New York: Basic Books.—The basis for the method explicated by H. E. Book. Luborsky's long and diligent research has given robust support to this formulation.

Messer, S. B., & Warren, C. S. (1995). *Models of brief psychodynamic therapy: A comparative approach*. New York: Guilford Press.—Very useful overview of those brief therapies that have been derived from psychoanalytic theories.

OVERVIEW OF PSYCHOTHERAPIES

Gurman, A. S., & Messer, S. B. (Eds.) (2003). *Essential psychotherapies: Theory and practice* (2nd ed.). New York: Guilford Press.—An edited volume with chapters by leading therapists representing different orientations and therapeutic modalities. Well written, scholarly, and readable. Authors were asked to include a case example representing reasonably good but not stellar work, lending a realistic quality to the discussion. Comprehensive and worth the not inconsiderable expense.

References

Abend, S. (1982). Serious illness in the analyst: Countertransference consider-ations. *Journal of the American Psychoanalytic Association, 30*, 365–379.

Ablon, S. L., Brown, D., Khantzian, E. J., & Mack, J. E. (Eds.). (1993). *Human feel-ings: Explorations in affect development and meaning*. Hillsdale, NJ: Analytic Press.

Adler, G. (1980). Transference, real relationship and alliance. *International Jour-nal of Psycho-Analysis, 61*, 547–558.

Allport, G. W. (1961). *Pattern and growth in personality*. New York: Holt, Rinehart & Winston.

Altman, N. (1993). Psychoanalysis and the urban poor. *Psychoanalytic Dialogues, 3*, 29–49.

Altman, N. (1995). *The analyst in the inner city: Race, class, and culture through a psy-choanalytic lens*. Hillsdale, NJ: Analytic Press.

Appelbaum, S. A. (2000). *Evocativeness: Moving and persuasive interventions in psy-chotherapy*. Northvale, NJ: Jason Aronson.

Aristotle. (n.d.). *Politics* (H. Rackham, trans.). Cambridge, MA: Harvard Univer-sity Press, 1997.

Arkowitz, H., & Messer, S. (Eds.). (1984). *Psychoanalytic therapy and behavior ther-apy: Is integration possible?* New York: Plenum Press.

Aron, L. (1991). The patient's experience of the analyst's subjectivity. *Psychoana-lytic Dialogues, 1*, 29–51.

Aron, L. (1996). *A meeting of minds: Mutuality in psychoanalysis*. Hillsdale, NJ: Ana-lytic Press.

Aron, L. (1997). Self-disclosure and the interactive matrix: Commentary on Ken-neth A. Franks' paper. *Psychoanalytic Dialogues, 7*, 315–318.

Atwood, G. E., Orange, D. M.., & Stolorow, R. D. (2002). Shattered worlds/psy-chotic states: A post-Cartesian view of the experience of personal annihila-tion. *Psychoanalytic Psychology, 19*, 281–306.

Atwood, G. E., & Stolorow, R. D. (1993). Faces in a cloud: Intersubjectivity in per-sonality theory. Northvale, NJ: Jason Aronson.

Bachrach, H. M. (1983). On the concept of analyzability. *Psychoanalytic Quarterly*, *52*, 180–203.

Bachrach, M. M., & Leaff, L. A. (1978). "Analyzability": A systematic review of the clinical and quantitative literature. *Journal of the American Psychoanalytic Association*, *26*, 881–920.

Bader, M. (1997). Cultural norms and the patient's experience of the analyst's business practices. *Psychoanalytic Quarterly*, *66*, 93–97.

Bashe, E. D. (1989). *The therapist's pregnancy: The experience of patient and therapist in psychoanalytic psychotherapy*. Unpublished doctoral dissertation, Rutgers University.

Beck, A. T. (1976). *Cognitive therapy and the emotional disorders*. New York: International Universities Press.

Beebe, B., Lachmann, F, & Jaffe, J. (1997). Mother–infant interaction structures and presymbolic self- and object representations. *Psychoanalytic Dialogues, 7*, 133–182.

Belsky, J. (1979). Mother–father–infant interaction: A naturalistic observational study. *Developmental Psychology, 15*, 601–607.

Benjamin, J. (1995). *Like subjects, love objects: Essays on recognition and sexual difference*. New Haven, CT: Yale University Press.

Benjamin, J. (1997). *The shadow of the other*. New York: Routledge.

Benjamin, J. (2002, January 19). [Discussion of papers presented by J. M. Davies and I. Z. Hoffman. Conference of the International Association for Relational Psychotherapy and Psychoanalysis, New York.]

Berger, L. (2002). *Psychotherapy as praxis: Abandoning misapplied science*. Victoria, BC: Trafford.

Bergin, A., & Garfield, S. (Eds.). (2000). *Handbook of psychological change: Psychotherapy processes and practices for the 21st century*. New York: Wiley.

Bergmann, M. S. (1982). Platonic love, transference love and love in real life. *Journal of the American Psychoanalytic Association, 30*, 87–111.

Bergmann, M. S. (1987). *The anatomy of loving: The story of man's quest to know what love is*. New York: Columbia University Press.

Bergmann, M. S. (1988). On the fate of the intrapsychic image of the psychoanalyst after the termination of the analysis. *Psychoanalytic Study of the Child, 43*, 137–153.

Bettelheim, B. (1983). *Freud and man's soul*. New York: Knopf.

Bion, W. R. (1962). *Learning from experience*. London: Karnac, 1984.

Bion, W. R. (1970). *Attention and interpretation*. New York: Jason Aronson.

Blagys, M. D., & Hilsenroth, M. J. (2000). Distinctive of short-term psychodynamic–interpersonal psychotherapy: A review of the comparative psychotherapy process literature. *Clinical Psychology: Science and Practice, 7*, 167–189.

Bleger, J. (1967). Psycho-analysis of the psycho-analytic frame. *International Journal of Psycho-Analysis, 48*, 511–519.

Blum, H. (1973). The concept of erotic transference. *Journal of the American Psychoanalytic Association, 21*, 61–76.

Bollas, C. (1987). *The shadow of the object*. New York: Columbia University Press.

Bollas, C., & Sundelson, D. (1995). *The new informants: The betrayal of confidentiality in psychoanalysis and psychotherapy*. Northvale, NJ: Jason Aronson.

Book, H. E. (1997). *How to practice brief psychodynamic psychotherapy: The core conflictual relationship theme method*. Washington, DC: American Psychological Association.

Bowlby, J. (1969). *Attachment and loss: Vol. 1. Attachment.* New York: Basic Books.

Bowlby, J. (1988). *A secure base: Parent–child attachment and healthy human development.* New York: Basic Books.

Brazelton, T. B. (1982). Joint regulation of neonate-parent behavior. In E. Tronick (Ed.), *Social interchange in infancy* (pp. 137–154). Baltimore: University Park Press.

Brazelton, T. B., & Als, H. (1979). Four early stages in the development of mother–infant interaction. *Psychoanalytic Study of the Child, 34*, 349–369.

Breger, L. (2000). *Freud: Darkness in the midst of vision: An analytical biography*. New York: Wiley.

Bretherton, I. (1990). Communication patterns, internal working models, and the intergenerational transmission of attachment relationships. *Infant Mental Health Journal, 11*, 237–257.

Bromberg, P. (1992). The difficult patient or the difficult dyad?—Some basic issues. *Contemporary Psychoanalysis, 28*, 495–502.

Brunswick, R. (1928). A supplement to Freud's "History of an Infantile Neurosis." *International Journal of Psycho-Analysis, 9*, 439–476.

Bucci, W. (2002). The challenge of diversity in modern psychoanalysis. *Psychoanalytic Psychology, 19*, 216–226.

Buckley, P. (2001). Ancient templates: The classical origins of psychoanalysis. *American Journal of Psychotherapy, 55*, 451–459.

Bugental, J. F. T. (1964). The person who is the psychotherapist. *Journal of Consulting Psychology, 28*, 272–277.

Cardinal, M. (1983). *The words to say it*. Cambridge, MA: VanVactor & Goodheart.

Casement, P. J. (1985). *Learning from the patient*. New York: Guilford Press.

Casement, P. J. (2002). *Learning from our mistakes: Beyond dogma in psychoanalysis and psychotherapy*. New York: Guilford Press.

Cassidy, J., & Shaver, P. R. (Eds.). (2002). *Handbook of attachment: Theory, research and clinical applications*. New York: Guilford Press.

Charles, M. (2003). On faith, hope, and possibility. *Journal of the American Academy of Psychoanalysis and Dynamic Psychiatry, 31*, 687–704.

Charles, M. (in press). *Learning from experience: A guidebook for clinicians*. Hillsdale, NJ: Analytic Press.

Chasseguet-Smirgel, J. (1992). Some thoughts on the psychoanalytic situation. *Journal of the American Psychoanalytic Association, 40*, 3–25.

Chernin, K. (1995). *A different kind of listening: My psychoanalysis and its shadow*. New York: HarperCollins.

Chessick, R. D. (1969). *How psychotherapy heals: The process of intensive psychotherapy*. New York: Jason Aronson.

Chodorow, N. (1999). *The power of feelings*. New Haven, CT: Yale University Press.

Clance, P. R., & Imes, S. A. (1978). The impostor phenomenon in high achieving women: Dynamic and therapeutic interaction. *Psychotherapy: Theory, Research, and Practice, 15*, 241–247.

Clarke-Stewart, K. A. (1978). And Daddy make three: The father's impact on mother and young child. *Child Development, 49*, 466–478.

Clarkin, J. F., Yeomans, F. E., & Kernberg, O. F. (1999). *Psychotherapy for borderline personality.* New York: Wiley.

Coates, S., & Moore, M. (1997). The complexity of early trauma: Representation and transformation. *Psychoanalytic Inquiry, 17*, 286–311.

Coen, S. (2002). *Affect intolerance in patient and analyst.* Northvale, NJ: Jason Aronson.

Cohn, J., Campbell, S., Matias, R., & Hopkins, J. (1990). Face-to-face interactions of post-partum depressed and nondepressed mother–infant pairs at 2 months. *Developmental Psychology, 26*, 15–23.

Comfort, A. (1972). *The joy of sex.* New York: Simon & Schuster.

Conners, M. E. (2001). Integrative treatment of symptomatic disorders. *Psychoanalytic Psychology 18*, 74–91.

Cooper, A. (1986). Some limitations on therapeutic effectiveness: The "burnout syndrome" in psychoanalysis. *Psychoanalytic Quarterly, 60*, 576–598.

Cooper, S. H. (2000). *Objects of hope: Exploring possibility and limit in psychoanalysis.* Hillsdale, NJ: Analytic Press.

Cortina, M., & Marrone, M. (Eds.). (2003). *Attachment theory and the psychoanalytic process.* London: Whurr.

Cozolino, L. (2002). *The neuroscience of psychotherapy: Building and rebuilding the human brain.* New York: Norton.

Crastnopol, M. (1997). Incognito or not?: The patient's subjective experience of the analyst's private life. *Psychoanalytic Dialogues, 7*, 257–280.

Csikszentmihalyi, M. (1990). *Flow: The psychology of optimal experience.* New York: Harper & Row.

Damasio, A. R. (1994). *Descartes' error: Emotion, reason, and the human brain.* New York: Grosset/Putnam.

Damasio, A. R. (2000). *The feeling of what happens: Body and emotion in the making of consciousness.* New York: Harcourt.

Davies, J. (1994). Love in the afternoon: A relational reconstruction of desire and dread in the countertransference. *Psychoanalytic Dialogues, 4*, 153–170.

Davies, J. M., & Frawley, M. G. (1994). *Treating the adult survivor of childhood sexual abuse: A psychoanalytic perspective.* New York: Basic Books.

DeCasper, A., & Fifer, W. (1980). Of human bonding: Newborns prefer their mothers' voices. *Science, 208*, 1174–1176.

DeCasper, A., & Spence, M. (1986). Prenatal maternal speech influences newborns' perception of speech sounds. *Infant Behavior and Development, 9*, 133–150.

Dewald, P. A. (1976). Transference regression and real experience in the psychoanalytic process. *Psychoanalytic Quarterly, 45*, 213–230.

Dewald, P. A. (1982). Serious illness in the analyst: Transference, countertransference, and reality responses. *Journal of the American Psychoanalytic Association, 30*, 347–363.

Dimen, M. (1994). Money, love and hate: Contradictions and paradox in psychoanalysis. *Psychoanalytic Dialogues, 4*, 69–100.

Doi, T. (1989). The concept of *amae* and its psychoanalytic implications. *International Review of Psycho-Analysis, 16*, 349–354.

Doidge, N. (2001). Diagnosing *The English Patient*: Schizoid fantasies of being skinless and of being buried alive. *Journal of the American Psychoanalytic Association, 49*, 279–309.

Doidge, N., Simon, B., Brauer, L., Grant, D. C., First, M., Brunshaw, J., et al. (2002). Psychoanalytic patients in the U.S., Canada, and Australia: 1. DSM-III-R disorders, indications, previous treatment, medications, and length of treatment. *Journal of the American Psychoanalytic Association, 50*, 575–614.

Duehrssen, A., & Jorswick, E. (1965). Empirical and statistical inquiries into the therapeutic potential of psychoanalytic treatment. *Der Nervenarzt, 36*, 166–169.

Ehrenberg, D. B. (1992). On the question of analyzability. *Contemporary Psychoanalysis, 28*, 16–31.

Eigen, M. (1981). The area of faith in Winnicott, Lacan and Bion. *International Journal of Psycho-Analysis, 62*, 413–433.

Eigen, M. (1992). *Coming through the whirlwind: Case studies in psychotherapy.* Wilmette, IL: Chiron.

Eigen, M. (1993). *The electrified tightrope.* Northvale, NJ: Jason Aronson.

Eigen, M. (2001). *Ecstasy.* Middletown, CT: Wesleyan University Press.

Eigen, M. (2002). *Rage.* Middletown, CT: Wesleyan University Press.

Eisenstein, A., & Regillot, K. (2002). Midrash and mutuality in the treatment of trauma: A joint account. *Psychoanalytic Review, 89*, 303–327.

Eissler, K. R. (1953). The effect of the structure of the ego on psychoanalytic technique. *Journal of the American Psychoanalytic Association, 1*, 104–143.

Ekstein, R., & Wallerstein, R. S. (1958). *The teaching and learning of psychotherapy.* Madison, CT: International Universities Press, 1971.

Ellman, S. J. (1991). *Freud's technique papers: A contemporary perspective.* Northvale, NJ: Jason Aronson.

Erle, J. B. (1979). An approach to the study of analyzability and analyses: The course of forty consecutive cases selected for supervised analysis. *Psychoanalytic Quarterly, 48*, 198–228.

Erle, J. B. (1993). On the setting of analytic fees. *Psychoanalytic Quarterly, 62*, 106–108.

Erle, J. B., & Goldberg, D. A. (1979). Problems in the assessment of analyzability. *Psychoanalytic Quarterly, 48*, 48–84.

Escalona, S. K. (1968). *The roots of individuality: Normal patterns of development in infancy.* Chicago: Aldine.

Escalona, S. K., & Corman, H. (1974). Early life experience and the development of competence. *International Review of Psycho-Analysis, 1*, 151–168.

Etchegoyen, R. H. (1991). *The fundamentals of psychoanalytic technique.* London: Karnac Books.

Fenichel, O. (1941). *Problems of psychoanalytic technique.* Albany, NY: Psychoanalytic Quarterly.

Ferenczi, S. (1932). *The clinical diary of Sandor Ferenczi* (J. Dupont, Ed.; M. Balint & N. Z. Jackson, Trans.). Cambridge, MA: Harvard University Press, 1988.

Field, T., Goldstein, S., & Guthertz, M. (1990). Behavior–state matching and synchrony in mother–infant interactions of depressed and nondepressed dyads. *Developmental Psychology, 26,* 7–14.

Fieldsteel, N. (1989). Analysts' expressed attitudes toward dealing with death and illness. *Contemporary Psychoanalysis, 25,* 427–431.

Fine, R. (1971). *The healing of the mind: The technique of psychoanalytic psychotherapy.* New York: David McKay.

Fiscalini, J. (1988). Curative experience in the analytic relationship. *Contemporary Psychoanalysis, 24,* 125–142.

Flournoy, O. (1992). Review of *Psychotic anxieties and containment: A personal record of an analysis with Winnicott. International Journal of Psycho-Analysis, 73,* 593–594.

Fonagy, P. (2000). *Attachment theory and psychoanalysis.* New York: Other Press.

Fonagy, P., Gergely, G., Jurist, E. L., & Target, M., (2002). *Affect regulation, mentalization, and the development of the self.* New York: Other Press.

Fonagy, P., Leigh, T., Steele, M., Steele, H., Kennedy, R., Mattoon, G., et al. (1996). The relationship of attachment status, psychiatric classification, and response to psychotherapy. *Journal of Clinical and Consulting Psychology, 64,* 22–31.

Fonagy, P., & Target, M. (1997). Perspectives on the recovered memories debate. In J. Sandler & P. Fonagy (Eds.), *Recovered memories of abuse: True or false?* (pp. 183–216). London: Karnac Books.

Fosha, D. (2000). *The transforming power of affect: A model for accelerated change.* New York: Behavioral Sciences Research Press.

Foster, R. P., Moskowitz, M., & Javier, R. A. (Eds.). (1996). *Reaching across boundaries of culture and class: Widening the scope of psychotherapy.* Northvale, NJ: Jason Aronson.

Fowler, J. W. (1981). *Stages of faith: The psychology of human development and the quest for meaning.* New York: HarperCollins.

Frank, J. D., & Frank, J. B. (1991). *Persuasion and healing: A comparative study of psychotherapy* (3rd ed.). Baltimore: Johns Hopkins Press.

Frank, K. A. (1992). Combining action techniques with psychoanalytic psychotherapy. *International Journal of Psycho-Analysis, 19,* 57–79.

Frattaroli, E. (2001). *Healing the soul in the age of the brain: Becoming conscious in an unconscious world.* New York: Viking Penguin.

Frawley-O'Dea, M. G., & Sarnat, J. E. (2001). *The supervisory relationship: A contemporary psychodynamic approach.* New York: Guilford Press.

Freedman, N., Hoffenberg, J. D., Vorus, N., & Frosch, A. (1999). The effectiveness of psychoanalytic psychotherapy: The role of treatment duration, frequency of sessions, and the therapeutic relationship. *Journal of the American Psychoanalytic Association, 47,* 741–772.

Freud, S. (1905). On psychotherapy. *Standard Edition, 7,* 257–268.

Freud, S. (1910). "Wild" psycho-analysis. *Standard Edition, 11,* 221–227.

Freud, S. (1912a). The dynamics of transference. *Standard Edition, 12,* 99–108.

Freud, S. (1912b). Recommendations to physicians practicing psycho-analysis. *Standard Edition, 12,* 111–120.

Freud, S. (1913). On beginning the treatment. *Standard Edition, 12,* 123–144.

Freud, S. (1914). On the history of the psycho-analytic movement. *Standard Edition, 14,* 7–66.

Freud, S. (1915). Observations on transference love. *Standard Edition, 12*, 159–171.

Freud, S. (1916). Some character types met with in psycho-analytic work. *Standard Edition, 14*, 311–333.

Freud, S. (1919). Lines of advance in psychoanalytic therapy. *Standard Edition, 17*, 159–168.

Freud, S. (1923). The ego and the id. *Standard Edition, 19*, 3–66.

Freud, S. (1926). The question of lay analysis. *Standard Edition, 20*, 183–250.

Freud, S. (1937). Analysis terminable and interminable. *Standard Edition, 23*, 209–254.

Frey, W. H., II (1985). *Crying: The mystery of tears*. Minneapolis: Winston Press.

Fromm, E. (1947). *Man for himself: An inquiry into the psychology of ethics*. New York: Rinehart.

Fromm-Reichmann, F. (1950). *Principles of intensive psychotherapy*. Chicago: University of Chicago Press.

Fromm-Reichmann, F. (1952). *Psychotherapy with schizophrenics*. New York: International Universities Press.

Furman, E. (1982). Mothers have to be there to be left. *Psychoanalytic Study of the Child, 37*, 15–28.

Gabbard, G. O. (1982). The exit line: Heightened transference–countertransference manifestations at the end of the hour. *Journal of the American Psychoanalytic Association, 30*, 579–598.

Gabbard, G. O. (Ed.). (1989). *Sexual exploitation in professional relationships*. Washington, DC: American Psychiatric Press.

Gabbard, G. O. (1994). Sexual excitement and countertransference love in the analyst. *Journal of the American Psychoanalytic Association, 42*, 1083–1106.

Gabbard, G. O. (1995). The early history of boundary violations in psychoanalysis. *Journal of the American Psychoanalytic Association, 43*, 1115–1136.

Gabbard, G. O. (1998). Commentary on paper by Jody Messler Davies. *Psychoanalytic Dialogues, 8*, 781–789.

Gabbard, G. O. (2000). On gratitude and gratification. *Journal of the American Psychoanalytic Association, 48*, 697–716.

Gabbard, G. O. (2002). *The psychology of* The Sopranos: *Love, death, desire, and betrayal in America's favorite gangster family*. New York: Basic Books.

Gabbard, G. O., & Lester, E. P. (1995). *Boundaries and boundary violations in psychoanalysis*. New York: Basic Books.

Gabbard, G. O., Peltz, M. L., & COPE Study Group on Boundary Violations. (2002). Speaking the unspeakable: Institutional reactions to boundary violations by training analysts. *Journal of the American Psychoanalytic Association, 49*, 659–673.

Gaston, L., Marmar, C. R., Gallagher, D., & Thompson, L. W. (1991). Alliance prediction of outcome beyond in-treatment symptomatic change in psychotherapy processes. *Psychotherapy Research, 1*, 104–113.

Gaylin, W. (1976). *Caring*. New York: Knopf.

Ghent, E. (1989). Credo—The dialectics of one-person and two-person psychologies. *Contemporary Psychoanalysis, 25*, 169–211.

Ghent, E. (1990). Masochism, submission, surrender—Masochism as the perversion of surrender. *Contemporary Psychoanalysis, 26,* 108–136.

Gill, M. M. (1994). *Psychoanalysis in transition: A personal view.* Hillsdale, NJ: Analytic Press.

Gill, S. (Ed.). (2002). *The supervisory alliance: Facilitating the psychotherapist's learning experience.* Northvale, NJ: Jason Aronson.

Gitelson, M. (1962). The curative factors in psycho-analysis. *International Journal of Psycho-Analysis, 43,* 194–205.

Glover, E. (1931). The therapeutic effect of inexact interpretation: A contribution to the theory of suggestion. In *The technique of psycho-analysis* (pp. 353–366). New York: International Universities Press, 1955.

Glover, E. (1955). *The technique of psycho-analysis.* New York: International Universities Press.

Goldstein, S., & Thau, S. (2003, April 4). *Couples, attachment, and neuroscience.* Paper presented at the 23rd annual spring meeting of the Division of Psychoanalysis (39) of the American Psychological Association, Minneapolis, MN.

Goleman, D. (1995). *Emotional intelligence.* New York: Bantam Books.

Good, G. E. (2001). Putting it into words: Developing a strategic marketing network. *American Psychoanalyst, 35*(3), 1, 6.

Gordon, K. (2004). The tiger's stripe . . . Some thoughts on psychoanalysis, gnosis, and the experience of wonderment. *Contemporary Psychoanalysis, 40,* 5–45.

Green, H. (1964). *I never promised you a rose garden.* New York: Holt, Rinehart & Winston

Green, M. R. (Ed.). (1964). *Interpersonal psychoanalysis: The selected papers of Clara Thompson.* New York: Basic Books.

Greenacre, P. (1959). Certain technical problems in the transference relationship. *Journal of the American Psychoanalytic Association, 7,* 484–502.

Greenberg, J. R. (1986). Theoretical models and the analyst's neutrality. *Contemporary Psychoanalysis, 22,* 87–106.

Greenberg, J. R. (1991). Countertransference and reality. *Psychoanalytic Dialogues, 1,* 52–73.

Greenberg, J. R. (2001). The analyst's participation: A new look. *Journal of the American Psychoanalytic Association, 49,* 359–381.

Greenberg, L. S. (1986). *Emotion in psychotherapy.* New York: Guilford Press.

Greenson, R. R. (1950). The mother tongue and the mother. In *Explorations in psychoanalysis* (pp. 31–43). New York: International Universities Press.

Greenson, R. R. (1954). About the sound "Mm . . . " In *Explorations in psychoanalysis* (pp. 93–97). New York: International Universities Press.

Greenson, R. R. (1966). That "impossible" profession. In *Explorations in psychoanalysis* (pp. 269–287). New York: International Universities Press, 1978.

Greenson, R. R. (1967). *The technique and practice of psychoanalysis.* New York: International Universities Press.

Greenson, R. R. (1971). The real relationship between the patient and the psychoanalyst. In *Explorations in psychoanalysis* (pp. 425–440). New York: International Universities Press.

Greenson, R. R. (1974). The decline and fall of the 50-minute hour. In *Explora-*

tions in psychoanalysis (pp. 407–503). New York: International Universities Press.

Greenspan, S. I. (1996). *Developmentally based psychotherapy.* New York: International Universities Press.

Grinker, R., Sr., Werble, B., & Drye, R. (1968). *The borderline syndrome: A behavioral study of ego functions.* New York: Basic Books.

Grosskurth, P. (1986). *Melanie Klein: Her world and her work.* New York: Knopf.

Grotjahn, M. (1954). About the relation between psycho-analytic training and psycho-analytic therapy. *International Journal of Psycho-Analysis, 35,* 254–262.

Grotstein, J. S. (2000). *Who is the dreamer who dreams the dream? A study of psychic presences.* Hillsdale, NJ: Analytic Press.

Gutheil, T. G., & Gabbard, G. O. (1993). The concept of boundaries in clinical practice: Theoretical and risk-management dimensions. *American Journal of Psychiatry, 150,* 188–196.

Gutheil, T. G., & Gabbard, G. O. (1998). Misuses and misunderstandings of boundary theory in clinical and regulatory settings. *American Journal of Psychiatry, 155,* 409–414.

Haas, L. J., & Malouf, J. L. (2002). *Keeping up the good work: A practitioner's guide to mental health ethics* (3rd ed.). Sarasota, FL: Professional Resource Press.

Hammer, E. (1990). *Reaching the affect: Style in the psychodynamic therapies.* New York: Jason Aronson.

Hatcher, R. (1973). Insight and self-observation. *Journal of the American Psychoanalytic Association, 21,* 377–398.

Hedges, L. E. (1983). *Listening perspectives in psychotherapy.* Northvale, NJ: Jason Aronson, 1995.

Hedges, L. E. (1996). *Strategic emotional involvement.* Northvale, NJ: Jason Aronson.

Hedges, L. E. (2000). *Facing the challenge of liability in psychotherapy: Practicing defensively.* Northvale, NJ: Jason Aronson.

Hellinga, G., van Luyn, B., & Dalewijk, H.-J. (Eds.). (2001). *Personalities: Master clinicians confront the treatment of borderline personality disorders.* Northvale, NJ: Jason Aronson.

Herman, J. L. (1992). *Trauma and recovery.* New York: Basic Books.

Hilsenroth, M. J., Ackerman, S. J., Clemence, A. J., Strassle, C. G., & Handler, L. (2002). Effects of structured clinician training on patient and therapist perspectives of alliance early in psychotherapy. *Psychotherapy: Theory/Research/Practice/Training, 39,* 309–323.

Hirsch, I. (1994). Countertransference love and theoretical model. *Psychoanalytic Dialogues, 4,* 171–192.

Hirsch, I. (1998). The concept of enactment and theoretical convergence. *Psychoanalytic Quarterly, 67,* 78–101.

Hoffman, I. Z. (1983). The patient as interpreter of the analysts's experience. *Contemporary Psychoanalysis, 19,* 399–422.

Hoffman, I. Z. (1992). Some practical implications of a social-constructionist view of the psychoanalytic situation. *Psychoanalytic Dialogues, 2,* 287–304.

Hoffman, I. Z. (1996). The intimate and ironic authority of the psychoanalyst's presence. *Psychoanalytic Quarterly, 65,* 102–136.

Hoffman, I. Z. (1998). *Ritual and spontaneity in the psychoanalytic process: A dialectical constructivist view.* Hillsdale, NJ: Analytic Press.

Hoffman, L. (2002). Psychoanalytic ideas and empirical approaches. *APA Review of Books, 47,* 728–731.

Holmqvist, R. (2000). Staff feelings and patient diagnosis. *Canadian Journal of Psychiatry, 45,* 349–356.

Hopkins, L. (1998). D. W. Winnicott's analysis of Masud Khan: A preliminary study of failures of object usage. *Contemporary Psychoanalysis, 34,* 5–47.

Hornstein, G. A. (2000). *To redeem one person is to redeem the world: The life of Frieda Fromm-Reichmann.* New York: Free Press.

Hovarth, A. O., & Symonds, B. D. (1991). Relation between working alliance and outcome in psychotherapy: A meta-analysis. *Journal of Counseling Psychology, 38,* 139–149.

Howard, K. I., Kopta, S. M., Krause, M. S., & Orlinsky, D. E. (1986). The dose–effect relationship in psychotherapy. *American Psychologist, 41,* 159–164.

Howard, K. I., Lueger, R. J., Maling, M. S., & Martinovich, Z. (1993). A phase model of psychotherapy: Causal mediation of outcome. *Journal of Counseling and Clinical Psychology, 61,* 678–685.

Howard, K. I., Moras, K., Brill, P., Martinovich, A., & Lutz, W. (1996). Evaluation of psychotherapy: Efficacy, effectiveness, and patient progress. *American Psychologist, 51,* 1059–1064.

Hurvich, M. S. (1989). Traumatic moment, basic dangers, and annihilation anxiety. *Psychoanalytic Psychology 6,* 309–323.

Isaacson, E. B. (1991). *Chemical dependency: Theoretical approaches and strategies working with individuals and families.* New York: Haworth Press.

Isay, R. (1991). The homosexual analyst: Clinical considerations. *Psychoanalytic Study of the Child, 46,* 199–216.

Jacobs, T. (1986). On countertransference enactments. *Journal of the American Psychoanalytic Association, 34,* 289–307.

Jacobson, J. (1994). Signal affects and our psychoanalytic confusion of tongues. *Journal of the American Psychoanalytic Association, 42,* 15–42.

Jeffery, E. H. (2001). The mortality of psychoanalysts. *Journal of the American Psychoanalytic Association, 49,* 103–111.

Jones, D. (1993). A question of faith. *Contemporary Psychoanalysis, 29,* 130–243.

Jones, E. (1957). *The life and work of Sigmund Freud, vol. 3: The last phase, 1919–1939.* New York: Basic Books.

Jordan, J. F. (1992). The transference: Distortion or plausible conjecture? *International Journal of Psycho-Analysis, 73,* 729–738.

Josephs, L. (1995). *Balancing empathy and interpretation: Relational character analysis.* Northvale, NJ: Jason Aronson.

Jung, C. G. (1945). The relations between the ego and the unconscious. In H. Read, M. Fordham, & G. Adler (Eds.), *The collected works of C. G. Jung* (Bollinger Series 20, Vol. 7, pp. 120–239). Princeton, NJ: Princeton University Press, 1953.

Jung, C. G. (1916). The transcendent function. In R. F. C. Hull (Trans.), *The collected works of C. G. Jung* (Vol. 8, pp. 67–91). Princeton, NJ: Princeton University Press, 1953.

Kandera, S., Lambert, M., & Andrews, A. (1996). How much therapy is really enough? A session-by-session analysis of the psychotherapy dose–effect relationship. *Journal of Psychotherapy Practice and Research, 4,* 132–151.

Kantrowitz, J. L. (1995). The beneficial aspects of the patient-analyst match. *International Journal of Psycho-Analysis, 76,* 299–313.

Kantrowitz, J. L., Paolitto, F., Sashin, J., Solomon, L., & Katz, A. L. (1986). Affect availability, tolerance, complexity, and modulation in psychoanalysis: Follow-up of a longitudinal, prospective study. *Journal of the American Psychoanalytic Association, 43,* 529–559.

Karon, B., & VandenBos, G. R. (1981). *Psychotherapy of schizophrenia: The treatment of choice.* New York: Jason Aronson.

Kassan, L. D. (1999). *Second opinions: Sixty psychotherapy patients evaluate their therapists.* New York: Jason Aronson.

Katz, J. N. (2001). *Love stories: Sex between men before homosexuality.* Chicago: University of Chicago Press.

Kernberg, O. F. (1975). *Borderline conditions and pathological narcissism.* New York: Jason Aronson.

Kernberg, O. F. (1984). *Severe personality disorders: Psychotherapeutic strategies.* New Haven, CT: Yale University Press.

Kernberg, O. F. (1986). Institutional problems of psychoanalytic education. *Journal of the American Psychoanalytic Association, 34,* 799– 834.

Kernberg, O. F. (1987, June 24). *Working with the borderline patient.* Paper presented at the University of Medicine and Dentistry of New Jersey, Piscataway, NJ.

Kernberg, O. F. (1995). *Love relations: Normality and pathology.* New Haven, CT: Yale University Press.

Kernberg, O. F. (2000). A concerned critique of psychoanalytic education. *International Journal of Psychoanalysis, 81,* 97–119.

Khan, M. M. (1970). Montaigne, Rousseau and Freud. In *The privacy of the self* (pp. 99–111). New York: International Universities Press, 1974.

Kirsner, D. (2000). *Unfree associations: Inside psychoanalytic institutes.* London: Process Press.

Klein, M. (1935). A contribution to the psychogenesis of manic–depressive states. In *Love, guilt and reparation and other works, 1921–1945* (pp.262–289). New York: Free Press, 1975.

Klein, M. (1957). Envy and gratitude. In *Envy and gratitude and other works 1946–1963* (pp. 176–235). New York: Free Press, 1975.

Klerman, G. L., Weissman, M. M., Rounsaville, B. J., & Chevron, E. S. (1984). *Interpersonal psychotherapy of depression.* New York: Basic Books.

Kogan, I. (1995). *The cry of mute children: A psychoanalytic perspective of the second generation of the Holocaust.* London: Free Association Books.

Kohut, H. (1959). Introspection, empathy and psychoanalysis. *Journal of the American Psychoanalytic Association, 7,* 459–483.

Kohut, H. (1968). The evaluation of applicants for psychoanalytic training. *International Journal of Psycho-Analysis, 49,* 548–554.

Kohut, H. (1971). *The analysis of the self: A systematic approach to the psychoanalytic treatment of narcissistic personality disorders.* New York: International Universities Press.

Kohut, H. (1977). *The restoration of the self.* New York: International Universities Press.

Kohut, H. (1979). The two analyses of Mr. Z. *International Journal of Psycho-Analysis, 60,* 3–27.

Kohut, H. (1984). *How does analysis cure?* (A. Goldberg, Ed., with P. Stepansky). Chicago: University of Chicago Press.

Koocher, G. P., & Keith-Spiegel, P. C. (1998). *Ethics in psychology: Professional standards and cases* (2nd ed.). New York: Oxford University Press.

Kristeva, J. (1987). *In the beginning was love: Psychoanalysis and faith.* New York: Columbia University Press.

Krystal, H. (1978). Trauma and affects. *Psychoanalytic Study of the Child, 33,* 81–116.

Krystal, H. (1988). *Integration and self-healing: Affect, trauma, alexithymia.* Hillsdale, NJ: Analytic Press.

Krystal, H. (1997). Desomatization and the consequences of infantile psychic trauma. *Psychoanalytic Inquiry, 17,* 126–150.

Kubie, L. (1952). Problems and techniques of psychoanalytic validation and progress. In E. Pumpian-Mindlin (Ed.), *Psychoanalysis as a science* (pp. 46–124). Palo Alto, CA: Stanford University Press.

Kuhn, T. S. (1962). *The structure of scientific revolutions.* Chicago: University of Chicago Press.

Kuhn, T. S. (1977). *The essential tension: Selected studies in scientific tradition and change.* Chicago: University of Chicago Press.

Laing, R. D. (1960). *The divided self.* New York: Pantheon.

Lamb, M. E. (1977). Father–infant and mother–infant interaction in the first year of life. *Child Development, 48,* 167–181.

Lane, R. E. (2000). *The loss of happiness in market democracies.* New Haven, CT: Yale University Press.

Langs, R. (1975). The therapeutic relationship and deviations in technique. *International Journal of Psychoanalytic Psychotherapy, 4,* 106–141.

Langs, R. (1979). *The therapeutic environment.* New York: Jason Aronson.

Lawner, P. (2001). Spiritual implications of psychodynamic therapy: Immaterial psyche, ideality, and the "area of faith." *Psychoanalytic Review, 88,* 525–548.

Lazarus, A. L., & Zur, O. (2002). *Dual relationships and psychotherapy.* New York: Springer.

Lear, J. (1990). *Love and its place in nature.* New York: Farrar, Straus & Giroux.

Lear, J. (2003). *Therapeutic action: An earnest plea for irony.* New York: Other Press.

LeDoux, J. E. (1992). Emotion as memory: Anatomical systems underlying indelible neural traces (pp. 269–288). In S.-A. Christianson (Ed.), *Handbook of emotion and memory.* Hillsdale, NJ: Erlbaum.

LeDoux, J. E. (1998). *The emotional brain: The mysterious underpinnings of emotional life.* New York: Simon & Schuster.

LeDoux, J. E. (2003). *Synaptic self.* New York: Penguin.

Leiblum, S. R., & Rosen, R. C. (Eds.). (2000). *Principles and practice of sex therapy* (3rd ed.). New York: Guilford Press.

Lepore, S. J., & Smyth, J. M. (Eds.). (2002). *The writing cure: How expressive writing promotes health and emotional well-being.* Washington, DC: American Psychological Association.

Lerner, H. G. (1989). *The dance of intimacy: A woman's guide to courageous acts of change in key relationships.* New York: Harper & Row.

Leuzinger-Bohleber, M., Stuhr, U., Ruger, B., & Beutel, M. (2003). How to study the "quality of psychoanalytic treatments" and their long-term effects on patients' well-being: A representative, multiperspective follow-up study. *International Journal of Psychoanalysis, 84,* 263–290.

Levenson, E. A. (1972). *The fallacy of understanding: An inquiry into the changing structure of psychoanalysis.* New York: Basic Books.

Levenson, E. A. (1978). Two essays in psychoanalytic psychology—I. Psychoanalysis: Cure or persuasion. *Contemporary Psychoanalysis, 14,* 1–17.

Levenson, E. A. (1982). Follow the fox: An inquiry into the vicissitudes of psychoanalytic supervision. *Contemporary Psychoanalysis, 18,* 1–15.

Levenson, E. A. (1988). The pursuit of the particular—On the psychoanalytic inquiry. *Contemporary Psychoanalysis, 24,* 1–16.

Levenson, E. A. (1992). Mistakes, errors, and oversights. *Contemporary Psychoanalysis, 28,* 555–571.

Levenson, E. A. (1996). Aspects of self-revelation and self-disclosure. *Contemporary Psychoanalysis, 32,* 237–248.

Levin, J. D. (1987). *Treatment of alcoholism and other addictions: A self-psychology approach.* Northvale, NJ: Jason Aronson.

Lichtenberg, J. (1998). Experience as a guide to psychoanalytic theory and practice. *Journal of the American Psychoanalytic Association, 46,* 17–36.

Linehan, M. M. (1993). *Cognitive-behavioral treatment of borderline personality disorder.* New York: Guilford Press.

Lipin, T. (1963). The repetition compulsion and "maturational" drive-representatives. *International Journal of Psycho-Analysis, 44,* 389–406.

Lipton, S. D. (1977). The advantages of Freud's technique as shown in his analysis of the Rat Man. *International Journal of Psycho-Analysis, 58,* 255–274.

Liss-Levinson, N. (1990). Money matters and the woman analyst: In a different voice. *Psychoanalytic Psychology, 7,* 119–130.

Little, M. (1951). Countertransference and the patient's response to it. *International Journal of Psycho-Analysis, 32,* 32–40.

Loewald, H. W. (1960). On the therapeutic action of psycho-analysis. *International Journal of Psycho-Analysis, 41,* 16–33.

Lohser, B., & Newton, P. M. (1996). *Unorthodox Freud: The view from the couch.* New York: Guilford Press.

Lothane, Z. (1987). Love, seduction and trauma. *Psychoanalytic Review, 74,* 83–105.

Lothane, Z. (2002). Commentary: Requiem or reveille. A response to Robert F. Bornstein (2001). *Psychoanalytic Psychology, 19,* 572–579.

Luborsky, L. (1984). *Principles of psychoanalytic psychotherapy: A manual for supportive/expressive treatment.* New York: Basic Books.

Luborsky, L., & Crits-Christoph, P. (1990). *Understanding transference: The CCRT method.* New York: Basic Books.

Luborsky, L., Diguer, L., Luborsky, E., Singer, B., & Dickter, D. (1993). The efficacy of dynamic psychotherapies: Is it true that everyone has won so all shall have prizes? In N. E. Miller, L. L. Luborsky, J. P. Barber, U J. Docherty (Eds.), *Psychodynamic treatment research: A handbook for clinical practice* (pp. 447–514). New York: Basic Books.

Luborsky, L., Rosenthal, R., Diguer, L., Andrusyna, T. P., Berman, J. S., Levitt, J. T., et al. (2002). The dodo bird verdict is alive and well—mostly. *Clinical Psychology: Science and Practice, 9*, 2–12.

Lueger, R., Lutz, W., & Howard, K. I. (2000). The predicted and observed course of psychotherapy for anxiety and mood disorders. *Journal of Nervous and Mental Disease, 188*, 127–134.

Luepnitz, D. A. (2002). *Schopenhauer's porcupines. Intimacy and its dilemmas: Five stories of psychotherapy.* New York: Basic Books.

Luhrman, T. M. (2000). *Of two minds: The growing disorder in American psychiatry.* New York: Knopf.

Main, M. (1998). Recent studies in attachment: Overview, with selected implications for clinical work. In S. Goldberg, J. Kerr, & R. Muir (Eds.), *Attachment theory: Social, developmental, and clinical perspectives* (pp. 407–474). Northvale, NJ: Analytic Press.

Main, M., & Hesse, E. (1990). Parents' unresolved traumatic experiences are related to infant disorganized attachment status: Is frightened and/or frightening parental behavior the linking mechanism? In M. Greenberg, D. Cicchetti, & E. M. Cummings (Eds.), *Attachment in the preschool years: Theory, research and intervention* (pp. 161–182). Chicago: University of Chicago Press.

Main, M., Kaplan, N., & Cassidy, J. (1985). Security in infancy, childhood and adulthood: A move to the level of representation. *Monograph of the Society on Research in Child Development, 50*(1–2 Serial No. 209), 65–104.

Main, M., & Solomon, J. (1991). Procedures for identifying infants as disorganized–disoriented during the Ainsworth Strange Situation. In M. T. Greenberg, D. Cicchetti, & E. M. Cummings (Eds.), *Attachment n the preschool years: Theory, research, and intervention* (pp. 22–31). Chicago: University of Chicago Press.

Mann, J. (1973). *Time-limited psychotherapy.* Cambridge, MA: Harvard University Press.

Marmor, J. (1979). Short-term dynamic psychotherapy. *American Journal of Psychiatry, 136*, 149–155.

Maroda, K. J. (1991). *The power of countertransference.* Northvale, NJ: Jason Aronson.

Maroda, K. J. (1999). *Seduction, surrender, and transformation: Emotional engagement in the analytic process.* Hillsdale, NJ: Analytic Press.

Maroda, K. J. (2002, March 23). *Issues in erotic countertransference: Origins, guilt and self-disclosure.* Paper presented at the annual spring meeting of the Institute for Psychoanalysis and Psychotherapy of New Jersey, Iselin, NJ.

Maroda, K. J. (2003). *Legitimate gratification of the analyst's needs.* Unpublished manuscript.

Masling, J. (2000, May 12). *Remarks to the American Psychoanalytic Association on the occasion of his honorary membership 89th annual meeting of members.* Retrieved February 1, 2002, from http://www.apsa.org/pubinfo/masling.htm.

Masterson, J. (1976). *Psychotherapy and the borderline adult: A developmental approach*. New York: Brunner/Mazel.

McDougall, J. (1985). *Theaters of the mind: Illusion and truth on the psychoanalytic stage*. New York: Basic Books.

McDougall, J. (1989). *Theaters of the body: A psychoanalytic approach to psychosomatic illness*. New York: Norton.

McGoldrick, M. (1996). Irish families. In M. McGoldrick, J. Giordano, & J. K. Pearce (Eds.), *Ethnicity and family therapy* (2nd ed., pp. 544–566). New York: Guilford Press.

McGuire, W. (Ed.). (1974). *The Freud/Jung letters: The correspondence between Sigmund Freud and C. G. Jung* (R. Manheim & R. F. C. Hull, Trans.). Princeton, NJ: Princeton University Press:

McWilliams, N. (1986). Patients for life: The case for devotion. *The Psychotherapy Patient, 3*, 55–69.

McWilliams, N. (1987) The grandiose self and the interminable analysis. *Current Issues in Psychoanalytic Practice, 4*, 93–107.

McWilliams, N. (1991). Mothering and fathering processes in the psychoanalytic art. *Psychoanalytic Review, 78*, 525–545.

McWilliams, N. (1994). *Psychoanalytic diagnosis: Understanding personality structure in the clinical process*. New York: Guilford Press.

McWilliams, N. 1998). Relationship, subjectivity, and inference in diagnosis. In J. W. Barron (Ed.), *Making diagnosis meaningful: Enhancing evaluation and treatment of psychological disorders* (pp. 197– 226). Washington, DC: American Psychological Association.

McWilliams, N. (1999). *Psychoanalytic case formulation*. New York: Guilford Press.

McWilliams, N. (2003). The educative aspects of psychoanalysis. *Psychoanalytic Psychology, 20*, 245–260.

McWilliams, N., & Weinberger, J. (2003). Psychodynamic psychotherapy. In G. Stricker & T. A. Widiger (Eds), *Comprehensive Handbook of Psychology, vol. 8: Clinical Psychology* (pp. 253–277). New York: Wiley.

Meissner, W. (1983). Values in the psychoanalytic situation. *Psychoanalytic Inquiry, 3*, 577–598.

Meissner, W. W. (1991). *What is effective in psychoanalytic therapy? The move from interpretation to relation*. Northvale, NJ: Jason Aronson.

Meissner, W. W. (1996). *The therapeutic alliance*. New Haven, CT: Yale University Press.

Meloy, J. R. (1988). *The psychopathic mind: Origins, dynamics, and treatment*. Northvale, NJ: Jason Aronson.

Meloy, J. R. (1998). (Ed.). *The psychology of stalking: Clinical and forensic perspectives*. New York: Elsevier Science.

Menaker, E. (1942). The masochistic factor in the psychoanalytic situation. *Psychoanalytic Quarterly, 11*, 171–186.

Messer, S. B., & Wampold, B. E. (2002). Let's face facts: Common factors are more potent than specific therapy ingredients. *Clinical Psychology: Science and Practice, 9*, 21– 25.

Messer, S. B., & Warren, C. S. (1995). *Models of brief psychodynamic therapy: A comparative approach*. New York: Guilford Press.

Messer, S. B., & Winokur, M. (1984). Ways of knowing and visions of reality in psychoanalytic theory and behavior therapy. In H. Arkowitz & S. B. Messer (Eds.), *Psychoanalytic therapy and behavior therapy: Is integration possible?* (pp. 63–100). New York: Plenum Press.

Messer, S. B., & Woolfolk, R. L. (1998). Philosophical issues in psychotherapy. *Clinical Psychology: Science and Practice, 5,* 251–263.

Michels, R. (1988). One psychoanalysis or many? *Contemporary Psychoanalysis, 24,* 359–371.

Miller, A. (1975). *Prisoners of childhood: The drama of the gifted child and the search for the true self.* New York: Basic Books.

Miller, A. (1979). The drama of the gifted child and the psycho-analyst's narcissistic disturbance. *International Journal of Psycho-Analysis, 60,* 47–58.

Mitchell, S. A. (1988). *Relational concepts in psychoanalysis.* Cambridge, MA: Harvard University Press.

Mitchell, S. A. (1993). *Hope and dread in psychoanalysis.* New York: Basic Books.

Mitchell, S. A. (1997). *Influence and autonomy in psychoanalysis.* Hillsdale, NJ: Analytic Press.

Mitchell, S. A. (2002). *Can love last? The fate of romance over time.* New York: Norton.

Mitchell, S. A., & Black, M. J. (1995). *Freud and beyond: A history of modern psychoanalytic thought.* New York: Basic Books.

Momigliano, L. (1987). A spell in Vienna: But was Freud a Freudian? An investigation into Freud's technique between 1920 and 1938, based on the published testimony of former analysands. *International Review of Psycho-Analysis, 14,* 373–389.

Money, J. (1986). *Lovemaps: Clinical concepts of sexual/erotic health and pathology, paraphilia, and gender transposition in childhood, adolescence and maturity.* New York: Irvington.

Morrison, A. L. (1997). Ten years of doing psychotherapy while living with a life-threatening illness: Self-disclosure and other ramifications. *Psychoanalytic Dialogues, 7,* 225–241.

Morrison, A. P. (1989). *Shame: The underside of narcissism.* Hillsdale, NJ: Analytic Press.

Moses, I. (1988). The misuse of empathy. *Contemporary Psychoanalysis, 24,* 577–593.

Mumford, E., Schlesinger, H. J., Glass, G. V., Patrick, C., & Cuerdon, T. (1984). A new look at evidence about reduced cost of medical utilization following mental health treatment. *American Journal of Psychiatry, 141,* 1145–1158.

Nacht, S. (1958). Variations in technique. *International Journal of Psycho-Analysis, 39,* 235–237.

Nacht, S. (1962). The curative factors in psycho-analysis. *International Journal of Psycho-Analysis, 43,* 206–211.

Nathanson, D. L. (Ed.). (1987). *The many faces of shame.* New York: Guilford Press.

Nathanson, D. L. (1996). *Knowing feeling: Affect, script, and psychotherapy.* New York: Norton.

Natterson, J. M. (2003). Love in psychotherapy. *Psychoanalytic Psychology, 20,* 509–521.

Norcross, J., Strausser-Kirtland, D., & Missar, C. (1988). The processes and outcomes of psychotherapists' personal treatment experiences. *Psychotherapy: Theory, Research, and Practice, 25,* 36–43.

Norcross, J., Geller, J., & Kurzawa, E. (2000). Conducting psychotherapy with psychotherapists: 1. Prevalence, patients and problems. *Psychotherapy: Theory, Research, and Practice, 37,* 199–205.

Nydes, J. (1963). The paranoid-masochistic character. *Psychoanalytic Review, 50,* 215–251.

Ogden, T. H. (1985). On potential space. *International Journal of Psycho-Analysis, 70,* 129–141.

Ogden, T. H. (1986). *The matrix of the mind: Object relations and the psychoanalytic dialogue.* Northvale, NJ: Jason Aronson.

Ogden, T. H. (1997). *Reverie and interpretation: Sensing something human.* Northvale, NJ: Jason Aronson.

Ogden, T. H. (2001). *Conversations at the frontier of dreaming.* Northvale, NJ: Jason Aronson.

Paolino, T. J. (1981). *Psychoanalytic psychotherapy: Theory, technique, therapeutic relationship and treatability.* New York: Bruner/Mazel.

Pearlman, L. A., & Saakvitne, K. (1995). *Psychotherapy with incest survivors.* New York: Norton.

Peebles-Kleiger, M. J. (2002). *Beginnings: The art and science of planning psychotherapy.* Hillsdale, NJ: Analytic Press.

Pennebaker, J. W. (1997). *Opening up: The healing power of expressing emotions* (rev. ed.). New York: Guilford Press.

Pennebaker, J. W., Kiecolt-Glaser, & Glaser, R. (1988). Disclosure of trauma and immune function: Health implications for psychotherapy. *Journal of Consulting and Clinical Psychology, 56,* 239–245.

Perry, J., Banon, E., & Ianni, R. (1999). Effectiveness of psychotherapy for personality disorders. *American Journal of Psychiatry, 156,* 1312–1321.

Person, E. S. (1991). Romantic love: Intersection of psyche and cultural unconscious. *Journal of the American Psychoanalytic Association, 39,* 383–412.

Phillip, C. E. (1993). Dilemmas of disclosure to patients and colleagues when a therapist faces a life-threatening illness. *Health Social Work, 18,* 13–19.

Pine, F. (1985). *Developmental theory and clinical process.* New Haven, CT: Yale University Press.

Pine, F. (1990). *Drive, ego, object, and self: A synthesis for clinical work.* New York: Basic Books.

Pine, F. (1998). *Diversity and direction in psychoanalytic technique.* New Haven, CT: Yale University Press.

Pinsker, H. (1997). *A primer of supportive psychotherapy.* Hillsdale, NJ: Analytic Press.

Pizer, B. (1997). When the analyst is ill: Dimensions of self-disclosure. *Psychoanalytic Quarterly, 66,* 450–469.

Pizer, S. (1996). The distributed self. Introduction to symposium on "The multiplicity of self and analytic technique." *Contemporary Psychoanalysis, 32,* 449–507.

Pope, K. S. (1986). Research and laws regarding therapist–patient sexual involvement: Implications for therapists. *American Journal of Psychotherapy, 40,* 564–571.

Putnam, F. W. (1989). *Diagnosis and treatment of multiple personality disorder.* New York: Guilford Press.

Racker, H. (1968). *Transference and countertransference* New York: International Universities Press.

Reich, W. (1932). *Character analysis.* New York: Farrar, Straus, and Giroux, 1972.

Reik, T. (1941). *Masochism and modern man.* New York: Farrar, Straus.

Reik, T. (1948). *Listening with the third ear: The inner experience of a psychoanalyst.* New York: Farrar, Straus.

Renik, O. (1995). The ideal of the anonymous analyst and the problem of self-disclosure. *Psychoanalytic Quarterly, 64,* 78–101.

Renik, O. (1996). The perils of neutrality. *Psychoanalytic Quarterly, 65,* 495–517.

Renshon, S. A. (1998). *High hopes: The Clinton presidency and the politics of ambition.* New York: Routledge.

Richards, H. J. (1993). *Therapy of the substance abuse syndromes.* Northvale, NJ: Jason Aronson.

Riding, A. (2001, July 14). Correcting her idea of politically correct. *New York Times,* pp. B9, 11.

Rieff, P. (1959). *Freud: The mind of the moralist.* New York: Viking Press.

Robbins, A. (Ed.). (1988). *Between therapists: The processing of transference/countertransference material.* New York: Human Sciences Press.

Robbins, A. (1989). *The psychoaesthetic experience: An approach to depth-oriented treatment.* New York: Human Sciences Press.

Rock, M. H. (Ed.). (1997). *Psychodynamic supervision: Perspectives of the supervisor and supervisee.* Northvale, NJ: Jason Aronson.

Rockland, L. H. (1992). *Supportive therapy: A psychodynamic approach.* New York: Basic Books.

Rodman, F. R. (2003). *Winnicott: Life and work.* Cambridge, MA: Perseus Books.

Roland, A. (1999). The spiritual self and psychopathology: Theoretical reflections and clinical observations. *Psychoanalytic Psychology, 16,* 211–233.

Roth, A., & Fonagy, P. (1996). *What works for whom?: A critical review of psychotherapy research.* New York: Guilford Press.

Roth, S. (1987). *Psychotherapy: The art of wooing nature.* Northvale, NJ: Jason Aronson.

Rothgeb, C. (1973). *Abstracts of the* Standard Edition of the Complete Psychological Works of Sigmund Freud (foreword by R. R. Holt). New York International Universities Press.

Rothschild, B. (2000). *The body remembers: The psychophysiology of trauma and trauma treatment.* New York: Norton.

Roughton, R. E. (2001). Four men in treatment: An evolving perspective on homosexuality and bisexuality, 1965 to 2000. *Journal of the American Psychoanalytic Association, 49,* 1187–1217.

Russell, P. L. (1998). Trauma and the cognitive function of affects. In J. G. Teicholz & D. Kriegman (Eds.), *Trauma, repetition, and affect regulation: The work of Paul Russell* (pp. 23–47). New York: Other Press.

Sacks, O. (1995). *An anthropologist on mars.* New York: Knopf.

Safran, J. D. (1993). Breaches in the therapeutic alliance: An arena for negotiating authentic relatedness. *Psychotherapy: Theory, Research, and Practice, 30*, 11–24.

Safran, J. D., & Muran, J. C. (2000). *Negotiating the therapeutic alliance: A relational treatment guide.* New York: Guilford Press.

Sandell, R., Blomberg, J., Lazar, A., Carlsson, J., Broberg, J., & Schubert, J. (2000). Varieties of long-term outcome among patients in psychoanalysis and long-term psychotherapy: A review of findings in the Stockholm outcome of Psychoanalysis and Psychotherapy Project (STOPP). *International Journal of Psycho-Analysis, 81*, 921–942.

Sass, L. A. (1992). *Madness and modernism: Insanity in the light of modern art, literature, and thought.* New York: Basic Books.

Schafer, R. (1974). Talking to patients in psychotherapy. *Bulletin of the Menninger Clinic, 38*, 503–515.

Schafer, R. (1976). *A new language for psychoanalysis.* New Haven, CT: Yale University Press.

Schafer, R. (1979). Character, egosyntonicity, and character change. *Journal of the American Psychoanalytic Association, 27*, 867–891.

Schafer, R. (1983). *The analytic attitude.* New York: Basic Books.

Schafer, R. (1999). Recentering psychoanalysis: From Heinz Hartmann to the contemporary British Kleinians. *Psychoanalytic Psychology, 16*, 339–354.

Schimek, J. G. (1975). A critical re-examination of Freud's concept of unconscious mental representation. *International Review of Psycho-Analysis, 2*, 171–187.

Schlesinger, H. J. (2003). *The texture of treatment: On the matter of psychoanalytic technique.* Hillsdale, NJ: Analytic Press.

Schneider, K. J. (1998). Toward a science of the heart: Romanticism and the revival of psychology. *American Psychologist, 53*, 277–289.

Schore, A. N. (1994). *Affect regulation and the origin of the self.* Mahwah, NJ: Erlbaum.

Schore, A. N. (2003a). *Affect dysregulation and disorders of the self.* New York: Norton.

Schore, A. N. (2003b). *Affect regulation and the repair of the self.* New York: Norton.

Schwartz, H. J., & Silver, A. S. (1990). *Illness in the analyst: Implications for the treatment relationship.* New York: International Universities Press.

Searl, M. N. (1936). Some queries on principles of technique. *International Journal of Psycho-Analysis, 17*, 471–493.

Searles, H. (1959). Oedipal love in the countertransference. In *Collected papers on schizophrenia and related subjects* (pp. 284–303). New York: International Universities Press, 1965.

Searles, H. (1975). The patient as therapist to his analyst. In *Countertransference and related Subjects: Selected papers* (pp. 380–459). New York: International Universities Press, 1979.

Sechehaye, M. A. (1960). *Symbolic realization: A new method of psychotherapy applied to a case of schizophrenia.* New York: International Universities Press.

Seinfeld, J. (Ed.). (1993). *Interpreting and holding: The paternal and maternal functions of the psychotherapist.* Northvale, NJ: Jason Aronson.

Seligman, M. (1995). The effectiveness of psychotherapy: The *Consumer Reports* study. *American Psychologist, 50,* 965–974.

Seligman, M. (1996). Science as an ally of practice. *American Psychologist, 51,* 1072–1079.

Semrad, E. V. (1980). *The heart of a therapist.* New York: Jason Aronson.

Shane, E. (2003, April 4). *Boundaries, boundary dilemmas, and boundary violations: A contemporary, non-linear dynamic systems perspective in the psychoanalytic situation.* Paper presented at the spring meeting of the Division of Psychoanalysis (39), American Psychological Association, Minneapolis, MN.

Shane, E., & Shane, M. (1996). Self psychology in search of the optimal: A consideration of optimal responsiveness, optimal provision, optimal gratification and optimal restraint in the clinical situation. *Progress in Self Psychology, 12,* 37–54.

Shane, E., & Shane, M. (Eds.). (2000). On touch in the psychoanalytic situation. *Psychoanalytic Inquiry, 20*(3).

Sharpe, E. F. (1930). The analyst. In *Collected papers on psycho-analysis* (pp. 9–21). New York: Brunner/Mazel, 1950.

Sharpe, E. F. (1947). The psycho-analyst. In *Collected papers on psycho-analysis* (pp. 109–122. New York: Brunner/Mazel, 1950.

Shaw, D. (2003). On the therapeutic action of analytic love. *Contemporary Psychoanalysis, 39,* 251–278.

Shedler, J., Mayman, M., & Manis, M. (1993). The *illusion* of mental health. *American Psychologist, 48,* 1117–1131.

Sifneos, P. (1973). The prevalence of 'alexithymic' characteristics in psychosomatic patients. *Psychotherapy and Psychosomatics, 22,* 255–262.

Silverman, L. (1984). Beyond insight: An additional necessary step in redressing intrapsychic conflict. *Psychoanalytic Psychology, 1,* 215–234.

Slavin, J. H. (1994). On making rules: Toward a reformulation of the dynamics of transference in psychoanalytic treatment. *Psychoanalytic Dialogues, 4,* 253–274.

Slavin, J. H. (2002, November 22). *Discussion of clinical presentation by Eric Sherman: Adventures in suburbia: The analyst, the patient, and the package in the waiting room.* Paper presented at the International Association for Relational Psychotherapy and Psychoanalysis Conference on Sexuality. New York.

Slavin, M., & Kriegman, D. (1992). *The adaptive design of the human psyche: Psychoanalysis, evolutionary biology, and the therapeutic process.* New York: Guilford Press.

Slavin, M., & Kriegman, D. (1998). Why the analyst needs to change: Toward a theory of conflict, negotiation, and mutual influence on the therapeutic process. *Psychoanalytic Dialogues, 8,* 247–284.

Slochower, J. A. (1997). *Holding and psychoanalysis: A relational perspective, vol. 5.* Hillsdale, NJ: Analytic Press.

Slochower, J. A. (1998). Illusion and uncertainty in psychoanalytic writing. *International Journal of Psychoanalysis, 79,* 333–347.

Smith, M., Glass, G., & Miller, T. (1980). *The benefits of psychotherapy.* Baltimore: Johns Hopkins University Press.

Snyder, C. R., & Ingram, R. E. (Eds.). (1994). *Handbook of psychotherapy and behavioral change* (4th ed., pp. 248–250). New York: Wiley.

Solms, M., & Turnbull, O. (2002). *The brain and the inner world: An introduction to the neuroscience of subjective experience.* New York: Other Press.

Spence, D. P. (1982). *Narrative truth and historical truth.* New York: Norton.

Spezzano, C. (1993). *Affect in psychoanalysis: A clinical synthesis.* Hillsdale, NJ: Analytic Press.

Stark, M. (1994). *Working with resistance.* Northvale, NJ: Jason Aronson.

Stark, M. (1999). *Modes of therapeutic action: Enhancement of knowledge, provision of experience, and engagement in relationship.* Northvale, NJ: Jason Aronson.

Steiner, J. (1993). Psychic retreats: *Pathological organizations in psychotic, neurotic and borderline patients.* London: Routledge, 1993.

Steingart, I. (1993). *A thing apart: Love and reality in the therapeutic relationship.* Northvale, NJ: Jason Aronson.

Sterba, R. (1934). The fate of the ego in analytic therapy. *International Journal of Psycho-Analysis, 15,* 117–126.

Stern, D. B. (1984). Empathy is interpretation (And whoever said it wasn't?). Commentary on papers by Hayes, Kiersky & Beebe, and Feiner & Kiersky. *Psychoanalytic Dialogues, 4,* 441–471.

Stern, D. B. (1988). Not misusing empathy. *Contemporary Psychoanalysis, 24,* 598–611.

Stern, D. B. (1997). *Unformulated experience: From dissociation to imagination in psychoanalysis.* Hillside, NJ: Analytic Press.

Stern, D. N. (1995). *The motherhood constellation: A unified view of parent-infant psychotherapy.* New York: Basic Books.

Stoller, R. S. (1997). *Splitting: A case of female masculinity.* New Haven, CT: Yale University Press.

Stolorow, R. D., & Atwood, G. E. (1997). Deconstructing the myth of the neutral analyst: An alternative from intersubjective systems theory. *Psychoanalytic Quarterly, 66,* 431–449.

Stolorow, R. D., Atwood, G. E., & Brandchaft, B. (1987). *Psychoanalytic treatment: An intersubjective approach.* Hillsdale, NJ: Analytic Press.

Stone, L. (1954). The widening scope of indications for psycho-analysis. *Journal of the American Psychoanalytic Association, 27,* 567–594.

Stone, L. (1961). *The psychoanalytic situation: An examination of its development and essential nature.* New York: International Universities Press.

Storr, A. (1990). *The art of psychotherapy* (2nd ed.). Woburn, MA: Butterworth-Heinemann.

Strachey, J. (1934). The nature of the therapeutic action of psycho-analysis. *International Journal of Psycho-Analysis, 15,* 127–159.

Strenger, C. (1991). *Between hermeneutics and science: An essay on the epistemology of psychoanalysis.* New York: International Universities Press.

Strenger, C. (1998). *Individuality, the impossible project: Psychoanalysis and self-creation.* New York: International Universities Press.

Strozier, C. B. (2001). *Heinz Kohut: The making of a psychoanalyst.* New York: Farrar, Straus & Giroux.

Strupp, H., Hadley, S., & Gomez-Schwartz, B. (1977). *Psychotherapy for better or worse: An analysis of the problem of negative effects*. New York: Jason Aronson.

Sue, D. W., & Sue, D. (1990). *Counseling the culturally different: Theory and practice* (2nd ed.). New York: Wiley.

Sullivan, H. S. (1947). *Conceptions of modern psychiatry.* New York: Norton.

Sullivan, H. S. (1953). *The interpersonal theory of psychiatry*. New York: Norton.

Symington, N. (1986). *The analytic experience*. New York: St. Martin's Press.

Szasz, T. S. (1956). On the experiences of the analyst in the psychoanalytic situation—A contribution to the theory of psychoanalytic treatment. *Journal of the American Psychoanalytic Association, 4*, 197–223.

Szasz, T. S. (1961). *The myth of mental illness: Foundations of a theory of personal conduct*. New York: Hoeber-Harper.

Szasz, T. S. (2003). The cure of souls in the therapeutic state. *Psychoanalytic Review, 90*, 45–62.

Tarasoff vs. Board of Regents of the University of California, 17 Cal. 3rd 425 (Cal. 1976).

Tessman, L. H. (2003). *The analyst's analyst within*. Hillsdale, NJ: Analytic Press.

Thompson, C. (1956). The role of the analyst's personality in therapy. *American Journal of Psychotherapy, 10*, 347–359.

Thompson, M. G. (1996). Freud's conception of neutrality. *Contemporary Psychoanalysis, 32*, 25–42.

Thompson, M. G. (2002). The ethic of honesty: The moral dimension to psychoanalysis. *fort da: The Journal of the Northern California Society for Psychoanalytic Psychology, 8*, 72–83.

Thomson, P. (2003, April 4). *Trauma, creativity, and neuropsychoanalysis: A dialectic interplay of hopelessness and hope.* Paper presented at the 23rd annual spring meeting of the Division of Psychoanalysis (39) of the American Psychological Association, Minneapolis, MN.

Tomkins, S. S. (1962). *Affect, imagery, consciousness: Vol. 1. The positive affects.* New York: Springer.

Tomkins, S. S. (1963). *Affect, imagery, consciousness: Vol. 2. The negative affects.* New York: Springer.

Tomkins, S. S. (1991). *Affect, imagery, consciousness: Vol. 3. The negative affects: Anger and fear.* New York: Springer.

Toronto, E. L. K. (2001). The human touch: An exploration of the role and meaning of physical touch in psychoanalysis. *Psychoanalytic Psychology, 18*, 37–54.

Tronick, E. (1989). Emotions and emotional communication in infants. *American Psychologist, 44*, 112–119.

Tyson, P. (1996). Object relations, affect management, and psychic structure formation. *Psychoanalytic Study of the Child, 51*, 172–189.

van der Kolk, B. A., McFarlane, A. C., & Weisaeth, L. (Eds.). (1997). *Traumatic stress: The effects of overwhelming experience on mind, body, and society.* New York: Guilford Press.

Vaughan, S. C. (1997). *The talking cure: The science behind psychotherapy*. New York: Grosset/Putnam.

Volkan, V. D. (1984). *What do you get when you cross a dandelion with a rose? The true story of a psychoanalysis*. New York: Jason Aronson.

Wachtel, P. L. (1977). *Psychoanalysis and behavior therapy: Toward an integration.* New York: Basic Books.

Wachtel, P. L. (1997). *Psychoanalysis, behavior therapy, and the relational world.* Washington, DC: American Psychological Association.

Waelder, R. (1937). The problem of the genesis of psychical conflicts in earliest infancy. *International Journal of Psycho-Analysis, 18,* 406–473.

Walker, L. E. (1980). *The battered woman.* New York: HarperCollins.

Wallerstein, R. S. (1986). *Forty-two lives in treatment: A study of psychoanalysis and psychotherapy.* New York: Guilford Press.

Wallerstein, R. S. (1988). One psychoanalysis or many? *International Journal of Psycho-Analysis, 69,* 5–19.

Wallerstein, R. S. (Ed.). (1992). *The common ground of psychoanalysis.* Northvale, NJ: Jason Aronson.

Wallerstein, R. S. (1998). *Lay analysis: Life inside the controversy.* Hillsdale, NJ: Analytic Press.

Wampold, B. E. (2001). *The great psychotherapy debate: Models, methods, and findings.* Mahwah, NJ: Erlbaum.

Washton, A. M. (Ed.). (1995). *Psychotherapy and substance abuse: A practitioner's handbook.* New York: Guilford Press.

Washton, A. M. (2004). *Substance abuse treatment in office practice.* New York: Guilford Press.

Weinberger, J. (1995). Common factors aren't so common: The common factors dilemma. *Clinical Psychology: Science and Practice, 2,* 45–69.

Weiss, J. (1993). *How psychotherapy works: Process and technique.* New York: Guilford Press.

Weiss, J., Sampson, H., & the Mt. Zion Psychotherapy Research Group. (1986). *The psychoanalytic process: Theory, clinical observation, and empirical research.* New York: Guilford Press.

Welch v. American Psychoanalytic Association, No. 85 Civ. 1651 (JFK), 1986 U. S. Dist. Lexis 27182 (S. D. N. Y., April 14, 1986).

Welch, B. L. (1999). Boundary violations: In the eye of the beholder. Interview in *Insight: Safeguarding psychologists against liability risks.* American Professional Agency.

Welch, B. L. (2003, November 15). *Safe practice: Legal and ethical dimensions* [Seminar on risk management], Philadelphia, PA.

Westen, D. (1998). The scientific legacy of Sigmund Freud: Toward a psychodynamically informed psychological science. *Psychological Bulletin, 124,* 333–371.

Wheelis, A. (1958). *The quest for identity: The decline of the superego and what is happening to American character as a result.* New York: Norton.

Wilson, A. (1995). Mapping the mind in relational psychoanalysis: Some critiques, questions, and conjectures. *Psychoanalytic Psychology, 12,* 9–30.

Winnicott, D. W. (1947). Hate in the countertransference. In *Collected papers* (pp. 194–203). New York: Basic Books, 1958.

Winnicott, D. W (1953). Transitional objects and transitional phenomena—A study of the first not-me possession. *International Journal of Psycho-Analysis, 34,* 89–97.

Winnicott, D. W. (1954). The depressive position in normal emotional development. In *Through paediatrics to psycho-analysis* (pp. 262–277). New York: Basic
Books, 1975.

Winnicott, D. W. (1955). Metapsychological and clinical aspects of regression
within the psycho-analytical set-up. *International Journal of Psycho-Analysis,
36*, 12–26.

Winnicott, D. W. (1958). The capacity to be alone. In *The maturational process and
the facilitating environment* (pp. 29–37). London: Hogarth Press, 1965.

Winnicott, D. W. (1960). Ego distortion in terms of true and false self. *The
maturational process and the facilitating environment* (pp. 140–152). New York:
International Universities Press, 1965.

Winnicott, D. W. (1963). Psychiatric disorder in terms of infantile maturational
processes. In *The maturational process and the facilitating environment* (pp. 37–
55). New York: International Universities Press, 1965.

Winnicott, D. W. (1971). *Playing and reality*. New York: Penguin.

Wolf, E. S. (1998). *Treating the self: Elements of clinical self psychology*. New York:
Guilford Press.

Wolpe, J. (Ed.). (1964). *The conditioning therapies: The challenge in psychotherapy*.
New York: Holt, Rinehart, & Winston.

Wurmser, L. (1981). *The mask of shame*. Baltimore: Johns Hopkins University
Press.

Yalom, I. D. (2002). *The gift of therapy: An open letter to a new generation of therapists
and their patients*. New York: HarperCollins.

Yeomans, F. E., Clarkin, J. F., & Kernberg, O. F. (2002). *A primer of transference-focused psychotherapy for the borderline patient*. Northvale, NJ: Jason Aronson.

Yogman, M. W. (1981). Games fathers and mothers play with their infants. *Infant
Mental Health Journal, 2*, 241–248.

Young, J. E., Klosko, J. S., & Weishaar, M. E. (2003). *Schema therapy: A practitioner's
guide*. New York: Guilford Press.

Young-Breuhl, E., & Bethelard, F. (2000). *Cherishment: A psychology of the heart.*
New York: Free Press.

Young-Eisendrath, P. (2001). When the fruit ripens: Alleviating suffering and increasing compassion as goals of clinical psychoanalysis. *Psychoanalytic Quarterly, 70*, 265–285.

Zetzel, E. (1956). Current concepts of transference. *International Journal of Psycho-
Analysis, 37*, 369–376.

Zetzel, E. (1970). *The capacity for emotional growth*. New York: International Universities Press.

Author Index

Subject Index

Superego, care of (*cont.*)
    family, doing right by, 298–299
    honesty, 303
    overview of, 298
    risk management, 299–301
Supervision
    exposing one's work and, 299
    getting most from, 53–60
    group for, 294
    reaction to, 50–52
Symptom, experience of in
        transference relationship, 232,
        233

T

Talking
    addressing resistance to self-
        expression, 141–142
    facilitating therapeutic process,
        139–141
    See also Expression
Teaching students
    approach to, xi–xii, xiv
    "classical" technique of
        psychoanalysis, 10–12
    See also Supervision
Technique, commonalities of, 135–
    136. *See also* Process of
    therapy
Terminating session, 113
Termination phase of treatment
    Donna, 236–237
    Molly, 214–217
Testimony, legal, giving, 109–111
Testing therapist, 102–104, 136
Theme of psychodynamic approach,
    1–3
"Theology" of psychoanalytic
    practitioner, 4
Therapeutic style
    influences of, 142–143
    patient characteristics and, 143–
        145
    personality of therapist and, 147–
        149
    phase of therapy and, 145–147

Therapist
    alliance between patient and, 41,
        73–76
    being alone in presence of, 132–
        133
    being oneself, 52–53
    characterological differences
        between patient and, 105–107
    as container of images and
        feelings, 134–135
    depressive dynamics in, 105–107,
        148–149
    first experience in role of, 46–47
    mistakes, making, 48–52
    paradox of, 47
    power in role of, 150–152, 155–156
    sense of safety of, 80–81
    testing, 102–104, 136
    therapy for, 60–69
    See also Supervision; Working
        alliance, establishing
Third-party reimbursement for
        psychotherapy, 7–8, 121, 290
Tikkun, 283
Time between sessions, 111
Tomkins, Sylvan, 20
Tone
    of book, xiv
    importance of, 219
    maternal versus paternal, 144–145,
        146–147
    of therapist, 143–144
Touch
    overview of, 189
    physical holding, 189–192
    sexual, 192–194
Tragic worldview, 28
Transference
    emergence of, 159
    experience of symptom in, 232, 233
    Freud's understanding of, 14, 15
    introducing work with, 94–96
    Molly case study, 210, 211
    negative, 83
    power and, 152
    processing of, 159–160
    toward supervisor, 57–59